STUTTERING

An Integrated Approach to Its Nature and Treatment

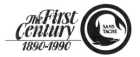

The First Century 1890-1990 · SANS TACHE

STUTTERING

An Integrated Approach to Its Nature and Treatment

Theodore J. Peters, Ph.D.
Professor
Department of Communication Disorders
University of Wisconsin-Eau Claire
Eau Claire, Wisconsin

Barry Guitar, Ph.D.
Professor and Chair
Department of Communication Science & Disorders
The University of Vermont
Burlington, Vermont

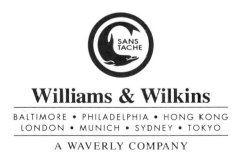

Williams & Wilkins

BALTIMORE • PHILADELPHIA • HONG KONG
LONDON • MUNICH • SYDNEY • TOKYO

A WAVERLY COMPANY

Editor: John P. Butler
Associate Editor: Linda Napora
Copy Editors: Clifford L. Malanowski, Jr., Stephen Siegforth
Designer: Wilma Rosenberger
Illustration Planner: Wayne Hubbel
Production Coordinator: Adèle Boyd
Cover Designer: Ginny Joyner

Printed in the United States of America

Library of Congress Cataloging-in-Publication Data

Peters, Theodore J.
    Stuttering, an integrated approach to its nature and treatment / Theodore J. Peters, Barry Guitar.
        p.   cm.
    Includes bibliographical references.
    Includes index.
    ISBN 0-683-06870-9
    1. Stuttering.   I. Guitar, Barry.   II. Title.
    [DNLM: 1. Stuttering—therapy.   WM 475 P483s]
    RC424.P48 1991
    616.85′54—dc20
    DNLM/DLC
    for Library of Congress   90-12509
                                                                      CIP

ISBN 0-683-06870-9

90000

96   97   98
    9   10

PREFACE

During the past 20 years, there has been controversy between the proponents of the two major current approaches to the treatment of stuttering. Ten years ago, in *Stuttering: An Integration of Contemporary Therapies* (Guitar & Peters, 1980), we referred to these two approaches as stuttering modification therapy and fluency shaping therapy, and we attempted to integrate these two approaches in order to retain the advantages of both. During the last 10 years, we have continued to experiment with better ways of combining stuttering modification and fluency shaping therapies, and we share the results of our more recent experiences in this present book. Besides discussing the integration of these two therapies, we have also added a major section on the integration of the current theoretical and research literature. We believe that an understanding of the etiology and development of the disorder is crucial in providing effective treatment.

We have written this book for the student who is studying to become a speech-language pathologist, as well as for the practicing clinician. The first section of this book covers the etiology and development of stuttering. With regard to the causes of the disorder, there are separate chapters on the predisposing or constitutional factors and the precipitating or developmental and environmental influences. There is another chapter devoted to the development of stuttering and the underlying processes accounting for it. In this first section, we have integrated the most recent theoretical and empirical information to provide the student or the clinician with a foundation on which to design her treatment. To help the reader more effectively use this book, each chapter is followed by study questions and suggested readings.

The second section of this book covers the assessment and treatment of stuttering. There is one chapter on the assessment and diagnosis of stuttering and separate chapters on each of the three levels—advanced, beginning, and intermediate stuttering. The treatment chapters are presented in this order because, most often, the treatment procedures for the intermediate stutterer are a modification of procedures for the advanced and beginning stutterer. Thus, understanding the treatment of the intermediate stutterer is easier if one first understands the treatment of the other two. In each of the three chapters, we describe the clinical procedures of a number of proponents of both stuttering modification and fluency shaping therapies. Each of these treatment chapters is followed by a chapter in which we discuss how we and other clinicians integrate these two approaches. Again, study questions and suggested readings follow each chapter.

In this book, we use masculine pronouns when referring to stuttering clients and female pronouns when referring to their clinicians. Because the majority of stutterers are male and most speech-language pathologists are female, we find this use of language to be very natural.

This book is a joint and equal effort by both authors. Since one of our ground rules was that we both needed to agree on a given point before it found its way into the book, we have made a number of trips and far too many telephone calls between Vermont and Wisconsin. This book has also required the patience and support of both of our wives, Karen and Carroll. We thank them both very much.

We thank our colleagues at our respective universities for their help and suggestions, and we acknowledge the University of Wisconsin-Eau Claire Faculty Sabbatical Leave Program for its support. We also thank Oliver Bloodstein, Brooklyn College of The City University of New York; Richard Curlee, University of Arizona; and Harold Luper, University of Tennessee for their critical review of our manuscript. Finally, we wish to thank the Speech Foundation of America for providing us with the opportunity to collaborate on our initial joint publication 10 years ago.

We would like to thank Ginny Joyner, our illustrator; she is gifted as an artist, sympathetic to our purpose, and perceptive in transforming our scribbled concepts into clear figures. Finally, we would like to express our gratitude to the many people at Williams and Wilkins who worked with us: John Butler, Linda Napora, Adele Boyd, Pamela Carras, and many others. Their support, enthusiasm, and guidance made this long labor bearable.

CONTENTS

NATURE OF STUTTERING

1

INTRODUCTION TO STUTTERING

Our aim in this book is to teach you to be the most effective stuttering therapist you can be. We believe that the best therapy is based on a thorough understanding of the disorder and the principles underlying its treatment. The first four chapters, therefore, are to help you develop this understanding. They will give you current knowledge about the etiology, onset, and development of stuttering. They will also teach you how stuttering is unwittingly maintained by the stutterer, even though he wishes to speak fluently. With this information about the nature of stuttering in mind, the logic of the later treatment chapters will be clear.

The second section of the book—on diagnosis and treatment—expands and updates ideas we presented in *Stuttering: An Integration of Contemporary Therapies* (Guitar and Peters, 1980). In this second section, we present the two major treatment approaches, stuttering modification and fluency shaping, and a method of integrating them. We begin with our diagnostic procedures, organized by the client's age: preschool, elementary school, and adolescent/adult. Then we describe treatment approaches, structured according to the level of the client. As explained in the Preface, they are presented in the following order: advanced, beginning, and intermediate. In these treatment chapters, we describe the therapies used by advocates of each approach. Then we describe our own integrated approach to the treatment of stuttering at each level.

OVERVIEW OF THE DISORDER

This section previews the next few chapters on the nature of stuttering and gives us a chance to reveal our own slant on the disorder. It is intended especially for readers who have not had a course in stuttering, and who may, therefore, know few details of its nature.

Stuttering is found in all parts of the world, in all cultures and races. It is indiscriminate of occupation, intelligence, and income; it affects both sexes and people of all ages, from toddlers to the elderly. It is an old curse; there is evidence that it appeared in Chinese, Egyptian, and Mesopotamian cultures more than 40 centuries ago.

What causes people to stutter? Researchers believe there are many influences that determine whether or not an individual will stutter. Neurophysiological, psychological, social, and linguistic factors all probably contribute to its onset and development. Stuttering's first appearance in a toddler, for example, may be determined by constitutional factors, such as a biologically inherited predisposition. Soon, other factors become more important. Stuttering in a young child may become progressively worse in response to family stresses, listener reactions, and even the task of learning speech and language. By the time a child is an adolescent, learned reactions influence many of the symptoms.[1] By now, the child has learned to anticipate stuttering and may thrash around wildly when he speaks, trying to escape and avoid it. By adulthood, the fear of stuttering and the desire to avoid it create a whole lifestyle. An adult stutterer often copes with stuttering by limiting his work, friends, and fun to those that put fewer demands on his speech.

Figure 1.1 gives an overview of many of the contributing factors in the development of stuttering. In this and the subsequent three chapters, we will describe in detail our current understanding of these influences.

Can stuttering be cured? Often, it cures itself. Some young children who begin to stutter recover without treatment. For other young stutterers, early intervention is needed to nurture the child's normal development of fluency and to prevent the development of a serious problem. Once stuttering has really taken hold, however, and the child has developed many learned reactions, a concerted treatment effort is needed. Good treatment of mild and moderate stutterers in their preschool and early elementary school years may leave a child with little trace of stuttering, except perhaps during stress, fatigue, or illness. Most severe stutterers, or those who are treated after puberty, will make only a partial recovery. They will learn to speak more slowly or to stutter more easily, and to be less bothered by it. Some stutterers will not improve, despite our best efforts. For reasons we don't understand, a few stutterers just don't change significantly in treatment.

Before we delve deeper into the nature and treatment of stuttering, we would like to touch briefly upon the personal side of the problem. Some of you may

---

[1] In the medical literature, the term "symptom" is often used for behavior that signifies a deeper underlying condition: a pain in the lower right abdomen may be a symptom of appendicitis. In the stuttering literature, however, symptom has often been used to denote a behavior that is an aspect of the disorder itself, such as multiple part-word repetitions. We will use the words symptom and "sign" interchangeably to indicate such behaviors.

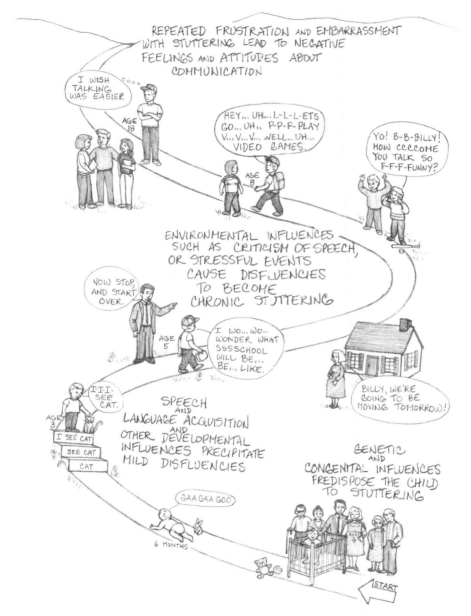

Figure 1.1. Factors contributing to the development of stuttering.

never have had a friend who stuttered or worked with a stutterer in treatment, so we want to present several examples of what stuttering can be like. If you are familiar with stuttering, you may want to read this section in order to expand your sense of what stuttering is like for the person who experiences it. These brief descriptions portray three stutterers who differ widely in age and in their accommodations to stuttering.

CASE EXAMPLES

Stuttering in an Adult

Tom is a 29-year-old botanist at a state university. He has stuttered since he was three, and his father and brother also stutter. Tom's speech was difficult to understand when he first began to speak, and he remembers his older brother interpreting for him when his parents kept asking him to repeat practically everything he said. Tom was told that his stuttering started as easy repetitions of sounds at the beginning of sentences. It gradually worsened during elementary and junior high school. Repetitions kept going on and on, and when he was stuck on a word, he began to push harder and harder to finish it. By the time he was an adult, Tom stuttered severely, sometimes struggling and contorting his face for what seemed to him like several minutes.

At present, he stutters frequently and with a great deal of tension when he talks in a group of people or to someone he doesn't know well, particularly on the first words in a conversation. He is embarrassed and frustrated by his stuttering. At times, he feels, he is unable to do what any child can do easily: just produce a single word. During his stutters, Tom knows what he is trying to say, but despite this, he feels his throat clamp shut, and he can't seem to say the word until, after he has struggled for many seconds, it just pops out.

Tom's stuttering varies. It is usually worse in formal situations, or when a listener is impatient or embarrassed, or when Tom is tired or ill. On the other hand, it is better if he is talking to his wife or children, or when he is talking to good friends, especially if there are only one or two of them together. There are also many times when the stuttering is unpredictable, which makes Tom feel he is woefully out of control.

Tom is very bright; he is nationally recognized for his achievements in botany. But he believes people think he is "dumb" as soon as they hear him stutter. This may be a perception left over from elementary school, where he was in the lowest reading group because he stuttered severely when reading aloud. He also thought his teachers regarded him as dumb because he would often answer "I don't know" when asked questions in class. He knew the answer but couldn't bear the teacher's impatience when he stuttered. Tom's embarrassment about his stuttering keeps him from presenting papers at professional conferences. He is also unwilling to teach courses because of his stuttering. For these reasons, he has a research appointment at the university, without the job security offered by a tenured teaching position.

Tom's case illustrates some of the hidden dimensions of stuttering. Tom's stuttering consists not only of the contortions he makes with his mouth, but also of the feelings and beliefs that years of stuttering have created in his mind. For example, his misperceptions and fears deter him from even trying to lecture in the classroom, when, in fact, many stutterers handle classroom teaching well.

Tom will probably never stop stuttering, but with treatment he can reduce its severity from a major problem in communication to a minor annoyance.

Stuttering in an Elementary School Child

Kendrick is a fifth grader. The speech-language pathologist in his school brought him to our clinic for help in planning treatment. Like many of his classmates, Kendrick is a study in extremes. He does well in school in every subject that he likes, and poorly in every subject that he hates. Sometimes he stutters severely; other times he is completely fluent. When he stutters, he says he has the sensation of his mouth bouncing out of control as sounds repeat themselves six or eight times. Recently, he has begun to tighten his throat and blink his eyes in an effort to get words out.

Kendrick talks a lot in class discussions, even though he often stutters. He is able to keep his speech flowing in this situation, despite frequent repetitions. What really throws him, however, is reading aloud. His teachers call on students to read by going down the rows. Anticipation builds as his turn comes nearer and nearer. He watches the clock as the teacher goes down the rows, hoping the period will end before he is called on. When it doesn't, and he hears the terrible sound of his name being called, his tongue seems to stick firmly to the roof of his mouth, and he is unable to utter a syllable. The child behind him takes great delight at this. He usually makes Kendrick's torment greater by slamming his desk against the back of Kendrick's chair and making little, stutter-like sounds, which are audible to everyone except the teacher.

Over the last several years, Kendrick's parents and teachers have been at a loss to help him. They have suggested that he think about what he wants to say before speaking, or that he slow down and take a breath whenever he thinks he might stutter. He has tried all of their suggestions. They seemed to work for a little while, but soon stopped working, and this resulted in feelings of failure and helplessness. Kendrick is regarded as someone with potential for going to college, but there is concern that his stuttering is becoming more severe and that he may begin to withdraw from class participation and become more self-conscious around his peers.

Kendrick's stuttering problem is not as severe as Tom's, but it is growing. On the surface, Kendrick's stuttering has changed relatively little since he started. He still repeats sounds, as he did when he was younger, although now he uses a lot more muscular tension to squeeze sounds out. The big change is Kendrick's sensitivity to his stuttering. He has grown self-conscious about it, as people have noticed it and responded with comments, advice, or impatience. Kendrick is at a crossroads. Proper treatment can reduce his stuttering and make it more likely that he will grow up without a sense that he is handicapped. Without treatment, Kendrick's stuttering is likely to get more severe, and he may feel more and more inhibited about speaking.

Stuttering in a Preschool Child

Sally is just shy of her fourth birthday. Her parents contacted us because they were worried about her speech. They were particularly concerned because Sally's uncle had stuttered throughout his childhood, although he has since recovered. Sally is the second of three children; she has an older sister, seven years old, and a new baby brother, six months old. About the time Sally's brother was born, Sally's parents were alarmed when they noticed that she was frequently repeating sounds. The repetitions often went on five or six times before she said the word. Sally continues to repeat sounds, particularly if she talks when she is excited or when she is exercising her rapidly expanding vocabulary. Although she usually repeats sounds only 3 or 4 times now, and her repetitions come and go, Sally's parents are concerned about it. Thinking back, they realized that Sally's sister had repeated sounds, but only one or two repetitions each time, and that she had stopped after several months. Sally doesn't seem to mind her repetitions, but her sister does and so do her grandparents. In fact, her grandmother once took Sally aside and gave her a little instruction about how to talk.

Sally can be treated very effectively, if her parents are willing to make some changes in their home. Her parents can discover, with a clinician's help, which of the many pressures in a normal home might be affecting Sally's speech. With several meetings devoted to discussing these factors and how to change them, and some direct work with Sally, Sally's fluency can be increased, and she can almost certainly be on her way again, developing normal speech and language.

These three cases should give you a glimpse of what stuttering can be like at different stages and for different people. They also echo our earlier overview of the nature of the disorder: stuttering may first appear as occasional, effortless repetitions of sounds, but soon, normal childhood experiences such as family stresses and the development of spoken language may increase its frequency and tension. The young stutterer's self-consciousness about his difficulty and about listener reactions contribute to his embarrassment and desire to avoid stuttering. This sets the stage for learned reactions that make the confirmed stutterer's problem so complex and make treatment so difficult.

Table 1.1.   Variables Suggested by Dalton and Hardcastle (1977) to Be Useful in Distinguishing between Fluent and Disfluent Speech

1. Presence of extra sounds, such as repetitions, prolongations, interjections, and revisions
   If a speaker says, "I-I-I nnnnneed to have uh my uh,well,I-I-I should get mmmmmy car fixed," he sounds disfluent.
2. Location and frequency of pauses
   If a speaker says, "Whenever I remember to bring my umbrella, (pause) it never rains," he sounds fluent. But if he says, "Whenever (pause) I remember to bring (pause) my (pause) umbrella, it never (pause) rains," he sounds disfluent.
3. Rhythmical patterning in speech
   English is typically spoken with stressed syllables at relatively equal intervals; in general, stressed syllables are followed by several unstressed syllables. When this pattern is deviated from markedly, as in cerebellar disease, when the speaker stresses all syllables equally, the speaker sounds disfluent.
4. Intonation and stress
   If a speaker does not vary intonation and stress, and is, therefore, monotonous, he may be considered disfluent. Abnormal intonation and stress patterns may also be considered disfluent.
5. Overall rate
   If a speaker has a very slow rate of speech, or if he has bursts of fast rate interspersed with slower rate, he may be considered disfluent.

DEFINITIONS

Fluency

By beginning with a definition of fluency, we will show you how many elements must be maintained in the speaker's flow of speech if he is to be considered fluent. It is an impressive balancing act; little wonder that everyone slips and stumbles from time to time when they talk.

Fluency is hard to define. In fact, most researchers have focused on its opposite, *dis*fluency.[2] One of the early researchers in fluency, Freida Goldman-Eisler, has shown that normal speech is filled with hesitations (Goldman-Eisler, 1968). Other researchers have acknowledged this and expanded the study of fluent speech by contrasting it with disfluent speech. Dalton and Hardcastle (1977), for example, distinguish fluent and disfluent speech by differences in the variables listed in Table 1.1.

Starkweather (1980, 1987) has suggested that many of these variables that determine fluency may reflect temporal aspects of speech production; that is, variables such as pauses, rhythm, intonation, stress, and rate are controlled by when and how fast we move our speech structures. Our temporal control determines our fluency. Starkweather also suggests that the rate of information flow,

---

[2] Throughout this book, we will use the term disfluency to apply both to stuttering and normal hesitancy, making it easier to refer to hesitations which could be either normal or abnormal.

not just sound flow, is an important aspect of fluency. Thus, a speaker who speaks without hesitations, but is slow, would not be considered entirely fluent.

In his description of fluency, Starkweather also includes the effort with which a speaker speaks. By effort, he means both the mental and physical work a speaker must do to speak. This is difficult to measure, but it may turn out to be a judgment that listeners can make reliably when they watch and listen to a speaker.

In essence, fluency can be thought of simply as a speaker's effortless flow of speech. Thus, a listener who judges a speaker to be "fluent" senses that he uses little effort to speak. The components of this effortless flow, however, are hard to pin down. As researchers analyze fluency more carefully, they may find that the appearance of excess effort may give rise to the judgment that a person is stuttering. The absence of other elements, such as rhythm or rate of information flow, may result in judgments that a person is a nonstuttering disfluent speaker. We will discuss aspects of fluency again when we relate dimensions of fluency to various therapy approaches.

Stuttering

GENERAL DEFINITION

Countless writers have tried to capture the essence of stuttering in a few sentences. The following definition is yet another attempt; it borrows most heavily from Andrews and Harris (1964) and Wingate (1964) but adds some of our own distinctions. Stuttering is characterized by an abnormally high frequency and/or duration of stoppages in the forward flow of speech. These stoppages usually take the form of (a) repetitions of sound, syllables, or one-syllable words, (b) prolongations of sounds, or (c) "blocks"[3] of airflow and/or voicing in speech. Individuals who stutter are usually aware of their stuttering and are often embarrassed by it. Moreover, they often use abnormal physical and mental effort to speak. Children who are just beginning to stutter may not always be highly conscious of it, but they usually show signs of tension and increased speech rate, which suggests they are at least minimally aware of their difficulty.

Another approach to defining stuttering involves specifying what it is not. For example, an important distinction must be made between the stuttering described above and normal hesitation. Normal children who are developing speech and language may show repetitions, revisions, and pauses—which are not stuttering. Neither are the momentary repetitions, revisions, and pauses in the speech of most normal adults, when the speaker is in a hurry or uncertain. In Chapter 4, we will describe the differences between normal disfluency and stuttering in more detail to prepare you for the task of differential diagnosis of stuttering in children.

A distinction should also be made between stuttering and certain other fluency disorders. Disfluency resulting from cerebral damage or disease, disfluency

---

[3] We will use the word "blocks" to denote stuttering behavior in which the speaker stops the flow of air or voice. This is different from historical usage wherein the writer would have been indicating any moment of stuttering.

resulting from psychological trauma, and cluttering all differ from stuttering and should be treated differently. These disorders will be discussed briefly in Chapter 6.

CORE BEHAVIORS

We have adopted the term "core behaviors" from Van Riper (1971, 1982), who uses it to describe the basic behaviors of stuttering, which include repetitions, prolongations, and blocks. These are the stuttering behaviors that seem involuntary to the stutterer, as though they were out of his control. They contrast with "secondary behaviors" that the stutterer has developed as a learned reaction to the basic core behaviors.

Repetitions are frequently the core behaviors of children who are just beginning to stutter.[4] They are simply a sound, syllable, or single-syllable word repeated several times. The speaker is apparently "stuck" on that sound and continues repeating it until the following sound can be produced. In children beginning to stutter, single-syllable word repetitions and part-word repetitions are more common than multisyllable word repetitions. Moreover, children who stutter will frequently repeat a word or syllable more than twice per instance (Yairi & Lewis, 1984; Yairi, 1983).

Prolongations of voiced or voiceless sounds also appear in the speech of children beginning to stutter. They may develop somewhat later than repetitions (Van Riper, 1982). We use the term prolongation to denote those stutters in which sound or air flow continues, but movement of one or more articulators is stopped. Prolongations may be as short as half a second and still be perceived as abnormal; in rare cases they may last as long as several minutes (Van Riper, 1982). In contrast to our use of the term, other writers (e.g., Conture, 1990; Van Riper, 1982; Wingate, 1964) include stutters with no sound or airflow, as well as stopped movement of articulators, in their definition of prolongations.

Repetitions and sound prolongations may also be part of the core behaviors of more advanced stutterers, as well as of children just beginning to stutter. Sheehan (1974) found that repetitive stutters occurred in the speech of every one of a sample of 20 adult stutterers. Indeed, 66% of their stutters were repetitions. Many of their stutters were also prolongations, although it is not clear how many, because Sheehan's definition of prolongations may differ from ours.

Blocks are typically the last core behavior to develop. They occur when the stutterer inappropriately stops the flow of air or voice, and often the movement of his articulators as well. Blocks may occur at any level of the speech mechanism—respiratory, laryngeal, or articulatory. A stutterer may block at one or more of these levels at the same time. There is some evidence, and much theorizing, that inappropriate muscle activity at the larynx characterizes many blocks (Conture, McCall, & Brewer, 1977; Freeman & Ushijima, 1978; Kenyon, 1942; Schwartz, 1974).

---

[4] Reviews of the stuttering behaviors reported by parents at the onset of the disorder can be found in Bloodstein (1987) and Van Riper (1982). Yairi's (1982) study details the behaviors that were reported by parents as the first signs of stuttering in a group of ten 2-3 year old children. The evidence suggests that part-word repetitions and, to a lesser extent, whole-word repetitions and sound prolongations are the most common first signs of stuttering.

As stuttering develops, we often see blocks grow longer and more tense. Tremors often become evident. These rapid oscillations, most easily observable in the lip or jaw, occur when the stutterer is blocked on a word. He closes off the airway, increases air pressure behind the closure, and squeezes his muscles particularly hard (Van Riper, 1982).[5] Stutterers vary considerably with regard to how frequently they stutter and how long their individual core behaviors last. Research indicates that an average stutterer stutters on about 10% of the words while reading aloud, although individuals vary greatly (Bloodstein, 1944, 1987). There are many mild stutterers who stutter on less than 5% of the words they speak or read, and a few severe ones who stutter on more than 50%. Durations of core behaviors vary much less. Stutters tend to average around one second in duration and are rarely longer than 5 seconds (Bloodstein, 1944, 1987).

SECONDARY BEHAVIORS

Stutterers don't enjoy stuttering. They react to their repetitions, prolongations, and blocks by trying to finish them quickly, if they can't avoid them altogether. These effortful reactions may begin as blind struggle, but soon turn into well-learned patterns.[6] We divide secondary behaviors into two broad classes: escape behaviors and avoidance behaviors, both of which we describe in greater detail in Chapter 4. We make this division rather than follow the traditional approach of dealing with secondary behaviors individually (as, for example, "starters" or "postponements"), because our treatment procedures are focused on the principles by which secondary behaviors are learned.

"Escape" and "avoidance" are terms from the behavioral learning literature. Briefly, escape behaviors occur when the speaker is stuttering and attempts to get out of the stutter and finish the word. Examples are eye blinks, head nods, or interjections of extra sounds, such as "uh." These often are followed by the termination of the stutter, and are thus rewarded. Avoidance behaviors, on the other hand, occur when a speaker anticipates stuttering. In an attempt to keep from stuttering, the speaker may change words, pause, or use an eye blink which is also an escape behavior. Avoidance behaviors are perpetuated because they sometimes prevent a stutter from occurring. The many subcategories of avoidances (such as postponements, starters, and timing devices, e.g., hand movements timed to saying the word) are described in Chapter 4.

FEELINGS AND ATTITUDES

A stutterer's feelings can be as much a part of the disorder as his speech behaviors. Feelings may precipitate stutters; conversely, stutters may create feelings, such as the shame a stutterer feels when he cannot say his name. In the beginning, a child's positive feelings of excitement or his negative feelings of fear may result in excess repetitions that alarm his listeners. Then, as the child stutters more frequently, he may become frustrated or embarrassed because he can't say what he

---

[5] You can duplicate these tremors by trying to say the word "By" while squeezing your lips together hard and building up air pressure behind the block. Imagine this happening to you unexpectedly whenever you tried to say "By".

[6] The learning processes responsible for secondary behaviors are described in Chapter 4.

wants to say as smoothly and quickly as others. These latter feelings that result from stuttering make speaking harder, because when the child is frustrated, he may put more effort into speaking, increasing the tension that holds back speech. Typical feelings about stuttering include not only frustration, but fear, embarrassment, shame, and hostility as well.

Attitudes are feelings that have become pervasive, part of the person's beliefs. As a stutterer experiences more and more stuttering, for example, he begins to believe he is a person who generally has trouble speaking. Adolescent and adult stutterers usually have many negative attitudes about themselves and their listeners that derive from years of stuttering experiences. Listeners probably play a major part in shaping the stutterer's attitude. Research has shown that most people, including classroom teachers and even speech pathologists, hold stereotyped views of stutterers as being tense, insecure, and fearful (Turnbaugh, Guitar, & Hoffman, 1979; Woods & Williams, 1976). Such listeners' stereotypes probably affect the way stutterers see themselves. Changing the stutterer's negative attitudes can be a major focus of treatment.

The three components of stuttering—core behaviors, secondary behaviors, and feelings and attitudes—are shown in Figure 1.2. The core behavior is simply the individual's blocks on the B in "Boston." The secondary behaviors consist of postponement devices such as "uh," "well," and "you know," and the substitution of "The Big Apple" for "New York." Feelings and attitudes are depicted as the individual's thoughts that he won't succeed in getting the word out fluently and his belief that his listener will think he is dumb because he stutters.

BASIC FACTS ABOUT STUTTERING AND THEIR IMPLICATIONS FOR THE NATURE OF STUTTERING

In this section, we will cover some of the best known "facts" about stuttering. These are often-replicated research findings that revolve around the occurrence and variability of stuttering in the population and in individuals. As we discuss these points, we will note what they suggest about the nature of stuttering. Thus, as you continue through the rest of this chapter, you will become increasingly aware of our perspective on the nature and treatment of stuttering.

Much has been made of the "heterogeneity" of stuttering; many authors have suggested that stuttering is not one disorder, but many. Researchers have made various divisions of stutterers, such as Van Riper's (1982) four "tracks" of stuttering development, and St. Onge's (1963) triad of speech-phobic, psychogenic, and organic stutterers. Our approach is to concentrate primarily on the vast majority of stutterers, whose stuttering begins during childhood, without an apparent link to a psychological or organic trauma. This most common type of stuttering has been called "developmental stuttering," because the symptoms usually appear gradually, during the period of greatest speech and language development. We will simply call it "stuttering." To distinguish other fluency problems, such as those that may be associated with psychological problems, brain damage, retardation, and cluttering, we will refer to them by their assumed etiology, such as "disfluencies associated with brain damage."

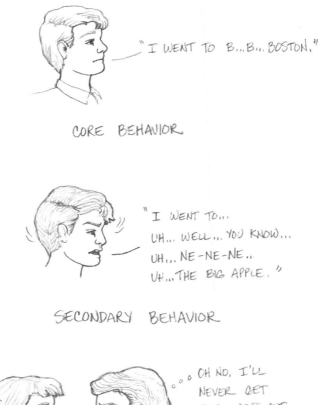

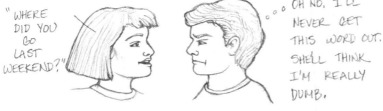

Figure 1.2.   Components of stuttering: core behaviors, secondary behaviors, and feelings and attitudes.

Onset

Our information about the onset of stuttering comes primarily from parents' reports. Because stuttering usually appears gradually, often emerging out of normal childhood disfluencies, parents' reports are frequently hazy about the exact time of onset and the particular symptoms that first came to their attention. Furthermore, onset is not easily identified, because stuttering usually comes and goes during its earliest stages. It may appear as an excess of normal disfluencies for a few days, then disappear for months, suddenly to reappear to stay. Which of these appearances was the true onset?

Despite these uncertainties, researchers generally agree that the onset of stuttering may occur at any time during childhood, between the beginning of multiword utterances (18 months) and puberty (11 or 12 years). It is most *likely* to occur, however, between ages 2 and 5 (Andrews, Craig, Feyer, Hoddinott, Howie, & Neilson, 1983). Because of this characteristic onset, stuttering seems not to be a disorder simply of making sounds, but a problem related to using spoken language in meaningful communication. Its onset often coincides, as we have said before, with the period of very intense speech and language learning.

Prevalence

The term "prevalence" is used to indicate the degree to which a disorder is widespread. Information about the prevalence of stuttering tells us how many people currently stutter. Accurate and up-to-date information on the prevalence of stuttering is difficult to obtain. The research literature shows many methodological differences among studies which are reflected in the wide differences in prevalence estimates. For example, the prevalence of stuttering varies considerably with age, and not all studies measure stuttering in the same age groups. Moreover, the definition of stuttering may vary from study to study. Some studies may include relatively normally disfluent individuals in their count; others may rule these out.

Bloodstein (1987) discusses these and other problems associated with measuring the prevalence of stuttering, and summarizes the results of 38 studies of schoolchildren in the U.S., Europe, Africa, Australia, and the West Indies. These studies show that the prevalence of stuttering is about 1%. Andrews et al. (1983) come to the same conclusion: about 1% of the school children world-wide can be considered stutterers at any given time. These authors add that there appear to be no reliable prevalence figures for stuttering in adults. However, both Bloodstein (1987) and Andrews et al. (1983) suggest that prevalence figures show a decline in stuttering after puberty. If the prevalence continued to decline, the figure for adults would be less than 1%.

Incidence

The incidence of stuttering is an index of how many people have stuttered at some time in their lives. Like the data on prevalence, incidence figures are not clear-cut, because different researchers use different definitions of stuttering. Some researchers report only stuttering that lasted six months or more, not wanting to include shorter episodes of disfluency. Others report any speech behaviors that informants or parents considered stuttering. Estimates of incidence, when reports of informants and parents are considered, are as high as 15%—a figure which includes those children who only stutter for a brief period (Bloodstein, 1987). When only stuttering that lasted longer than 6 months is included, the incidence appears to be about 5% (Andrews et al., 1983). We think the latter estimate may more accurately reflect the chronic disorder we call stuttering, but the former emphasizes how close are perceptions of normal disfluency and stuttering. Incidence figures tell us another thing about the nature of stuttering. The difference between incidence (5%) and prevalence (1%) suggests that most individuals who stutter at some time in their lives recover from it, and we know that prevalence begins to decline after puberty. Thus, unless treatment alone is responsible for remissions, some aspect of growth or maturation allows many individuals to recover from stuttering.

Recovery Without Treatment

Studies suggest that a large number of stutterers have recovered without professional treatment (Andrews & Harris, 1964; Bloodstein, 1987). Our knowledge about how many stutterers recover is based, to a large extent, on retrospective reports of adults who say they used to stutter but overcame it without treatment. This information is likely to be somewhat unreliable, because the adults who were surveyed may have been told by their parents they stuttered, but were actually no more disfluent than many normal children. Moreover, some of these individuals may still have stuttered when they were surveyed, but disguised it fairly well.

Bloodstein (1987), who reviewed the retrospective studies and their weaknesses, indicated a recovery range of from 36 to 79%. The longitudinal study by Andrews and Harris (1964) avoided many of the problems of self-reporting by following a group from onset of stuttering to their teenage years. These researchers report a recovery rate of 79%, but it should be noted that this figure includes all individuals who ever stuttered, even for very brief periods of time. The recovery rate from all available studies varies from 23 to 80% (Andrews et al., 1983). The lower recovery rates could be explained by the fact that, if children who stutter are observed for only a few years, fewer will have had a chance to recover.

In summary, there appears to be no single figure that pinpoints the percentage of stutterers who will recover without treatment. It depends on many factors—the accuracy with which stuttering is differentiated from normal disfluency, whether the study is retrospective or longitudinal, and the size of the group studied, among other things. In general, we can say that between 50 and 80% of children who stutter will recover with or without professional treatment, most before puberty. Factors that may be related to recovery include: a less severe stuttering problem, some change in the way the stutterer is speaking (especially slowing speech rate), and being a female. We will now consider this last variable, the sex factor, in more detail.

Sex Ratio

Studies of the sex ratio in stuttering were first published in the 1890s, and have been published every decade since. With this steady stream of information, we ought to have reliable data on this phenomenon. In fact, we do. The results of these studies of stutterers at many ages and in many cultures put the ratio at about 3 male stutterers to every female stutterer. There is strong evidence, however, that the ratio increases as children get older. For example, Yairi (1983) reported that of 22 children between the ages of 2 and 3 whose parents perceived they were stutterers, 11 were boys and 11 were girls.[7] Bloodstein's (1987) review indicates that the sex ratio is about 3:1 by the first grade and 5:1 by the fifth grade. It appears that girls may begin to stutter a little earlier (Yairi, 1983), but also may recover earlier (Andrews et al., 1983). Thus, female stutterers who don't recover by adulthood may be an interesting sub-population to study. They may have inherited a substantial predisposition toward stuttering, or may have been subjected to strong environmental pressures on their speech, or both (Andrews et al., 1983). Alternately, they may lack the "recovery factor" that most young female stutterers have.

Variability and Predictability of Stuttering

Another important piece of background information about stuttering is how it varies. Despite the fact that it seems so inconsistent and so disorganized, stuttering is surprisingly predictable in its occurrence. This lawfulness is an important clue to its nature. As we trace the research on stuttering's variability, we can see how this information reflects changing theoretical perspectives on the disorder.

Before the 1930s, stuttering had been commonly regarded as a medical disorder. Lee Edward Travis, the first person to be trained as a Ph.D. to work with speech and hearing disorders, set up a laboratory at the University of Iowa in 1924 to study stuttering from a neurophysiological perspective. To Travis and his fellow researchers, the variability of stuttering behaviors was seen as part of a disease process, and an unimportant part at that. Far more relevant were the stutterer's brain waves, heart rate, and breathing pattern. But in the 1930s, psychologists at Iowa, as elsewhere, were taking a keen interest in behavioral approaches to the study of human subjects. This enthusiasm spilled over into research on stuttering, and scientists who had been trying to understand the neurophysiology of stuttering gradually began trying to fathom the social, psychological, and linguistic factors that govern its occurrence and variability (Bloodstein, 1987).

Anticipation, Consistency, and Adaptation

Much of the early research into behavioral aspects of stuttering focused on how stuttering varies in predictable ways. Researchers found, for example, that when stutterers were asked to read a passage aloud, many stutterers could forecast—with a high degree of accuracy—which words they would stutter on.[8] Researchers also discovered that when stutterers read a passage aloud several times, many tended to stutter on the same words each time (Johnson & Knott, 1937; Johnson & Inness, 1939). They found that when stutterers read a passage repeatedly, their stuttering usually occurred less and less often (Johnson & Knott, 1937;

---

[7] Note that these stutterers were not diagnosed by expert clinicians, but by parents. Thus this 1:1 sex ratio must be accepted tentatively. However, other researchers have also reported sex ratios close to 1:1 in preschool stutterers (Glasner and Rosenthal, 1957).

[8] Johnson & Solomon, 1937; Knott, Johnson, & Webster, 1937; Milisen, 1938; Van Riper, 1936.

Van Riper & Hull, 1955).[9] These findings, called anticipation, consistency, and adaptation, respectively, changed some assumptions about the disorder. Stuttering, it seemed, was not simply a neurophysiological disorder. It had aspects of learned behavior.

LANGUAGE FACTORS

One of this group of Iowa researchers, Spencer Brown, pushed this investigation of the predictability of stuttering into the realm of language. In seven studies completed over a stretch of ten years, Brown found that stuttering varied lawfully with several grammatical factors.[10] He showed that most adult stutterers stutter more frequently (*a*) on consonants, (*b*) on sounds in word-initial position, (*c*) in contextual speech (versus isolated words), (*d*) on nouns, verbs, adjectives, and adverbs (versus articles, prepositions, pronouns, and conjuctions), (*e*) on longer words, (*f*) on words at the beginnings of sentences, and (*g*) on stressed syllables. Evidently, stuttering is highly influenced by the language the stutterer uses.[11]

These studies not only changed the view of stuttering; they also opened the door on new treatment possibilities. If much of stuttering is learned, it may be unlearned. The challenge, then, was to determine how much is learned, and how to help the stutterer develop new responses. Many of the treatment approaches we will discuss later in the book were developed using this orientation.

FLUENCY-INDUCING CONDITIONS

One of the researchers at the University of Iowa, Oliver Bloodstein, wrote his Ph.D. dissertation on "Conditions under which Stuttering is Reduced or Absent" (Bloodstein, 1948, 1950). In studying the speech of stutterers in 115 conditions, Bloodstein found that, in many of these conditions, stuttering is markedly decreased. Some of these are: speaking when alone, when relaxed, in unison with another speaker, to an animal or an infant, in time to a rhythmic stimulus or singing, in a dialect, while simultaneously writing, and swearing. In later studies, additional conditions which were found to reduce stuttering included: speaking in a slow prolonged manner, speaking under loud masking noise, speaking while listening to delayed auditory feedback, shadowing another speaker, speaking with reinforcement for fluent speech, as well as others. Various explanations have been

---

[9] These studies were usually carried out by giving the stutterer a passage and asking him to read it out loud. If the experimenter were studying consistency, for example, he would have his own copy of the passage upon which he would mark every word the stutterer stuttered on Then he would ask the stutterer to read it again, and the experimenter would again mark the words stuttered on in the second reading. From this he could calculate the percentage of words stuttered on in two (or more) readings.

[10] These findings were reported in the series of papers Brown published from 1935 to 1945 (Brown, 1937, 1938a, b, c, 1943, 1945; Brown & Moren, 1942; Johnson & Brown, 1935). However, only four of the factors (phonetic type, grammatical class, sentence position, and word length) are usually cited as "Brown's factors." The remaining three are brought out in the excellent discussion of Brown's work in Chapter 3 of Wingate's *The Structure of Stuttering* (1988)

[11] In his recent book, Wingate (1988) reinterpreted many of the above findings, and suggested that stuttering is a neurological dysfunction of utterance planning and assembly. His work is indicative of a recent trend to integrate neurological, linguistic, and learning explanations of the disorder.

given for the impact of all these conditions. Most are compatible with the idea that stuttering has a substantial learned component and is affected by external stimuli such as communicative pressure. Recently, however, new explanations have appeared,[12] reflecting a new trend of thought about stuttering. It has been suggested that "reduced stuttering is associated with conditions in which the neurophysiological demands of speech motor control and language formulation are reduced" (Andrews, Howie, Dozsa, & Guitar, 1982). Thus, the earlier view of stuttering as a neurophysiological disorder has not been forgotten. It has reappeared with a new sophistication that acknowledges a learning component and incorporates some understanding of speech and language production.

This updated view is essentially the model of stuttering presented in this book. We see stuttering as a disorder of the neuromotor control of speech, influenced by the interactive processes of language production, and intensified by complex learning processes. The next few chapters will expand upon this theme, and prepare you to use this information in diagnosis and treatment.

SUMMARY

Stuttering appears in all cultures and has been a problem for humankind for at least 40 centuries. It can be defined as a high frequency or severity of stoppages that impede the forward flow of speech. It begins in childhood and usually becomes more severe with age, unless the child recovers with or without formal treatment.

Core behaviors of stuttering are repetitions, prolongations, and blocks. Secondary behaviors are the result of attempts to escape or avoid core behaviors. They may be physical concomitants of stuttering, such as eye blinks, or verbal concomitants, such as word substitution. Feelings and attitudes can also be an important component of stuttering. They are the stutterer's emotional reactions to the experience of being unable to speak fluently and to listener responses to their stuttering. Feelings are the immediate reactions, and include such emotions as fear and embarrassment. Attitudes crystallize more slowly, from repeated stuttering experiences with negative feelings. An example is a stutterer's belief that listeners think he is stupid when they hear him stuttering.

The onset of stuttering is usually gradual. It may occur any time between 18 months and puberty, but onset is most likely to be reported between 2 and 5 years of age. Prevalence of stuttering is about 1%. Incidence is about 5%. Recovery rate without professional treatment is between 50 and 80% of children who ever stuttered. The larger percentage is probably a result of including children who were very mild stutterers or who stuttered for a very brief time. The sex ratio is generally considered to be 3:1 (males to females). There is, however, some indication that the sex ratio may be similar at onset, and that more females recover during childhood, increasing the proportion of males with the disorder after puberty.

---

[12] Among many who have proposed new explanations of fluency-inducing conditions are: Andrews, Howie, Dozsa, & Guitar (1982); Martin & Haroldson (1979); Perkins, Rudas, Johnson, & Bell (1976); and Wingate (1969, 1970).

Many stutterers have been shown to be able to predict which words in a reading passage they will stutter on with a high degree of accuracy (anticipation). In addition, most tend to stutter on the same words each time in repeated reading of a paragraph (consistency). On the other hand, stuttering frequency decreases for most stutterers when they read a passage over many times (adaptation). It has been shown that stuttering occurs more frequently with certain grammatical categories. Research has also revealed that a variety of conditions reduce the frequency of stuttering. Their effect may be attributable to changes in speech pattern, reduction in communicative pressure, or both. Research on these fluency-inducing conditions has recently suggested that stuttering may be diminished by reducing the demands of speech motor control and language formulation.

STUDY QUESTIONS

1/ What are the differences between "core" and "secondary" behaviors in stuttering?

2/ When stuttering is defined, what other kinds of hesitation must it be distinguished from?

3/ What are some feelings and attitudes a stutterer might have, and where do these come from?

4/ What is the age range for the onset of stuttering (what are the youngest and oldest ages at which onset is commonly reported)?

5/ What is the difference between "incidence" and "prevalence"?

6/ What problems do researchers encounter when they try to determine how many stutterers recover without treatment?

7/ Why does the sex ratio of male to female stutterers change?

8/ In what ways is stuttering predictable? In what ways does it vary?

Suggested Readings

Johnson, W. and Leutenegger, R. (1955). *Stuttering in children and adults.* Minneapolis: University of Minnesota Press.

These authors have compiled the research papers from one of the most productive research efforts ever applied to stuttering. These studies, conducted between the 1930s and 1950s at the University of Iowa, uncovered many of the basic facts we have about the variability and predictability of stuttering. The first chapter, "The Time, the Place, and the Problem," gives a historical perspective on this research.

Shields, D. (1989). *Dead languages.* New York: Knopf.

This is a novel about a young boy who stutters. It conveys the feelings associated with being a stutterer in a world that prizes spoken language. It is recommended for students who would like to understand a child who stutters.

Wingate, M. (1988). *The structure of stuttering—A psycholinguistic analysis.* New York: Springer-Verlag.

Wingate builds a logical case for the explanation of stuttering as a neurological disorder whose overt symptoms are the result of dysynchrony in utterance planning and assembly. It reflects the current thinking that stuttering has an important language component.

2

CONSTITUTIONAL FACTORS

ROLE OF HEREDITY

One of the best known facts about stuttering is that it usually runs in families. Because it passes from generation to generation, many researchers believed that stuttering is transmitted genetically. Others argued that stuttering is not biologically inherited but learned. It runs in families, they suggested, because a critical attitude toward hesitations and repetitions has been handed down from one generation to the next. A child whose parents were critical of his normal disfluencies would grow afraid and would "hesitate to hesitate." This would start a spiral of more hesitations leading to greater fear, and so on.

For many years researchers clustered on one side of this argument or the other. In the last two decades, however, a version of the genetic hypothesis has become widely accepted. In part, this may be due to new evidence about heredity in stuttering, but it is probably also due to a less deterministic view of heredity. Stuttering, asthma, migraine, and certain other disorders are seen as the result of both heredity and environment, acting together, with elements of chance thrown in (Kidd, 1984).

We will review two approaches to heredity and stuttering in this chapter: family studies and twin studies. These are quite different ways of gathering evidence, but both suggest that stuttering, like most other behaviors, is in part transmitted genetically.

Family Studies

FAMILY STUDIES OF STUTTERERS

Researchers gather evidence for the inheritance of stuttering by looking at the family trees of stutterers. They interview family members to find out which, if any, of the stutterers' first-degree relatives also stutter. At the same time, a control group of nonstutterers is formed of persons matched with the stutterers for age, sex, and other important characteristics. Researchers construct family trees for the control group, and compare the two groups to determine if stutterers have more first-degree stuttering relatives than nonstutterers. They also search for patterns of occurrence of stuttering that will rule out non-hereditary explanations such as imitation and family attitudes.

One of the first studies to report evidence of genetic transmission of stuttering was an interim report on an ongoing study of a thousand families in Newcastle, England (Andrews and Harris, 1964). With the help of genetic researchers Roger Garside and David Kay, Gavin Andrews & Mary Ann Harris investigated the family histories of 80 stuttering children. They found that (*a*) stutterers had far more stuttering relatives than nonstutterers, (*b*) males in this group were more at risk than females to develop stuttering, and (*c*) females who stuttered were more likely to have stuttering relatives than were male stutterers.

A geneticist at Yale University, Kenneth Kidd, and his coworkers followed up the British study by looking for familial patterns of stuttering in the United States (Kidd, 1977; Kidd, Reich, & Kessler, 1973; Kidd, Kidd, & Records, 1978). They first reexamined the Andrews and Harris (1964) data, combined with evidence they gathered themselves, and used statistical models to predict the pattern of inheritance. In this and subsequent studies they were able to predict with remarkable accuracy which first-degree relatives of stutterers would also have the disorder. Males were more likely to stutter than females; females who stuttered were more likely to have first-degree relatives who stuttered. Kidd and his associates concluded that the patterns of stuttering are best explained by an interaction between the environment and a combination of several genes.

We are still not completely sure how the transmission patterns of stuttering result in the sex ratios found in many studies. The finding that the incidence of stuttering is higher in males than females may indicate that males are more vulnerable to stuttering and females more resistant to it. But why should there be more stutterers among relatives of female stutterers? The answer may be that if females are more resistant to stuttering, only those females who have inherited a large amount of "genetic predisposition" will actually stutter. These must, then, be females with many ancestors who stutter. Furthermore, if they have considerable genetic predisposition, they will be likely to pass it on to their offspring.

In summary, family studies have provided evidence that many stutterers have inherited a predisposition for stuttering. Research has not shown what that predisposition is. In other words, no one has discovered exactly what physical differences exist in stutterers that may give rise to the symptoms of stuttering.[1]

FAMILY STUDIES OF STUTTERING AND CLUTTERING

A different perspective on the inheritance of stuttering has been given by researchers looking at the relationship between stuttering and cluttering. Cluttering is primarily a disorder of speech rate and intelligibility. Clutterers talk rapidly and often slur; they speak in short bursts, putting in many fillers such as "uh." They have many false starts and hesitations. A number of studies have shown that stuttering and cluttering often occur in the same families (Van Riper, 1982). Some writers have speculated that a subgroup of stutterers—those who stutter but also talk rapidly, in short spurts with many fillers, in addition to their usual symptoms of stuttering—may be more likely to have inherited their stuttering (Van Riper, 1982; Weiss, 1964). This introduces an idea that recurs frequently in stuttering research—that there may be several different types of stutterers, based on different etiologies. One of these subtypes may have a neurological predisposition toward both stuttering and cluttering.

Twin Studies

Inheritance of stuttering can also be investigated by comparing the incidence of stuttering in fraternal and identical twins. Identical twins (also called monozygotic twins) have identical genes. Fraternal twins (dizygotic) may share only half their genes, like any other siblings. Any greater similarity in the traits of identical twins compared to those of fraternal twins is generally attributed to inheritance. Twin studies of stuttering have shown that stuttering occurs more often in both members of identical twin pairs than in both members of fraternal twin pairs (Andrews, Morris-Yates, Howie, & Martin, 1990; Howie, 1981; Luchsinger, 1944; Seeman, 1937). To use the vocabulary of genetics, there is higher "concordance" for stuttering in identical twins than in fraternal twins. This supports the hypothesis that stuttering is inherited. But it doesn't reveal specifically what is inherited. How does a gene (or several genes) affect a child's speech so that stuttering results? No one is sure. Later in this chapter, we will describe several "educated guesses" about how an inherited difference might result in stuttering.

In addition to evidence of genetic factors in stuttering, twin studies demonstrate that heredity does not work alone. In one of the twin studies described above, although there was more concordance for stuttering among identical twins, some of the identical twin pairs were discordant (Howie, 1982); that

---

[1] Genetic differences between stutterers and nonstutterers may be extremely subtle, and not evident in the child at birth. Researchers have found, for example, that heredity may govern the extent to which an individual may be classically conditioned to fear. Such genetically determined tendencies appear only if and when environmental conditions are right for learning a fear-induced response.

is, in 6 of 16 identical twin pairs, one twin stuttered, but the other didn't. This finding suggests that environmental factors, as well as genetic factors, are at work to create stuttering, at least in some individuals. Environmental influences appear to have interacted differentially with genetic predisposition to produce stuttering for one member of the twin pair and not the other in these 6 cases. An estimate of the proportion of genetic and environmental influences has been suggested by a recent twin study involving 3810 unselected twin pairs (Andrews, Morris-Yates, Howie, & Martin, 1990). Analysis of these data suggested that 71% of the variance (the probability of whether or not one would stutter) is accounted for by environmental factors, and 29% is accounted for by the individual's unique environment (including factors influencing the fetus, as well as factors after birth). We hope that future research will reveal the critical aspects of the environment that have this effect. Many environmental factors—which can be influenced in early treatment—have been under scrutiny for some time. These will be discussed in the next chapter.

In general, researchers who conduct family studies and those who conduct twin studies agree that stuttering is not the product of a single inherited trait. Stuttering is likely to be the result of several inherited (or congenital) factors and several environmental factors interacting, as well as combining, in different proportions for different individuals (see, for example, Cox, Seider, and Kidd, 1984).

Summary

Studies of stutterers' families indicate that relatives of stutterers are at greater risk for stuttering than relatives of nonstutterers. Females appear to be more resistant than males to stuttering, but relatives of female stutterers are more likely to be stutterers. Twin studies show more concordance for stuttering in identical twins than in fraternal twins. Some identical twin pairs, however, are discordant, suggesting an environmental influence, as well as a genetic one. Some unknown factor appears to be inherited, creating a predisposition. There may, in fact, be several predisposing factors, which can act singly or together. In some cases, environmental factors may trigger stuttering in children who have this predisposition. In other cases, the predisposition may be there, but the environment may nurture fluency. These children may never develop stuttering.

DIFFERENCES BETWEEN STUTTERERS AND NONSTUTTERERS

Pinpointing the predisposing factors in stuttering will be difficult. To find the cause of a disorder, a researcher must be able to manipulate the conditions that create it. For example, some of the causes of cleft palate have been discovered because researchers have selectively bred animals to produce cleft palate in the animals' offspring. But there is nothing exactly like stuttering in animals. And obviously, selective breeding or destructive brain surgery to create stuttering is not an option in humans. Researchers, therefore, have turned to more indirect approaches. They compare stutterers and nonstutterers in tasks which might be related to speech fluency. If they find, again and again, that stutterers and nonstutterers perform differently in certain tasks, they may have a clue about the disorder.

Such indirect research is complicated because the differences might be a *result* of stuttering, not a cause of it. For example, in a study of how quickly subjects can say a word flashed upon a screen, the results might find that stutterers are slower than nonstutterers. This difference, however, might be the result of stutterers saying words slowly to keep from stuttering. Even if a difference were not the result of trying not to stutter, it might be caused by a distantly related factor: some stutterers may have slower responses because the cerebral processes responsible for motor reactions affect not only speech, but also other motor responses. It's like finding that taller people have larger shoe sizes than shorter people. The tallness doesn't directly cause a large shoe size. Instead both are related to genetically determined bone size.

In the following section we will review some of the findings from studies comparing stutterers and nonstutterers. The research literature, however, has many inconsistent findings, as scientists repeat each others' experiments to verify their results. One study finds a difference, but another study reports it isn't there. Often the conflict between two studies occurs because there are small differences in the way the studies are done. One study, for example, may use a 1000 Hz tone for a stimulus, and another may use a recording of the word "Go." Despite these conflicts in the results of studies, there are certain areas of agreement among researchers. In the following sections, we will summarize findings in several important areas where stutterers and nonstutterers have been compared. In many cases, researchers agree that an important difference between stutterers and nonstutterers has been found. Yet no one has completely put together the pieces of the puzzle to explain why stutterers stutter.

Intelligence

Several early studies of stutterers' intelligence showed that they were close to the norm or only slightly below it (Berry, 1937; Darley, 1955; Johnson et al., 1942; Schlinder, 1955; West, 1931). These studies, however, were plagued by lack of control groups of nonstutterers, in some cases, and highly selected groups of subjects, in others.[2] The slightly lower IQs of the stuttering group, found by a few studies, were usually dismissed as the result of stuttering, not the cause of it. Researchers assumed that stutterers might often be reluctant to give a correct answer because they were afraid of stuttering.

More recent studies have shown that both verbal and nonverbal intelligence is slightly lower in stutterers as a group. This suggests that even when stutterers don't have to answer a question verbally, they may still score slightly

---

[2] The studies of Darley (1955) and Johnson et al. (1942) were conducted with children from the University of Iowa community. This sample is unlikely to be representative of the general population, and so it doesn't tell us much about the disorder of stuttering per se.

lower. One study found stutterers to be poorer than nonstutterers on language-related subtests. Another found stutterers poorer on subtests requiring motor skills. This evidence suggests that stuttering might be linked to some inadequacy in linguistic and/or motor processes (Bloodstein, 1987). One might guess that, the greater the deficit one had in cerebral resources in general, the greater would be the chances of stuttering. And indeed, Van Riper observes that among those who are mentally retarded, the less intelligent have a higher incidence of stuttering than the more intelligent (Van Riper, 1982). In this population, those who are more retarded undoubtedly have the possibility of greater deficits in all cerebral resources, including those underlying both linguistic and motor performance. Their increased stuttering, then, would reflect the fact that deficits in linguistic ability, motor ability, or both, increase the likelihood of stuttering.

School Performance

Studies have shown that stutterers perform slightly below average in school. Stutterers are more likely than their peers to be a grade behind and their achievement test scores are lower (Schlinder, 1955). At least two factors may contribute to stutterers' poorer school achievement. One is their difficulty in talking, simply because of stuttering. Many stutterers, including both of the authors during their school days, would answer "I don't know" to a teacher's question rather than risk stuttering. The other factor is a deficit in language-related skills, as shown by various standardized tests (Williams, Melrose, & Woods, 1969). Consider how much of school involves reading, as well as both oral and written verbal expression. In such a verbal environment as this, both of these factors would put stutterers at some disadvantage.

Speech and Language Development

We have reported that stutterers don't do as well as their peers on measures of school achievement and IQ. Both of these findings may be related in part to stutterers' poorer language skills. Further evidence of the importance of a language factor comes from research which shows that stutterers lag behind nonstutterers in speech and language development. When assessed on such measures as the age at which they produced their first word and their first sentence, level of receptive vocabulary, mean length of utterance, and expressive and receptive syntax, children who stutter often score lower than their peers (Andrews & Harris, 1964; Berry, 1938; Kline & Starkweather, 1979; Murray & Reed, 1977; Wall, 1980).

Stutterers have also been shown to have difficulty with articulation. In the clinic, we often observe children in the early stages of stuttering who have multiple articulation or phonological problems and are consequently difficult to understand. Research has repeatedly confirmed the finding that stutterers have roughly two and a half times the incidence of articulation disorders as that found in nonstutterers (Andrews & Harris, 1964; Bloodstein, 1958; Kent & Williams, 1963; Berry 1938).

These findings about articulation and language performance in stutterers can be interpreted in several ways. Some authors have suggested that a child who has difficulty with articulation or language will start to believe that speaking is difficult. The anticipation of difficulty is hypothesized to lead to hesitation and struggle, and then to stuttering (Bloodstein, 1987). An alternate view is that stuttering, language disorders, and articulation errors all come from a common deficit. This may be the deficit that is passed on genetically in stutterers. Because circumscribed areas of the brain are responsible for speech and language related functions, a delayed development of (or damage to) these areas may result in language, articulation, or fluency problems, in any combination. Small differences in how the brain processes such functions could tip the balance toward any of these disorders.

Sensory-Motor Coordination

CENTRAL AUDITORY PROCESSING

In their search for the physiological basis of stuttering, researchers have investigated many different parts of the speech mechanism, including the auditory system. It is known that learning to speak involves both the motor processes of speaking and the sensory processes of feeling and hearing oneself speak. Some researchers have suspected that stuttering may be the result of errors in how stutterers hear themselves speak. In exploring this hypothesis, researchers have measured how stutterers' central nervous systems handle various sounds, including speech. Assessment tools developed to detect tumors and other lesions in the auditory system, such as the Synthetic Sentence Identification Test, have been applied to stutterers with interesting results. Several studies have shown that stutterers, as a group, perform more poorly than nonstutterers on tasks requiring discrimination of small time differences in signals (Hall & Jerger, 1978; Toscher & Rupp, 1978; Kramer, Green, & Guitar, 1987).[3] One of the tasks which has shown group differences between stutterers and nonstutterers is the Masking Level Difference test. This requires the listener to detect the onset and offset of a tone under conditions of masking noise. When the masking noise is played in the same ear as the tone, there are fewer cues for the listener to use to "filter out" the masking noise and "filter in" the tone. The listener must use very subtle temporal cues to detect the tone, and it is under these conditions that stutterers, as a group, perform most poorly.

Researchers have speculated that timing of incoming signals is the particular weakness of the stutterers who perform poorly on central auditory tests. Researchers have tried to link this deficit to stuttering by suggesting that a single mechanism in the brain may control timing for both incoming and outgoing signals (for example, Kent, 1983). Faulty timing of incoming signals would give rise to stutterers' poorer performance on central auditory tests. Faulty timing of outgoing signals would result in stuttering.

---

[3] A review of the research on stutterers' auditory functioning can be found in D.B. Rosenfield and J. Jerger, "Stuttering and Auditory Function" in R. Curlee and W. Perkins (eds.) *Nature and Treatment of Stuttering*, San Diego: College-Hill Press (1984).

Right Hemisphere Processing

Researchers have also theorized that stutterers' faulty input and output timing may be related to which half of their brain is dominant for speech. Normal speakers use both right and left hemispheres of the brain for speech, but the left is usually dominant. Scientists speculate that the left hemisphere of the brain is more specialized for speech and language because it can process rapidly changing signals (like the quick shift of /t/ into /o/ in the word "toe") better than the right hemisphere (Liberman, Cooper, Shankweiler, & Studdert-Kennedy, 1967). The right hemisphere, by contrast, is specialized for more slowly changing signals, such as music, environmental sounds, and the intonation patterns of speech (Hammond, 1982). Some experimenters who have found that stutterers are poorer at tests of central auditory processing suggest that this deficit may occur because stutterers do not use their left hemispheres for speech as efficiently as nonstutterers. Instead, they suggest, stutterers use their right hemispheres for speech processing to a greater extent than nonstutterers (Moore, 1984; Moore and Haynes, 1980).

Further evidence of stutterers' right hemisphere processing has been gathered by researchers measuring brain function during speech. Records of electrical and chemical activity in the brain have shown more activity in the stutterers' right hemispheres during speech when they are stuttering (McFarland and Moore, 1982; Wood, Stump, McKeehan, Sheldon, and Proctor, 1980). The implication is that stutterers may be using a less effective part of the brain for timing speech—at least when they are stuttering. Richard Curlee (personal communication, 1990) has suggested another interpretation of the increased activity of the right hemisphere during stuttering. He notes that right hemisphere activity is usually associated with emotional expression (e.g., Sackeim and Gur, 1978), and that the findings of greater right hemisphere activation during stuttering could be a correlate of greater emotionality during stuttered speech. This suggestion also has implications for the onset of stuttering in childhood, when many functions, presumably including speech and emotion, appear to be bilateralized. Fluency may be especially vulnerable to emotional disruption then because of "crosstalk" between speech and emotional expression.

Reaction Time

Stutterers' poorer abilities in decoding and encoding the rapidly changing components of speech may explain the next group of experimental findings. Research has shown that stutterers, as a group, are slower in their reaction times. Many studies have measured how fast stutterers can push a button when they hear a buzzer or how rapidly they can say a word that is flashed upon a screen. These reaction time tasks assess the sensory (input) and motor (output) systems working together. The first experiments compared vocal reaction time in stutterers and nonstutterers, and found that stutterers were slower in starting and stopping a sound such as "ahhh" when they heard a buzzer (Adams and Hayden, 1976; Starkweather, Hirschman, and Tannenbaum, 1976). Gradually researchers broadened their focus. They discovered that stutterers were slower in reacting with respiration (exhalation) and articulation (lip closing). They found that stutterers are slower than nonstutterers whether they are responding to an auditory signal or a visual one. They found that children who stutter also have slower reaction times (Cross and Luper, 1979; Cullinan and Springer, 1980;[4] Till, Reich, Dickey, and Sieber, 1983). They discovered that stutterers are slower in "tracking" a tone that goes up and down in pitch (Neilson, Quinn, and Neilson, 1976; Nudelman, Herbrich, Hoyt, and Rosenfield, 1987).

In this area of research, as in many others, the results of many studies conflict. Despite the confusion, the majority of studies show groups of stutterers react more slowly than groups of nonstutterers. Furthermore, in spite of dozens of studies, none show stutterers, as a group, to be faster than nonstutterers. There are, however, many individual differences. In most experiments, some stutterers are faster than many nonstutterers, and some nonstutterers are slower than many stutterers. Thus, slow reaction times themselves are not *sufficient* to create stuttering (since some nonstutterers are also slow). And slow reaction times are not *necessary* to create stuttering (since some stutterers don't have slow reaction times). Oliver Bloodstein (1987) has pointed out that the differences between stutterers and nonstutterers have shown themselves to be neither necessary nor sufficient to create stuttering.

ACOUSTIC STUDIES OF FLUENT SPEECH

Reaction time responses, such as lip closing or saying "ahhh," are relatively indirect measures of speech. Researchers have been able to make a more direct assessment by examining the speed and coordination of stutterers' speech movements when they are talking fluently. Even when they are fluent, stutterers, on the average, have longer vowel durations, slower transitions between consonants and vowels, and delayed onsets of voicing after voiceless consonants (Colcord and Adams, 1979; DiSimoni, 1974; Hillman and Gilbert, 1977; Starkweather and Myers, 1979).[5] These results of acoustic studies have been supported by "kinematic" research which has measured the movements of speakers' speech structures (Alfonso, Story, and Watson, 1987; Zimmerman, 1980). As a group, stutterers have been found to move some of their speech structures more slowly than nonstutterers, even in fluent speech (e.g., Zimmerman, 1980).

But what does this mean? Why might many stutterers speak more slowly than normal when they are fluent? Some researchers think that this finding reflects a basic delay in processing incoming and outgoing signals. Stutterers may be unable to send the neural signals fast enough to make the rapid, precise

---

[4] This study actually found that significant differences from nonstuttering children were found only in children who stuttered *and* had language, articulation, and learning problems.

[5] There are several sources that review both reaction time studies and acoustic studies of stutterers' fluent speech. Woodruff Starkweather, for example, reviews both areas in his monograph *Stuttering and Laryngeal Behavior: A Review*, Rockville, Maryland: American Speech-Language-Hearing Association (1982). He also reviews these studies in his more recent chapter, Laryneal and articulatory behavior in stuttering: Past and future, in Peters, H. and Hulstijn, W. (eds.) (1987), *Speech Motor Dynamics in Stuttering*, New York: Springer-Verlag.

movements used in normal conversational speech, especially at times when they are under the stress of planning a complex sentence or competing with other talkers. Their delays in voicing onset or slower transitions in their fluent speech may simply reflect a stutterer's slower mechanism working at its normal rate. A different view, suggested by more skeptical researchers, is that the delays in fluent speech reflect only the way stutterers have learned to talk to avoid stuttering. They have developed a slow and cautious style of speaking that keeps them from stuttering.

Yet another interpretation is that the slower movements are the result of heightened tension in all speech muscles (Starkweather, 1987). The increased tension would affect muscles that move a structure forward (agonists), as well as muscles that hold it back (antagonists). Tension in agonist and antagonist pairs of muscles would make movement considerably slower. It would be as if two people were pulling a rope in opposite directions. Even if one were stronger, their progress in pulling the rope would be slow because they would be pulling against the other person.

The slowed movements of stutterers' speech structures would account for not only slow reaction times, but the longer durations and the delays in their fluent speech as well. A number of studies have suggested that stutterers excessively contract both the agonist and antagonist muscles of the laryngeal (Freeman and Ushijima, 1975; Shapiro, 1980) and articulatory (Guitar, Guitar, Neilson, O'Dwyer, and Andrews, 1988) muscle groups during speech.[6] These studies, like Starkweather's (1987) review, have noted that heightened tension in agonist and antagonist muscles appears in the fluent speech of stutterers. This finding has led many researchers to the position that stuttering is not an "all or nothing" event (Adams and Runyan, 1981; Bloodstein, 1987). Sometimes, stutterers may speak entirely freely, without a trace of excess tension. At other times, they may have a degree of excess tension that isn't heard by the listener as stuttering. At still other times, the tension may be so great that both the stutterer and the listener notice stuttering. This continuum of fluency reflects the subjective impression of many stutterers, including the present authors.

Summary

There is substantial evidence that, as a group, stutterers differ from nonstutterers on cognitive, linguistic, and motor tasks. Moreover, children who stutter perform slightly poorer on IQ tests. They show poorer school achievement, are delayed in language development, and are more likely to have articulation errors. Stutterers also appear to perform more poorly on central auditory processing tasks, perhaps more so when fine discrimination of temporal information is needed. Stutterers may not have the normal degree of left hemisphere dominance for speech, but instead may use their right hemisphere, which may be

---

[6] Note, however, that like most findings, this evidence is disputed by other studies. Caruso (1988), McClean, Goldsmith and Cerf (1984), and Smith (1989) have reported absence of co-contraction of opposing muscles during stuttering.

specialized for slower signals than the left. Finally, stutterers' reaction times are slower than those of nonstutterers, and they have slower speech movements, even during fluent speech.

What do these differences between stutterers and nonstutterers mean? Are they symptoms of a constitutional predisposition that causes stuttering? We don't know the answer to this, but it is unlikely that any of these differences directly cause stuttering. Studies reveal that many stutterers don't show such differences, and many nonstutterers perform as deviantly as stutterers. Thus, these differences appear to be neither necessary nor sufficient to cause stuttering. One possible explanation, mentioned earlier, is that they may be simply the result of some general differences in brain development that also provide the fertile ground in which stuttering grows. That is, they may be causally unrelated to stuttering. Another possibility, which we suggested in the section on speech and language differences, is that some of these differences may give rise to communication problems which, through the frustration and failure they engender, produce stuttering. They may be causally related to stuttering, but indirectly.[7] These are, of course, speculations. The differences between stutterers and nonstutterers remain intriguing contrasts which await a unifying theory that relates them to stuttering.

SPECULATIONS ABOUT CONSTITUTIONAL FACTORS IN STUTTERING

There are no formal theories of stuttering, with carefully delineated postulates, hypotheses, and corollaries. Instead, researchers have made various speculations about stuttering, usually based on models of other disorders, or extrapolated from current understanding of normal speech processes. They pull together current evidence to explain stuttering from a particular point of view, guide further research, and, in some cases, influence how stutterers are treated. These explanations change every few years, as more data come in and as new models in related disciplines are developed. Doubtless, the explanations of stuttering we summarize in this section will be superseded by others in a few years.

We have chosen three contemporary views of constitutional factors to discuss briefly below. Although these three views are different, they are not mutually exclusive. Linked together, they provide us with some interesting notions about what might be inherited and how that might result in stuttering.

Stuttering as a Disorder of Cerebral Localization

Although normal speakers use both right and left halves of their brains for speech and language, evidence suggests that, for most speakers, the left hemisphere is dominant. Studies of normal subjects have demonstrated this with a

---

[7] The reader is encouraged to read Chapter 10, "Inferences and Conclusions" in Bloodstein (1987) for a full description of this view.

wide variety of techniques.[8] Studies of brain-damaged patients have also confirmed left hemisphere dominance for speech, finding far more speech and language impairment with left hemisphere damage than with right.

Stutterers may deviate from this pattern of left hemisphere dominance,
according to the cerebral dominance theory of stuttering, developed at the University of Iowa in the 1920s. In an atmosphere of intense scientific curiosity and
collaboration among researchers, Samuel Orton, a neurologist, and Lee Edward
Travis, a psychologist and speech pathologist, observed that many stutterers
seemed to have been left-handers whose parents changed them into right-
handers. This change, they suspected, led to a conflict of hemispheric control of
speech in which neither side was fully in charge. This in turn, it was hypothesized, created neuromotor disorganization and mistiming for speech, which led
to stuttering. The treatment was simply to switch stutterers back to being left-
handers. As you might guess, this simple treatment was fruitless. Furthermore,
evidence was never found that most stutterers were originally left-handers. Consequently, the original cerebral dominance theory of stuttering languished for
many years. But in the 1960s data started to trickle in suggesting that stutterers
may not, after all, have normal left hemisphere dominance for speech. In the
1970s and early 1980s, more studies were published supporting this finding. In
1985, a new version of the cerebral dominance theory of stuttering was proposed. Two neurologists, Norman Geschwind and Albert Galaburda, published a
theory which suggested that many disorders, including stuttering, dyslexia, and
autism, are the result of a delay in left hemisphere growth during fetal development (Geschwind and Galaburda, 1985). Such a delay, in these male-related disorders, is thought to be caused by a male-related factor. Geschwind and
Galaburda hypothesized that the delay might be the result of excess secretion of
the hormone testosterone. So far, no evidence has been found to support their
hypothesis about testosterone, but their theory is still of great interest.

Geschwind and Galaburda's theory suggests that a delay in left hemisphere development may affect speech and language for the following reasons.
Various structures which evolve in the left hemisphere during embryonic development appear to be especially suited for speech and language functions. As
these structures develop, specialized nerve cells, which are destined to sprout
the neural connections for speech and language processes, disperse from their
point of creation in the "neural tube" (where the central nervous system is
formed). These nerve cells normally migrate to the structures in the left hemisphere which are appropriate for their function. But if development of left hemisphere structures is delayed, the cells, somehow detecting this delay, may
migrate across the brain to establish themselves in right hemisphere structures
which are further developed than those on the left. These right hemisphere

---

[8] Among the methods that have demonstrated left hemisphere dominance for speech are brain
wave and blood flow studies, electrical stimulation of the brain, measures of response to linguistic
stimuli delivered to each half of the brain, and anesthetization of each hemisphere with sodium
amytal.

structures and the organization of their interconnections, however, may not be ideally suited for speech and language. Speech and language developing there may be delayed or deviant.

To grasp this concept clearly, imagine the Geschwind-Galaburda theory in terms of a telecommunication system in a new building under construction for a large corporation. The establishment of speech and language networks in the brain is comparable to a centralized communication network being installed in this new building. If the communications equipment arrives before the central room is ready, the network may have to be operated from a less appropriate room. Communication functions may be impaired. Like stuttering, which occurs most often in conditions of linguistic or psychological stress, the dysfunction of the telephones, fax machines, and computer networks may not be apparent until many of the lines are connected and a multitude of messages are going through at once.

Although the Geschwind/Galaburda hypothesis about stuttering suggests how abnormal localization of speech and language functions might occur, the way in which stuttering behaviors result from abnormal localization is another question, requiring other theories.

2. Stuttering as a Disorder of Timing

Several authors have concluded that the known facts about stuttering point toward a disorder of timing. Van Riper (1982), for example, has suggested that, "when a person stutters on a word, there is a temporal disruption of the simultaneous and successive programming of muscular movements required to produce one of the word's integrated sounds . . . " (p. 415). In a recent book chapter, Raymond Kent, a speech scientist, reviewed the evidence of differences between stutterers and nonstutterers and suggested they might correspond to differences between males' and females' abilities to process temporal and verbal information (Kent, 1984). He speculated that the deficit that may arise from inappropriate localization of speech and language is an inability to create the precise timing patterns needed for efficiently perceiving and producing speech. These hypothesized timing patterns might be likened to a timing belt on a car. This belt regulates the order of firing of the cylinders and the rate at which they fire. A more appropriate metaphor may be the conductor of a symphony orchestra. In directing the orchestra, he must regulate when each section plays, as well as the speed or beat of their playing. The timing patterns for speech may determine the rate at which we speak and the order of movements to produce sequential sounds. Like an orchesra conductor integrating the timing of several sections, the brain must coordinate complex timing relationships for phrases, syllables, phonemes, and segments.

The inability to create the proper timing programs, Kent suggests, may stem from the fact that a stutterer's left hemisphere is not as developed as his right hemisphere. Since the left hemisphere is typically more adept than the right at creating temporal programs for fine motor control of verbal output, a stutterer may be at a disadvantage in timing regulation at the speed or frequency required for speech. The central timing device, it is suggested, must not only regulate left hemisphere aspects of speech production, but must integrate timing between rapid left hemisphere segments and slower prosodic elements.

Kent also notes that emotion may play an important role in the disruption of timing in stuttered speech. As we indicated earlier, the right hemisphere is thought to be heavily involved in the expression of emotion. The stutterer's deficit, then, may be that his processes of timing regulation for speech are functionally arranged so that they are (*a*) not as efficient as a nonstutterer's and (*b*) vulnerable to interference by right hemisphere activity during increased emotion. How this deficit causes the repetitions we hear in the beginning stutterer's speech is not dealt with in this theory.

3. Stuttering as Reduced Capacity for Internal Modeling

Another theory of constitutional factors in stuttering has been advanced by researchers studying motor control of speech and other movements. Megan Neilson and Peter Neilson have suggested that the repetitions of beginning stutterers are the result of a deficit in their ability to make and use "inverse internal models of the speech production system" (Neilson and Neilson, 1987). This rather complicated sounding theory can be easily understood if we go back to an assumption about how children learn to speak. During their first year, children store up perceptions of the speech sounds they hear around them. They also coo and babble and learn what movements make what sounds. In other words, they build up both a store of perceptual targets they will aim for when they speak, and a model of the relationship between their motor movements and the sensory consequences. This might be called a sensory-motor model for speech or an inverse internal model of the speech production system. It's called "inverse" because it inverts the sensory targets into the motor commands needed to achieve them. As they learn to produce the sounds they hear, children constantly use their sensory-motor model for speech. They plan a word or sentence on the basis of what it should sound like, then they load their sensory-motor model, and generate motor commands based on the sensory or perceptual target they are trying to hit.

This process of learning to speak is like learning to drive a car. At first, keeping the car on the road requires your constant vigilance. But as you learn the relationships between turning the wheel, stepping on the accelerator, and going where you want, the linkage becomes automatic. Moreover, the linkage is refined as you encounter different driving conditions and different cars—cars, for example, with loose steering wheels and sticky accelerators. This is a sensory-motor model of driving. Children develop a sensory-motor model of speaking.

Figure 2.1 depicts a schematic of how the brain may transform desired sensory (perceptual) targets into motor commands for speech. In the figure, the Desired Output (the word or phrase, for example, that a child intends a listener to hear) is fed into the Inverse Internal Model of the Speech Production System. Here, the desired output enters as sensory code (the expected auditory and kin-

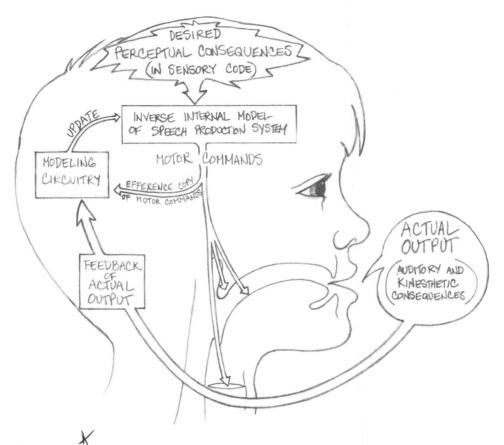

Figure 2.1. A schematic of the inverse internal model theory of speech production.

esthetic results), is "inverted" by the model, and exits as motor code or motor commands. Experience, practice, and vocal play have helped a child learn to make these inversions or transformations. Moreover, this internal model is continually updated as a child learns more and as a child's system changes with age. The motor commands exiting the internal model are sent to the muscles of the speech production system, which produces the planned utterance; feedback of the actual output is sent to the Modeling Circuitry. Retracing our steps for a moment, when the motor commands are sent to muscles, a copy of these commands (called "efference copy" by motor physiologists) is also sent to the Modeling Circuitry. Here, the efference copy is transformed into hypothetical output (a model of what the output would be expected to be, based on these commands). This hypothetical output is then compared to the feedback of the actual output and, if necessary, the Inverse Internal Model is updated so that future motor commands will more accurately produce the desired output. These components of the speech production process are assumed to be the cortico-cerebellar structures and pathways commonly described in neural models of speech output (see, for example, Neilson and Neilson, 1987 and Neilson, Neilson, and O'Dwyer, 1989).

The Neilsons and their co-workers used this model of speech to understand performance of stutterers in their experiments (Neilson, Quinn, and Neilson, 1976). In research referred to earlier, they tested stutterers on their ability to track an auditory tone that changed unpredictably. In one ear, subjects heard the changing "target" tone, and in the other ear, they heard a changing "cursor" tone, which they regulated with a hand-held device. Their task was to track the target tone with the cursor tone. The Neilsons' experiments showed that stutterers were poorer than nonstutterers at tracking an auditory tone that went up and down in pitch. Stutterers were even poorer after practicing the task. These results suggested that stutterers might have some weakness in learning relationships between the sounds they want to say and the movements required to say them. They have difficulty in making sensory-to-motor and motor-to-sensory transformations.[9] This deficit doesn't always produce stuttering. When situations don't call for a large amount of the brain capacity available in the speech and language area, stutterers can compensate for their slight weakness. When, on the other hand, a large portion of capacity might be allocated for language tasks such as choosing new words or making complex sentences, the deficit can't be compensated for, resulting in more repetitions. As these researchers have put it, "whether one will become a stutterer depends on one's neurological capacity for these sensory-to-motor and motor-to-sensory transformations and the demands posed by the speech act (Andrews et al., 1983)."

How do these intermittent deficits in available brain capacity result in the symptoms of stuttering? This theory attempts to account only for the core behaviors of early stuttering—repetitions and prolongations. According to the theory, repetitions and prolongations are the result of inadequate transformations of sensory targets, transformations which should generate the motor commands for speech. The speaker with reduced capacity can begin to speak, but is often unable to plan and carry out the rest of his utterance. The repetition or prolongation may occur while the speaker tries to push ahead with speech while waiting for his brain to plan the following syllables and link them to the initial sound.

Integrating the Theories

We have presented three views about the constitutional basis of stuttering. Each of them organizes the facts in a slightly different way. We shall now try to integrate these views so they can be seen as parts of a larger picture of stuttering.

First, consider localization of speech and language in stutterers. The Geschwind/Galaburda view suggests that conditions for stuttering may be created when speech and language structures in the left hemisphere are slow to ma-

---

[9] A recent study using electrical and chemical techniques of mapping brain activity suggests that a number of stutterers show an abnormal pattern of activity in a sensorimotor integration area of the brain (Freeman, 1988).

ture, causing speech and language functions to develop in the right hemisphere. We would like to clarify this view to emphasize that many conditions could delay the development of left hemisphere speech and language structures. One influence on the delay would be inheritance, of course, but another might be brain damage (from slight to severe) occurring before, during, or just after birth. The high frequency of stuttering associated with brain damage, mentioned earlier, can be accounted for by this view. We would also like to fine-tune the Geschwind/Galaburda view by suggesting that, when speech and language structures are delayed in development or damaged, a range of localization of speech and language functions can occur. Depending on when the delay or damage occurs and how much occurs, three outcomes are possible. Speech and language functions may develop in the damaged or delayed left hemisphere, they may develop in the right hemisphere, or they may develop in both hemispheres. These additions to the localization view of stuttering allow for different etiologies to result in somewhat similar problems.

This may be clearer if we return to our earlier analogy comparing speech and language functions to a telecommunications system placed in a building under construction. Imagine that the planned location for central control of the network is like the left hemisphere structures in the brain suited to speech and language development. For a telecommunications control room, the ideal location would have plenty of space and the proper interconnections to permit communication throughout the building. If the room were still under construction, but the telecommunications network were centralized there anyway, the half-finished space and poor connections would result in communication problems, at least until construction could be finished. Analogously, children may begin to stutter if their speech and language functions are centralized in a slow-to-develop left hemisphere, and they may recover if their left hemisphere development catches up.

In a second case, when rooms designed for the telecommunications equipment are unavailable because of construction delays, the equipment may have to be set up in another room designed for something else, perhaps the custodial closet. Without the proper space, plugs, and cable ducts, the equipment may function poorly, particularly under heavy communication traffic and intense custodial activity. Analogously, when speech and language functions migrate to the right hemisphere, communication problems may result, especially if the child is highly stimulated with much input and output and is also emotionally aroused.

The third inappropriate localization suggested above is development of speech and language in both left and right hemispheres. In the example of the telecommunications network, it would be as if the central network control room were only partly built when the network was installed. Some equipment might go in the intended room, some in another room. The function of the telecommunications network would be less effective in this case, because the equipment was designed to work with each piece in close proximity. The controllers might have delays as they passed messages back and forth as well as kept the network running. Once again, if speech and language processes are in divided locations, processing may be slowed and disrupted, especially under high levels of stress.

These three possiblities for the localization of speech and language processes are shown in terms of the telecommunications network analogy in Figure 2.2.

These imagined situations may not accurately reflect the constitutional predisposition for stuttering, but they convey an impression we have about the multiple origins of stuttering. Many different pathologies may give rise to the symptoms of stuttering, but at the same time, affect IQ, school achievement, reaction times, and other functions to very different degrees. This theme will be expanded as we integrate this with other theories of stuttering.

The two other theories of stuttering, as a disorder of timing and as reduced capacity for sensory-motor transformations, may fit into one or another of the above descriptions of speech and language localization. As Kent and others have pointed out, the right hemisphere is specialized for handling slower signals than the left, as well as being a source of emotional expression. If part or all of the speech and language functions in stutterers are in the right hemisphere, timing problems may be the basis for stuttering symptoms, especially during emotional arousal.

When speech and language functions remain in the left hemisphere, but that hemisphere is damaged or delayed, stuttering may result from inadequate neuronal space to handle the rapid sensory-motor processing that takes place as the child is learning to talk. This problem—reduced capacity in the part of the brain serving speech and language—is most acute when the stutterer is under heavy demand for other speech and language tasks besides speech production. When the child who is predisposed to stutter is trying to use newly acquired language constructions or trying to communicate complex ideas, he may be more likely to stutter. Under these conditions, he may be overloading his speech-language capacity. Stuttering may appear because fluent speech production is a weak link in the chain and the first to give way under stress.

In some cases of inherited or acquired abnormal brain development, speech and language functions may develop in both the right and left hemispheres. Some specialized cells may have migrated to the right hemisphere, some to the left. This bilateralization of speech and language may put the system under strain because processing of speech in two locations may require more time for integration. The structures located in the right hemisphere probably need to share information with the structures in the left, for both speaking and listening. These individuals, like those with complete right hemisphere localization of speech, may be vulnerable to stuttering if they are trying to speak at a faster rate than their systems can easily handle.

Summary

In this section on theories of constitutional factors, we have described 3 attempts to unify many of the findings about stuttering. None of these leads us, sure-footedly, from a specific inherited deficit through details of neurophysiology for speech to repetitions, prolongations, and blocks. Current knowledge hasn't progressed this far.

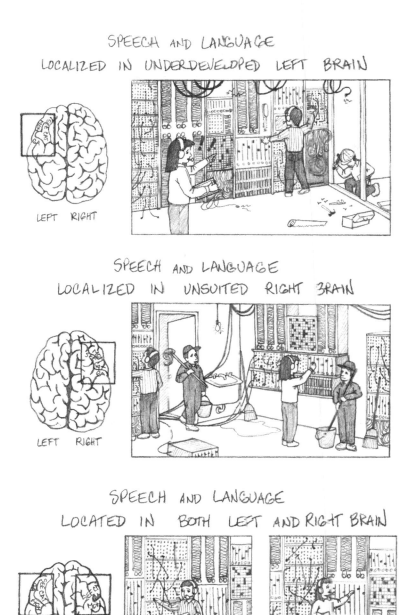

Figure 2.2. The location of a telecommunications center is depicted as an analogy for central localization of speech and language processing in stutterers. Three inefficient localizations are depicted.

We have, instead, small pieces of the puzzle. Geschwind and Galaburda propose that normal left hemisphere growth is delayed during fetal development, causing speech and language functions to be localized inappropriately. Kent (1983) and Van Riper (1982) suggest that the disturbance of stuttering is the product of mistiming in the pattern of neuromuscular commands for speech. Neilson and Neilson (1987) suggest that stuttering results from inadequate neuronal resources to make the necessary sensory-to-motor transformations for fluent speech.

Our attempt at integrating these views is to suggest that delayed development of left hemisphere structures for speech may have a number of outcomes. Three simple possibilities are that: speech and language processes (*a*) become established in left hemisphere structures that have reduced capacity because of slow development, (*b*) migrate to right hemisphere structures where temporal patterning is slower, (*c*) are divided between right and left hemispheres which creates a time delay in processing. The first outcome allows the possibility of outgrowing stuttering as capacity is increased; the second and third outcomes suggest that recovery depends on the individual's ability to reorganize or compensate neurologically. The combinations and permutations for speech and language localizations are many. Thus, the wide variability we see among stutterers is not unexpected, nor are the concomitant articulation and language problems.

These views will be outdated as more studies fill in the huge gaps in our knowledge about stuttering. They are meant only to give the reader an impression of the possible basis for stuttering. These are the constitutional attributes with which the developmental and environmental factors, considered in the next chapter, interact to create the first symptoms of stuttering.

STUDY QUESTIONS

1/ What evidence is there that stuttering is inherited?

2/ Researchers have found many differences between groups of stutterers and nonstutterers. Discuss why we cannot say that these differences "cause" stuttering.

3/ What findings suggest that many stutterers have deficits in speech and language functions other than stuttering?

4/ What are the three theories of the constitutional basis of stuttering described in this chapter?

5/ What do family studies tell us about who is most at risk for inheriting stuttering (which children of which parents)?

6/ Do any of these theories suggest why the early symptom of stuttering is repetitions of syllables?

7/ Name four findings of differences between stutterers and nonstutterers that reflect a possible speech or language deficit.

8/ Name four measures of sensory-motor functioning which have shown stutterers to perform more poorly, to have more errors, or to respond more slowly than nonstutterers.

9/ How might delays in speech and language development in stutterers be related to their poorer sensory-motor coordination?

10/ In the Geschwind/Galaburda theory of right hemisphere localization of speech and language, why have these functions migrated to the right hemisphere?

11/ In Kent's view of stuttering as a timing disorder, why would right hemisphere localization of speech and language disrupt timing?

12/ In the theory of stuttering as the result of inadequate sensory-to-motor transformations, why would learning new vocabulary interfere with fluency?

Suggested Readings

Andrews, G., Craig, A., Feyer, A.-M., Hoddinott, S., Howie, P., and Neilson, M. (1983). Stuttering: A review of research findings and theories circa 1982. *J. Speech Hearing Dis.* 48, 226–246.

This article distills the research about stuttering into a small number of "facts"—those findings that have been replicated by more than one study. Although the model of stuttering at which the authors arrive is controversial, the review is very worthwhile in its summary of a great body of research. It is also worthwhile to read the responses to this article in the commentaries on the subsequent pages of this issue of the journal.

Bloodstein, O. (1987). *A handbook on stuttering.* Chicago: National Easter Seal Society.

This book, which we frequently cite in our references, contains a critical review of research in practically every area of stuttering. Bloodstein has been producing a new edition of this handbook every 5 years.

Kidd, K. (1984). Stuttering as a genetic disorder. In R.F. Curlee and W.H. Perkins (Eds.). *Nature and treatment of stuttering: New directions.* San Diego: College-Hill Press, Inc.

This is a good review of the genetic research in stuttering. Kidd is a geneticist, but his writing is clearly understandable to those who are not.

Starkweather, C.W. (1987). *Fluency and stuttering.* Englewood Cliffs, N.J.: Prentice Hall.

This is a useful description of facts about various aspects of stuttering, including the relationship between language and stuttering, differences between stutterers and nonstutterers, and the variability of stuttering. Starkweather takes these facts in each area and relates them to theory in a coherent way.

Van Riper, C. (1982). An attempted synthesis. In *The nature of stuttering.* Englewood Cliffs, N.J.: Prentice Hall. (pp. 415–453)

Van Riper brings together the information he has reviewed throughout this text, and formulates a theory of stuttering as a disorder of timing. A very readable author.

3

DEVELOPMENTAL AND ENVIRONMENTAL INFLUENCES ON STUTTERING

Many factors both within the child and in his environment create the conditions under which stuttering first emerges and then grows progressively worse. Some of these factors seem to be part of normal childhood development, such as the child's explosive growth of speech and language skills during his preschool years. Other factors may be very common situations which most children take in stride as they grow up; for example, competition with siblings for attention and speaking time in a busy home. These factors, which we will call developmental and environmental influences, rarely work alone. In most cases, they interact with constitutional factors such as those discussed in the previous chapter. Figure 3.1 depicts the interaction of constitutional factors, which predispose the child to stuttering, with developmental and environmental factors, which precipitate the stuttering during the busy and sometimes stressful years of childhood.

Probably because constitutional predisposition frequently plays a part in the first appearance of stuttering and its effect is gradual, the conditions at the onset of stuttering are typically not dramatic. The child is usually not under great

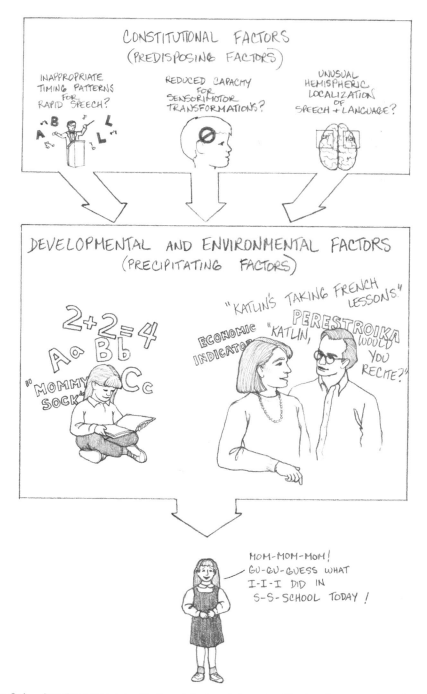

Figure 3.1. Predisposing constitutional factors interact with developmental and environmental factors to precipitate or worsen stuttering.

stress, nor has he just experienced some traumatic event. The ordinariness of the environment when stuttering first appears is reflected in this observation by Van Riper (1973):

In the great majority of children we have carefully studied soon after onset, we were unable to state with any certainty . . . what precipitated the stuttering. In most instances there simply were no apparent conflicts, no illnesses, no opportunity to imitate, no shocks or frightening experiences. Stuttering seemed to begin under quite normal conditions of living and communicating (p.81).

Because the child's situation is so ordinary when stuttering first emerges, research to determine critical developmental and environmental factors affecting the onset and progress of stuttering has not produced substantial results. As you can see from our opening statements above, this is a domain of educated guesses and tentative conclusions. Evidence for developmental factors is inferred from the fact that the onset of stuttering almost always occurs when children are growing rapidly, physically and mentally, in their preschool years (Andrews et al., 1983; Wingate, 1983). Evidence for the influence of the environment comes in part from clinical reports of particular stresses often associated with the onset of stuttering, and its remission when these stresses are lessened. Environmental factors are also implicated by the higher prevalence of stuttering in those cultures that are more achievement and conformity oriented (Bloodstein, 1987).[1] Finally, some sources of evidence for genetic factors in stuttering are also evidence for environmental factors. Studies by Andrews, Morris-Yates, Howie, and Martin (1990) and Kidd, Kidd, and Records (1978), for example, indicate that both genetic and environmental influences contribute to the occurrence of stuttering. This evidence, however, does not suggest what the environmental factors might be. Because of the paucity of hard data on specific developmental and environmental factors, this chapter will be more speculative than the last. Wherever we can, however, we will try to tie our speculations to facts.

In the following pages, we have divided developmental and environmental factors into separate sections, but they do not operate independently. Rather, they are intertwined in their effect. As an example, consider how much more vulnerable a child may be to environmental pressure for rapid speech when his speech development is still in an early stage.

DEVELOPMENTAL FACTORS

Our view of how developmental factors affect fluency in children assumes that the brain must share its resources to cope with many demands.[2] Like a com-

---

[1] It has been argued that genetic influences, which also are somewhat responsible for marked differences in cultures, may just as easily explain these results.

[2] This sharing of resources by a limited capacity system is similar to assumptions of the "Reduced Capacity for Internal Modeling" view of stuttering, described in Chapter 2. It is essentially the same as the Capacities and Demands model of developmental and environmental factors, described later in this chapter.

puter, the brain can work on several things at once. Like a computer, the more tasks it does simultaneously, the slower and less efficiently it does each one. Unlike a computer, however, if the tasks are dissimilar (such as driving your car and talking about the weather) there is less interference between them. But if they are similar (such as rubbing your stomach while patting your head) there is more interference between them (Kinsbourne and Hicks, 1978). The problem of shared resources is more acute, of course, in children, because their immature nervous systems have less processing capacity to share (Hiscock and Kinsbourne, 1977; 1980). Some children are especially at risk for strain on their developing resources. They may be delayed in the development of speech or language skills, yet have to compete in a highly verbal environment. Or their language development may surge ahead of their speech development, giving them much to say, but a limited capacity to express themselves articulately. These children may become excessively disfluent as other developmental demands outpace their more limited ability to coordinate the complex movements of rapid, articulate speech. We recently evaluated a four year old girl whose uncle and grandmother stuttered. Her parents were concerned because for a year and a half, this child had been repeating words and sounds excessively, sometimes up to 20 times per instance. However, her language development was well above average: she began to talk with single words at 9 months and to produce sentences intelligibly at 12 months. Her motor development lagged somewhat behind; she had not walked until 18 months. We think it possible that her disfluencies may be emerging as a result of the high proportion of resources used for language (and an urge to express that language) in the face of reduced capacity for motor activities, including fluent speech. In other words, the disparity between language facility and motor ability may be an important contributor to her stuttering.

Physical Development

Between the ages of one and six, children grow by leaps and bounds. Their bodies get bigger. Their nervous systems develop new pathways and new connections. Their perceptual and motor skills improve with practice and maturation. This intensive growth is a two-edged sword for children predisposed to fluency problems. Neurological maturation may provide more "functional cerebral space," which supports fluency. But neurological maturation may also spur the development of other motor tasks, which compete with fluency for available neuronal resources. An example of such competition is the common observation that children learn to walk first or talk first, but not both at the same time. Netsell (1981) says of this trade-off: "The practice of walking *or* talking seems sufficient to 'tie up' all the available sensorimotor circuitry because the Toddler seldom, if ever, undertakes both activities at once." (p. 25, italics the author's). We have also found that children who are learning a new motor skill may become temporarily more disfluent.[3]

---

[3] Adults also sometimes find they have temporary disfluency if they need to reorganize motor movements, as, for example, when an adult breaks his right arm and must write with his left hand. This anecdotal evidence suggests the possibility that demands associated with neural reorganization for non-speech tasks may increase childhood disfluencies.

Physical development is also related to fluency because speaking is a physical (motor) skill. If a child's fine motor skills are slow in developing, speech production may be more difficult for him. We would speculate that a notable delay in fine motor skills for speech in relation to a strong urge to communicate and rapidly developing language may set the stage for disfluency. There is some evidence to support the contention that children who stutter are delayed in development of fine motor coordination[4] but the many conflicting results suggest that this is not a simple issue.

Another way in which physical development may affect speech is when physical growth of the whole body, including the vocal tract, occurs rapidly. This may require the child to learn new sensory-to-motor and motor-to-sensory transformations as he tries to produce an intended sound with a recently changed speech mechanism. This explanation was suggested by Stark, Tallal, and McCauley (1988) as one of several hypotheses to interpret their finding that above average height and weight are strong correlates of articulation impairment.

In Table 3.1 below, we have listed some motor skills that all normal children have mastered by the ages given. These landmarks, taken from the *Denver Developmental Screening Test* (Frankenburg and Dodds, 1967), will give you some idea of the rapid physical growth that occurs during the early preschool years.

Cognitive Development

We use the phrase "cognitive development" to refer to the development of processes of perceiving, reasoning, imagining, and problem solving (Zimbardo, 1985) that subserve speech and language but are separate from it. This is a difficult area, with more questions than answers. We don't know, for example, where to draw the dividing line between language and cognition, or even if such a division makes sense.

The relationship between cognition and fluency is also complex. On the one hand, we know that individuals with cognitive deficits, such as those who are retarded, have an increased amount of stuttering (Van Riper, 1982). This appears to suggest that a deficit in cognitive ability may cause a deficit in fluency. On the other hand, as Starkweather (1987) suggests, stuttering in retarded individuals may result from their delay in learning speech and language—an issue we will discuss later in this chapter.

Table 3.1. Items Mastered by Most Normal Children at the Ages Given

Age	Physical Skill
15 months	Playing pat-a-cake, walking, drinking from a cup
2 years	Walking up stairs, building a tower of four cubes, kicking a ball forward
3 years	Imitating the experimenter after he or she draws a vertical line, throwing a ball overhand, pedaling a tricycle
4 years	Balancing on 1 foot, building a tower of 8 cubes, dressing self

[4] See Starkweather, 1987, p.220ff. and Van Riper, 1982, p.405ff.

To the extent that cognition and language are separate, some aspects of cognitive development may compete with speech and language development for the same neuronal resources and thereby jeopardize fluency. Consider the stages of cognitive development described by the Swiss psychologist Jean Piaget. He suggested that, from birth to 2 years, infants go through the Sensorimotor Period, in which their cognitive growth is fostered by sensory and motor activities. From 2 to 6, children progress through the Preoperational Period, in which they understand numbers, classify, and reason. Perhaps in the span from 2 to 6, children are occupied with higher level cognitive development, at the expense of such sensorimotor processes as the expression of language with newly emerging motor speech skills. This age span, interestingly, is just the time when normal disfluency is greatest and when most stuttering onsets occur.

Our understanding of the relationship between fluency and cognition is tenuous, but we have some idea of the questions that need to be asked. We need research on the extent and type of cognitive deficits in retarded individuals and the stuttering they manifest. We also need research on the potential disparity between cognitive development and motor speech development in stutterers of normal intelligence.

Social and Emotional Development

Social and emotional development may also contribute to normal disfluency and stuttering. In early childhood, a child's immature nervous system may permit "cross-talk" or interference between the limbic system, structures and pathways involved in the regulation and expression of emotion, and structures and pathways used for speech and language. This may even be truer for children predisposed to stuttering, whose speech and language functions are not optimally localized, as we discussed in the preceding chapter. Thus, when such children are emotionally aroused, fluency may suffer because neural signals for properly timed and sequenced muscle contractions may be degraded in some way. We see evidence of this when we ask parents when their child first began to stutter. Parents frequently tell us they first noticed it when their child was highly excited about something and wanted to talk. Excitement is also mentioned in the literature as a common stimulus for disfluency. Starkweather (1987), for example, notes that " . . . all children speak more disfluently during periods of excitement." Dorothy Davis (1940), who conducted one the first studies of normal disfluency, reported that of the ten situations in which children showed repetitions in their speech, "excitement over own activity" was the situation in which children most frequently repeated sounds and words. Johnson and Associates (1959) asked parents of children identified as stutterers to describe the situation in which they first observed the child's stuttering. Conditions most often reported to be associated with the first appearance of stuttering were when the child was in a hurry to tell something, and when the child was in a state of excitement. Thus, we see that both stuttering and normal disfluency seem to be associated with states of transitory emotional arousal.

Some stages of development may provide more social and emotional stress than others. The processes of separation and individuation, for example, may be such a time. After the child passes his second birthday, he strives harder toward autonomy, creating the conflict of the "terrible twos." Parents gradually relinquish control and, at the same time, help the child learn limits to his freedom. In some cases, the change from a dependent infant to an independent preschooler may be too rapid for a parent or a child. If the child is pushed toward independence faster than he wants to be, he may feel frustrated and insecure as his mother seems less nurturing. A mother may be alarmed if she isn't ready for the child's quest for independence. She may respond by restraining him. He may conform on the surface but feel angry and hostile underneath. Yet, he cannot easily express anger at someone he depends upon so much. The result may be disfluency in those interactions where the ambivalence of anger and fear create an emotional conflict, which may spill over to affect motor control of speech (Lidz, 1968).

As the child grows older, other members of the family play a part in social and emotional changes. On the one hand, the child's father and brothers and sisters provide a wider support system. On the other hand, the child's resentment at having to share his mother's attention may provoke feelings of anger, aggression, and guilt. If these feelings are punished or ignored, they may provoke temporary disfluency, or they may make stuttering more severe.

One of the most common provocations for feelings of resentment is the birth of a sibling. We will refer to the effect of a sibling's birth on fluency again when we discuss environmental factors, but it is worth mentioning here too, because the child's strong feelings are often a product of his developmental level as well as the environmental event. Theodore Lidz (1968), a developmental psychiatrist with an interest in speech and language, describes a good (but very psychoanalytically oriented) example:

Psychoanalytically oriented play therapy with children also indicates that many of their forbidden wishes and ideas have relatively simple access to consciousness. A six-year-old boy who started to stammer severely after a baby sister was born was watched playing with a family of dolls. He placed a baby doll in a crib next to the parent dolls' bed and then had a boy doll come and throw the baby to the floor, beat it, and throw it into a corner. He then put the boy doll into the crib. In a subsequent session, he had the father doll pummel the mother doll's abdomen, saying, "No, no!" At this point of childhood, even though certain unacceptable ideas cannot be talked about, they are still not definitely repressed. (p.246)

Although we feel, with Lidz, that stuttering may be triggered by the birth of a sibling, our belief about the underlying cause is not so Freudian. Many threats to feelings of security create emotional stress, and may interfere with speech in children who are predisposed. As will be evident in our treatment section, we have found that therapy strategies that increase the child's sense of security and help him learn to speak more fluently will usually suffice.

The development of self-consciousness, which begins during the child's second year, is another source of social and emotional stress. This is the growing awareness by the child of how he is performing in relation to adult standards. Although this concept is not thoroughly understood, Jerome Kagan presents an interesting description of the process in his book, *The Second Year* (1981). In a relevant example, Kagan suggests that the self-corrections the child makes in his speech are evidence of this self-awareness. Taking this further, we might surmise that this increasing self-awareness, in a child who is excessively disfluent, might lead to self-corrections that worsen the problem.

Before we leave this section, we want to comment on stutterers' psychological adjustment in general. Sometimes, people who have little exposure to stuttering believe that stutterers are essentially nervous people, or that stuttering is a sign of neurosis. If this were true, we would find evidence of psychological maladjustment and excessive anxiety in stutterers, particularly when the disorder first begins in childhood. Reviews of the research on stutterers' personality and adjustment find no convincing evidence that stutterers are different from nonstutterers (Bloch and Goodstein, 1971; Bloodstein, 1987; Van Riper, 1982). There are a few findings that suggest that stutterers are not quite as socially well-adjusted as nonstutterers, but this can probably be attributed to the influence of stuttering on social experiences (Bloodstein, 1987).

Summarizing the effect of social and emotional development on fluency, we have suggested that many of the normal social and emotional stresses that children experience may produce disfluencies, though our evidence is mostly anecdotal. Moreover, children who may be neurophysiologically vulnerable to stuttering may be especially prone to difficulty when social conflicts and emotions create extra "noise" in their neural circuitry for speech. Children who stutter appear to be as psychologically well-adjusted as nonstutters.

Speech and Language Development

Stuttering usually begins when speech and language are developing most rapidly (Van Riper, 1982; Bloodstein, 1987). Consider how much pressure this rapid growth applies to fluent speech. In the first place, the child is having to learn to control a speech mechanism that is continuously changing size and shape, because he is growing rapidly. He is also having to synchronize his speech to the rates and rhythms of parents and siblings with whom he has a growing urge to communicate. In addition, his speech motor skills must accommodate his burgeoning linguistic abilities. In the single year between ages 2 and 3, the child's vocabulary jumps from 50 to 250 words; in fact, toward the end of this year he is learning between 5 and 7 new words a day (Studdert-Kennedy, 1987). At the same time, his utterances are developing from successive single word pairs with sentence-like intonations and durations into multiword sentences (Branigan, 1979).[5] As he is expanding his sentences, the child is also overhauling his lexical storage strategy. At first he stocks his lexical shelves with whole words in the form of articulatory routines or gestural patterns; then he changes strategies and stores, not whole words, but segments which can be combined variously into a multitude of words (Kent, 1985; Stemberger, 1982; Nittrouer, Studdert-Kennedy, and McGowan, 1989). Dur-

---

[5] This mode of sentence development may be yet another reflection of the fact that language planning leads speech production ability.

ing these same early preschool years, he is also progressively learning active, negative, and passive constructions; present, future, and past tenses. At the same time, he
is increasing the length of his sentences and, concomitantly, the rate of his utterances.[6] This multitude of tasks must inevitably take its toll on a preschooler's fluency. To imagine how this might happen, remember the metaphor we are using in
this chapter: the child is a system with a finite amount of resources which must be
parceled out to tasks he is engaged in. Rapid acquisition of language competes with
available resources for the task of speech production. However, as more language is
acquired and utterances become longer, speech rate usually increases. But in a system with finite resources, there must be a speed-accuracy trade-off; that is, if speed
increases, accuracy decreases. Thus, if the child, already burdened with increasing
complexity of language, succumbs to producing his utterances more quickly, before
his available resources can meet that demand, he may become less accurate in his
productions. Depending on the child, this inaccuracy may manifest itself as stuttering, decreased intelligibility, or some combination thereof.

The notion that development of speech and language may diminish fluency is not new. Peggy Dalton and W. J. Hardcastle (1977), for example, commented that "It is tempting to see the ever-increasing demands on linguistic
competence and articulatory proficiency as a major factor in the onset of some
disfluency." Joseph Sheehan (1975) put it this way: "The age of onset of stuttering
is consistently related to certain stages in the developmental sequence. Most notably, the 'period of resonance,' or high readiness in language learning, noted by Len-
neberg . . . is also the period during which stuttering develops and flourishes."
Andrews et al. (1983) pointed to the demand placed on speech by rapidly developing language by saying, " . . . stuttering [has] a maximal frequency of onset at a
time when an explosive growth in language ability outstrips a still-immature
speech-motor apparatus."

The reduction in fluency with development of speech and language may
be another similarity between normal disfluency and the early stutterer. Bloodstein (1987) has noted that there is considerable evidence of a connection between
language development and stuttering, and that part of this evidence is the tendency
for many children, both stutterers and nonstutterers, to become more disfluent
during certain stages of intense language development. In addition, experimental
studies show that both stutterers (Bernstein-Ratner and Sih, 1987; Stocker and
Usprich, 1976) and nonstutterers (Gordon, Luper, and Peterson, 1986; Haynes
and Hood, 1978; Pearl and Bernthal, 1980) show increased disfluencies as language complexity is increased. Unfortunately, there is little longitudinal research
directly on the question of how and when emerging language is associated with
disfluency. One of the few descriptive studies of this phenomenon was the analysis
of disfluencies in 4 nonstuttering children, carried out by Norma Colburn using
data originally gathered by Lois Bloom for her work on normal language development. The published reports of this analysis (Colburn and Mysak, 1982a,b) suggest that normal disfluencies appeared not when these children first learned a new

---

[6] The connection between increasing length of utterance and increasing rate is discussed by many
authors, including Malecot, Johnston, and Kizziar, 1972; Starkweather, 1987; and Umeda, 1975, 1977.

language construction, but after they began to master it and started to use it regularly. Suggested explanations for this result include the possibility that the child has incompletely automatized the construction, and allocates fewer than necessary resources for production (Kent and Perkins, 1984) and the idea that, having been mastered, the constructions were produced with an increased rate, straining capacity (Starkweather, 1987). These suggestions, along with other hypotheses derived from resource theory, should be used to explore the relationship between syntax acquisition and normal disfluencies. In spite of numerous clinical observations and theoretical views, relatively little is actually known about the appearance of either normal disfluency or stuttering in relation to speech and language acquisition.

Earlier we suggested that the increased incidence of stuttering among the retarded may be explained by the fact that their acquisition of speech and language is delayed, or more to the point, their learning period is longer than normal. They may be trying to acquire language from infancy to adulthood, increasing the risk period for developing stuttering. Our own clinical experience confirms this, and suggests, more specifically, that competition for neuronal resources may explain why fluency suffers when speech and language are learned. Recently, a mother of a Down syndrome child told us that her son's stuttering increased dramatically in frequency and severity when he made great gains in vocabulary and syntax. This suggests some aspect of acquiring language may make a child vulnerable to stuttering. In individuals with more limited capacity, the strain placed on resources by language learning may be particularly great.

ENVIRONMENTAL FACTORS

Some children predisposed to stuttering may show the first signs of stuttering as a result of developmental pressures alone, but most children who will become stutterers are probably also affected by environmental pressures. These are factors outside of these children. Typically, they are attitudes or events that occur in their homes. One way they affect children's fluency is by pressuring them to speak at a level beyond their developmental capacity. For example, children who are at an early stage of speech development may encounter a listener's impatience when they're speaking slowly and haltingly. Responding to the listener's impatience, they may begin to stutter because they try to speak at a rate beyond their capacity. Or they may begin to stutter because the listener's response creates stress in children that disrupts their motor coordination. Other environmental factors inside and outside children's homes, besides speech and language pressures, influence their fluency. However, these environmental effects on children's speech probably work somewhat differently than developmental effects. Our earlier metaphor, of a computer overloaded because it must work on several tasks at once, was well-suited to describe developmental effects. We now ask you to imagine that anything that creates uncertainty or insecurity, or that calls for greater speed or greater complexity, may result in less efficiency in the computer, and that this, in turn, creates fluency breakdowns in the vulnerable child. These environmental pressures also worsen the symptoms of stuttering, as we shall describe in Chapter 4.

We begin this section by reviewing the research on the most important factor in the environment, the parents of stutterers.

Parents

In the 1930s at the University of Iowa, Wendell Johnson developed the "diagnosogenic" theory of stuttering. This theory, which will be described more fully in a later section, suggests that a child's parents erroneously diagnose his normal disfluency as stuttering. Their reaction to the "stuttering" then causes the child to struggle and avoid, in a way that becomes real stuttering. Johnson's diagnosogenic theory generated a great deal of research on parents of stutterers. Were they different from the parents of nonstutterers? Were they unusually critical? Did they have unreasonably high standards of speech?

One of the first studies of parents of stutterers was conducted by John Moncur (1952). Moncur interviewed the mothers of stutterers and the mothers of nonstutterers about their parenting practices. He found that mothers of stutterers tended to be more critical, more protective, and more domineering toward their children than mothers of nonstutterers. Not long afterward, Frederick Darley, a student of Wendell Johnson at the University of Iowa, investigated the attitudes of stutterers' parents in more detail. Using interview techniques based on the famous sex studies of Alfred Kinsey, Darley (1955) questioned the parents of 50 stutterers and 50 nonstutterers. Although there was a great deal of overlap in the parental attitudes of these two groups, the parents of the stutterers showed significantly higher standards and expectations, particularly with regard to speech. They believed in early intervention with nonfluencies; they had greater sensitivity to speech deviations; their overall drive and domination was greater. Darley's study was expanded by Wendell Johnson and his research associates (1959). This study looked at parents of 150 stuttering children and parents of 150 nonstuttering children, and again found there was much overlap between parents of stutterers and parents of nonstutterers. But again, stutterers' parents were found to be more perfectionistic and to have higher standards of behavior than other parents. These studies by Moncur, Darley, Johnson and others are probably responsible for the widespread belief that parents are a key factor in the onset of stuttering. Parents may transmit the culture's "competitive pressure for achievement or conformity" which may be the environmental factor most likely to be causally linked with stuttering (Bloodstein, 1987). We should emphasize, however, that there are many conflicting findings in this literature and that parents of stutterers, if they are different from parents of nonstutterers, are only slightly different. We note also that these are group differences; many parents of stuttering children are more accepting and less competitive than parents of nonstuttering children, and vice-versa.

Parents' high standards and perfectionism alone do not produce stuttering. After all, the stutterer's brothers and sisters may thrive under this influence. And as we have suggested, the children of many demanding parents do not become stutterers. But for a child who is vulnerable—constitutionally predisposed to stuttering—it may be just the thing he doesn't need. One can imagine a child feeling self-conscious in a family that strives for perfection, especially in speech. Such a child could be so concerned about minor disfluencies that he tries too hard to be perfectly fluent and produces labored, struggled speech. Some children who become stutterers may not be highly vulnerable and may have only slight constitutional predisposition, but may encounter overwhelming environmental pressures. For example, a child without evident disfluencies may gradually develop stuttering under relentless pressure to perform at maximum levels socially, academically, or athletically.

Let us digress for a moment away from the Iowa studies which showed competitive pressure to be common in the homes of stutterers. Quite different results were found in England. Gavin Andrews and Mary Ann Harris (1964), whose work we have described in Chapter 2, collected and analyzed data from an ongoing study of families in Newcastle, England. Combining medical records and home visits, Andrews and Harris compared the parents of stutterers and nonstutterers. They found both groups were generally similar in personality, but differed in some key traits. The parents of stutterers were lower in intelligence, had poorer school records when they were younger, had poorer work histories, and provided poorer housing for their children. There was no evidence that parents criticized or pressured their children. This finding is a far cry from the evidence of excessively high standards in the stutterers' homes in Iowa.

Why are these results so different from those of the Iowa studies? There may be many reasons, but two come easily to mind. The first is that stuttering may emerge in children under any stress. In industrial England, the greatest stress may have come from social and economic disadvantage, but in Iowa, the greatest stress may have been the high standards of upwardly mobile parents. A second reason for the difference in these studies may be a difference in the researchers' expectations and biases of two decades ago. Americans tended to believe all men are created equal. American researchers, especially those in the heartland of the United States, looked for influences not in heredity, but in the stutterers' environment. On the other hand, many Britons believed inheritance plays the major role in determining life outcome. Researchers in Britain looked for causes of stuttering in the parents' intelligence and social class.

The hypothesis that lower class homes can provide stress on stutterers is not new in Great Britain. John Morgenstern (1956), who investigated stuttering in Scottish children, found that stuttering was most prevalent in relatively lower class homes (skilled manual weekly wage earners). This, however, was a stratum that in Scotland was upwardly mobile and may have expressed their ambitions through high speech standards for their children. Here we have a combination of forces, if Morgenstern's hypothesis is correct. The stress of lower class homes is not their deprivation, but the pressure to perform well to rise above humble beginnings.

There are other studies of stutterers' parents, some of which suggest they are more rejecting or anxious than parents of nonstutterers (Flugel, 1979; Zenner, Ritterman, Bowen, and Gronhovd, 1978), and some of which suggest that there are very small differences or no differences between parents of the two groups (Goodstein, 1956; Goodstein and Dahlstrom, 1956). The evidence in this area is not clear, but as we have indicated above, some research depicts stutterers' parents as critical listeners with high standards of speech performance, but much of the research does not. It isn't surprising to us that the differences that are seen are subtle. We do not believe that many stutterers' home environments cause stuttering. Instead, as we have said before, stuttering seems to be the result of several factors acting together. Home environment is only one, and may not be a factor at all for some stutterers.

Speech and Language Environment

Clinical observation and research suggest that more stuttering occurs when children use more advanced forms of speech and language. Two writers have presented models that emphasize the demands placed on the speech production skills of stutterers as higher levels of language are used. Crystal (1987) proposed an "interactive" view of many speech and language disorders which suggested that demands made by one level of language production (e.g., syntax) may deplete resources for other levels (e.g. prosody or phonology), resulting in breakdown. His supporting data nicely illustrated how stuttering in particular may be exacerbated by production of advanced language. He recorded evidence that the more complex the syntax and semantics a child used, the more he stuttered. Starkweather (1987), describing a demands and capacities view of stuttering, commented that, " . . . the production of speech and the formulation of language place a simultaneous demand on the young person. If the demands in either of these two dimensions are excessive, performance in the other dimension may be reduced." These two views imply that stuttering may increase when an individual uses longer words, less frequently occurring words, more information-bearing words, and longer sentences. Stuttering may also increase when the individual is uttering a more linguistically complex sentence.[7] Because a preschool child's speech and language are so heavily influenced by the speech and language around him, especially that of his parents, the speech and language used by others may be an important source of pressure on the stuttering child. As the child tries to imitate adult models of speech and language, to use longer words and longer sentences, to try less familiar words, and to pack more meaning into his utterances, he will be more likely to stutter. Van Riper (1973) suggests the child may be vulnerable to this pressure when he is most rapidly developing language: "Stuttering usually begins at the very time that great advances in sentence construction occur, and it seems tenable that, when the speech models provided by the parents or siblings of the child are too difficult for him to follow, some faltering will ensue." (p. 381).

What do we know about the speech and language of stutterers' parents?[8] Unfortunately, very little. One study focused directly on speech of parents. Susan

---

[7] The interested reader should consult pages 175–176 of Starkweather's *Fluency and Stuttering* (1987) for more discussion of these phenomena and for the references to this research.

[8] Kasprisin-Burrelli, Egolf, and Shames (1972) studied the parent-child interactions of parents of stutterers and parents of nonstutterers. They found that parents of stutterers tended to make a much higher proportion of negative statements in their conversations than did parents of nonstutterers. Although these findings do not tell us about the models of speech, per se, they suggest that stuttering children may be under more negative emotional pressure in talking with their parents.

Meyers and Frances Freeman (1985a,b) compared the speech of mothers of stutterers and mothers of nonstutterers. They found that mothers of stutterers spoke more rapidly than mothers of nonstutterers. This may be critical, since a mother's high speech rate has the potential to make a child try to speak faster than his optimal speed (e.g., Jaffe and Anderson, 1979). The possibility that a rapid speech rate may lead to stuttering is supported by Johnson and Rosen's (1937) finding that adult stutterers were more likely to stutter when they spoke more rapidly than normal. Children who stutter may be even more vulnerable than adults who stutter to breakdown during rapid speech, by virtue of the fact that children's natural rate of speech is slower and their temporal coordination less (e.g., Kent, 1981).

Meyers and Freeman (1985a) also studied mothers' interruptions of children's speech. Both mothers of stutterers and mothers of nonstutterers interrupted children more than usual whenever the children were disfluent. It seems possible that these interruptions, which may have been elicited by the child's disfluencies, may in turn elicit changes in the child's speech. One might predict that some children would increase tension and rate and thereby develop the struggled behaviors of stuttering. Other children might be able to suppress disfluencies to avoid interruptions and eventually be "taught" by their parents not to be disfluent.

Besides the modicum of research cited above, there is a wealth of clinical material that suggests that the speech and language environment of the child is an important influence on his fluency. In *The Treatment of Stuttering*, for example, Van Riper cites nine references in which clinicians point to parental speech models as a major source of stress on a child's fluency (pp. 380–383). This stress includes not only the parents' speech and language, but also the conditions under which the child tries to speak. Advice for parents of stutterers, given by clinicians with experience treating young stutterers (e.g., Fraser and Perkins, 1987; Starkweather, 1986; and Van Riper, 1973), often includes observing and, where appropriate, changing the speech and language environment in the home. In their publications, clinicians have noted that the speech and language stresses listed in Table 3.2 are likely to increase stuttering:

The above conditions appear to pressure many children with average speech abilities, to the point that they become mildly disfluent. But what about the child who is also experiencing difficulty with fine motor coordination for speech or is delayed in language? This child may be especially vulnerable to speech and

Table 3.2. Speech and Language Stresses

Stressful Adult Speech Models	
Rapid speech rate	Complex syntax
Polysyllabic vocabulary	Use of two languages in home

Stressful Speaking Situations for Child	
Competition for speaking	Hurried when speaking
Frequent interruptions	Frequent questions
Demand for display speech	Excited when speaking
Loss of listener attention	Many things to say

language stresses in the home. Fluency may break down as he struggles to produce speech and language at a rate and complexity far beyond his reach. He may also be vulnerable because he is frequently misunderstood: a child who misarticulates several sounds or is notably delayed in language may develop a conviction that talking is hard and he is an inadequate speaker. Bloodstein (1987) cites several accounts of the appearance of stuttering in children with delayed language development or articulation problems; their parents' models of speech and language and their attempts to improve the child's speech appear to have contributed to the child's stuttering. Research by Merits-Patterson and Reed (1981) may also be relevant. They found that children receiving language therapy had more stuttering-type disfluencies (part-word repetitions, word repetitions, prolongations, and fixations) than either children with language delay who were not receiving treatment or normal children. Although their findings are somewhat weakened by the fact that they could not demonstrate that the two groups of language-delayed children were equal in disfluencies before treatment, this study suggests that the communicative pressure created by treatment may result in an increase in stuttering-type disfluencies. It may not be stretching the point too far to suggest that language delayed children in a home with fast and complex language may be experiencing pressure somewhat similar to those in treatment.

Life Events

Certain events in a child's life can deliver a blow to the child's stability and security. When this happens, stuttering may suddenly appear out of nowhere, or previously easy repetitions may be transformed into hard, struggled blocks. To have someone close to you die, to be hospitalized for an operation, or to have your parents divorce is difficult for any of us, but especially difficult for children. Obviously, many children go through these events and adapt to them without major problems. But children who may be vulnerable to stuttering will often show the effects of these events in their speech.

There is little research on the relationship of difficult life events to stuttering, but many authors have observed the connection. Starkweather (1987), for example, says, "All children speak more disfluently during periods of tension—when moving or changing schools, when their parents divorce, or after the death of a family member." This increased disfluency could easily result in the onset of stuttering or increased stuttering in those children who are most vulnerable. Johnson and Associates (1959) noted that among 16 situations in which parents first noticed their child's stuttering were these: (a) child's physical environment changed (e.g., moving to new house), (b) child ill, (c) child realized his mother was pregnant, (d) arrival of new baby. Van Riper (1982), in discussing the onset of stuttering, acknowledges that various studies have found no differences in the amount of emotional conflict in the homes of children who developed stuttering, versus those who didn't. "Nevertheless," says Van Riper, "we have studied individual cases in which stuttering did seem [to be] triggered by such conflicts, and it is difficult for us to ignore these experiences."

Our own clinical experience is similar. For example, in the past several years, we've encountered four children in four different families who began to stutter when their parents were in the early stages of divorce. However, this turmoil was not the only factor in the stuttering. Three of the children had relatives who stuttered, and the father of the fourth child was a clutterer. Moreover, all four were preschoolers, experiencing various growth and development pressures. But for all of them, their parents' divorce appeared to us to be the added factor that pushed them over the line from normal speech to stuttering.

In rare cases, traumatic life events appear to precipitate stuttering in children (and adults) who have no predisposition. These unusual onsets will be discussed when we explore "psychogenic stuttering" in a later chapter. But more commonly, we see children who are already showing some signs of stuttering, and when they encounter a stressful life event, their stuttering increases dramatically. The list in Table 3.3 contains some of the life events that, we have found, are stressful to children's fluency.

THEORIES ABOUT DEVELOPMENTAL AND ENVIRONMENTAL FACTORS

The three views we will present in this section represent three different concepts of how developmental and/or environmental stresses may contribute to stuttering. One view (Diagnosogenic) takes normal disfluency as a starting point, and assumes that stuttering develops as a response to it. The other two look more broadly at situations from which stuttering might arise. One of these (Communicative Failure and Anticipatory Struggle) suggests that some form of communication difficulty precipitates stuttering, and the other (Capacities and Demands) suggests that almost any developmental or environmental pressure may be the stimulus. As you read this section, keep in mind that these three views are different not only in their concept of the role of development and environment, but also in their degree of specificity. The first (Diagnosogenic) proposes particular elements that create stuttering; the last (Capacities and Demands) suggests general principles by which variables may interact to produce stuttering; the middle view (Communicative Failure) falls between the specific and general.

Table 3.3. Stressful Life Events That May Increase a Child's Disfluency

1. The child's family moves to a new house, a new neighborhood, or a new city.
2. The child's parents separate cr divorce.
3. A family member dies.
4. A family member is hospitalized.
5. The child is hospitalized.
6. A parent loses his or her job.
7. A baby is born or another child adopted.
8. An additional person comes to live in the house.
9. One or both parents go away frequently or for a long period of time.
10. Holidays or visits occur, which cause a change in routine, excitement, or anxiety.

Diagnosogenic Theory

In the 1930s, Wendell Johnson and other researchers at the University of Iowa were studying the onset of stuttering in children. As Johnson examined the speech of young stutterers and nonstutterers, he noticed a similarity. He saw that the most common disfluencies for both groups were repetitions. As Johnson contemplated this evidence, he was struck by the possibility that these children all had the same disfluencies to begin with, but those who were stutterers developed more serious disfluencies by over-reacting to their repetitions. Why? Their parents or other listeners may have mislabeled their repetitions as "stuttering." In so doing, they may have made the children so self-conscious that they tried hard to speak without disfluencies. This effort to avoid disfluencies may have become, with the help of further negative listener reactions, what we generally regard as stuttering.

Johnson's hypothesis, which came to be called the Diagnosogenic Theory (meaning that the disorder begins with its diagnosis, or in this case, misdiagnosis) was the most widely accepted explanation of stuttering throughout the 1940s and 1950s. It was a strong indictment of environmental factors in the onset of the disorder. It placed the blame solely on the negative reactions of parents and other listeners and implied that constitutional predisposition for stuttering played little part.

Johnson and his associates continued gathering data on the disfluencies of stuttering children and their normally disfluent peers to further support the Diagnosogenic Theory. The results of several studies were summarized in a landmark book, *The Onset of Stuttering* (Johnson and Associates, 1959). Table 3.4, taken from this book, gives an overview of similarities and differences between the stutterers' and nonstutterers' disfluencies.

It is immediately evident that certain types of disfluencies were far more common in the stuttering children than in the nonstuttering children. Syllable repetitions, sound prolongations, and complete blocks occurred more frequently in stut-

Table 3.4. Percentage of Parents of Stutterers and Nonstutterers Who Reported Child Was Performing Each Speech Behavior when They First Thought Child Was Stuttering[a]

Group	Repetition			Sound Prolonga-tion	Silent Intervals	Interjec-tions	Complete Blocks
	Syllable	Word	Phrase				
Control (Nonstutterers)							
Fathers	4	59	23	3	36	30	0
Mothers	10	41	24	4	41	21	0
Experimental (Stutterers)							
Fathers	57	48	8	15	7	8	3
Mothers	59	50	8	12	3	9	3

[a]From Johnson, W. and Associates. (1959). *The onset of stuttering.* Minneapolis: University of Minnesota Press. Copyright © 1959 by the University of Minnesota. © 1987 Edna Johnson. Reprinted by permission of the University of Minnesota Press.

tering children. Phrase repetitions, pauses, and interjections occurred more frequently in the control group. What does this mean? Other authors have interpreted these findings as evidence that these two groups of children were different at the onset of their disfluencies.[9] Johnson, on the other hand, emphasized the similarity of the groups. He pointed out that both groups had at least some samples of each type of disfluency. The same disfluency types that some parents considered normal in their children were categorized by other parents as the earliest signs of stuttering in their children. This left him still convinced that part of the problem was the parents' interpretation of their child's disfluencies. Or as Johnson often put it, "the problem was not in the child's mouth but in the parent's ear." However, Johnson and his associates also observed that the stuttering children had significantly more sound/syllable repetitions, complete blocks, and prolonged sounds. Johnson acknowledged that some of the problem might be more than parents' abnormal reactions. His modified view depicted stuttering as a result of interaction among these three factors: (*a*) the extent of the child's disfluency, (*b*) the listener's sensitivity to that disfluency, and (*c*) the child's sensitivity to his own disfluency and to the listener's reaction. This revision of the Diagnosogenic Theory still implicates the environment as a potent influence on the development of stuttering. But it also acknowledges the important contribution of factors within the child.

To illustrate the Diagnosogenic view, we will take an example from a masters' thesis Johnson directed (Tudor, 1939). At that time, the Diagnosogenic Theory had not been formally proposed, but undoubtedly Johnson and others must have entertained the possibility that labeling a child a stutterer would create more hesitancy in his speech. The thesis was an exploration of that idea. Johnson's student, Mary Tudor, screened all the children at a nearby orphanage for speech and language disorders. Selecting six who were normal speakers, she told these children that they should speak more carefully because they were making errors when they talked. They had symptoms of stuttering. She also warned their caregivers that these children should be watched closely for speech errors and corrected when they slipped up. After several months, Tudor went back to the orphanage and found that a number of the selected students showed stuttering-like behaviors. Although she tried to treat them, at least one was reported to continue stuttering for some time thereafter (Silverman, 1988). The experimenters were, of course, remorseful about the results, and regretted this experiment. But nonetheless, it gave Johnson the strong conviction that he held throughout his career: that if a child is made self-conscious about his normal disfluencies, they may develop into stuttering.

Communicative Failure and Anticipatory Struggle

This theory, developed by Oliver Bloodstein (1987), suggests that stuttering may develop when a child experiences frustration and failure when trying to talk. The child's original difficulty in talking need not be disfluency. Many types of

---

[9] McDearmon (1968) has shown these differences between stuttering and control children at onset to be statistically significant. He argues that the data from Johnson and Associates' study suggest stutterers' typical first disfluencies (e.g., repetitions of syllables, sound prolongations) are categorically different from normals' first disfluencies (e.g., repetitions of phrases, pauses).

Table 3.5.   Experiences that May Make Some Children Believe that Speaking Is Difficult

1. Normal disfluencies criticized by significant listeners
2. Delay in speech or language development
3. Speech or language disorders, including articulation problems, word finding difficulty, cerebral palsy, and voice problems
4. Difficult or traumatic experience reading aloud in school
5. Cluttering, especially if listeners frequently say "Slow down" or "What?"
6. Emotionally traumatic events during which child tries to speak

communication failure may cause the child to anticipate future difficulty with speech. It is common, Bloodstein noted, to find articulation problems, language deficits, cluttering, and many other speech problems in the histories of children who begin to stutter. Table 3.5 lists some of the circumstances which Bloodstein suggests may cause some children to experience speech as difficult. If a child cannot make himself understood or is penalized for the way he talks, he may well begin to tense his speech muscles and fragment his speech. These are the core behaviors of stuttering; they soon become part of the speaking difficulty that the child learns to dread.

Other aspects of the "internal" and "external" environments play important parts also. The child's personality may be perfectionistic or he may harbor a need to live up to parental expectations. His family may have high standards for speech or intolerance of any speech abnormality or may otherwise pressure the child to conform to standards beyond his reach. The presence or absence of such environmental pressures may be what cause some children to interpret their articulation difficulty, language problem, or disfluency as a failing, while others would shrug it off.

This perspective on stuttering accounts for the wide variability of disfluency among children. Most normal children experience enough temporary frustration when learning to talk to produce the mild fragmentation of speech we associate with normal disfluency. Children who stutter for just a few weeks may be those who encounter unusual difficulty when first learning to talk but soon master the fundamentals and feel successful. Children who become chronic stutterers may be those who repeatedly experience communication failure and grow up in an environment fraught with communicative pressure.

Here is a case that illustrates some of the environmental pressures that often surround children who begin to stutter. Susan M. grew up in the oil fields of Oklahoma, where her parents set themselves apart from the rest of the community by their aloof manner and by their precision of speech. They raised their children to feel they were more cultured than their neighbors; in fact, Susan's father would often say, "We speak better than other people." Unfortunately, Susan was delayed in beginning to talk. When she did begin to speak, her parents couldn't understand her, so her older sister interpreted what she was saying to her parents. When she was 3, her mother became pregnant, miscarried, and plunged into a depression. Looking back as an adult, Susan remembers thinking that her mother's silence and depression were disapproval of her speech. Her unintelligible speech soon became stuttering. She escalated from repetitive stutters to tightly squeezed blocks within the course of a year. For the next twenty-five years she felt deeply ashamed of her stuttering.

Although we have no way of knowing for sure, Susan's critical home may have been a major factor in the onset of her stuttering. Many other children go through a period of unintelligible speech in their second and third years, but don't develop stuttering. On the other hand, her delayed speech, perhaps an inherited or congenital deficit, was also an important factor. Neither may have been sufficient by themselves to create stuttering, but combined they may have been enough to tip the balance.

Capacities and Demands

A third interactional view of stuttering onset is the "Capacities and Demands Theory." This view suggests that disfluencies as well as real stuttering emerge when the capacities of the child for fluency are not equal to the demands of the environment for speech performance. We briefly discussed this view in Chapter 2, in our description of the Reduced Capacity for Internal Models theory of stuttering. Andrews et al. (1983) suggested that, " . . . whether one will become a stutterer depends on one's neurological capacity . . . and the demand posed by the speech act."[10] They indicated that some demands come from the rapid development of language between ages 3 and 7. Others may come from fast-talking parents whose speech rates may be hard for a child to keep up with. Demands for speech performance are sometimes from within the child and sometimes from outside stimuli.

Joseph Sheehan (1970; 1975) developed an early variation of the capacities and demands view in his belief that "a child who has begun to stutter is probably a child who has had too many demands placed on him while receiving too little support." The demands which Sheehan pinpointed are primarily those of parents who have high standards and high expectations for their child's behavior. Sheehan also acknowledged developmental factors, such as "differences in the rate of maturation," which result in a greater incidence of stuttering in males. Moreover, he believed "there are persisting reasons for retaining the possibility that some kind of physiological predisposition for stuttering exists." Thus Sheehan, who, ironically, is best known for a theory that stuttering is strictly a learned behavior, in fact professed the view that stuttering in children is precipitated by the demands of the environment interacting with the limitations of the child's rate of development and his predispostion to stuttering.

Starkweather (1987) has added considerable detail to the concept of capacities and demands as an explanation of stuttering onset. The normal child's capacities, he points out, include the potential for rapid movement of speech structures in well-planned and well-coordinated sequences, with the rhythms of his language. Demands on the child include those of his internal environment, such

---

[10] The reader interested in further references on the topic of capacities for information processing should seek out Neilson and Neilson (1987), as well as the references in that article.

as increasingly complex thoughts to be expressed, and increasingly sophisticated phonology, syntax, semantics, and pragmatics with which to express them. The external environment often forces its demands on the child's fluency through parents' interactions. They may ask questions rapidly, interrupt frequently, and use complex sentences choked with big words. They may show impatience with the child's normal disfluencies. They may make the child feel that he or she meets their expectations only when he's performing at a high level. These interactions can stress any child, but they are likely to push a slow-developing child beyond his capacity for fluency.

Because a child's capacity develops as he grows and because environmental demands fluctuate daily, stuttering waxes and wanes. A younger child, for example, with an immature nervous system may be more likely to stutter when surrounded by fast-talking adults than when speaking to peers. As he grows older, the increased capacity of his more mature nervous system will help him compensate for any constitutional predisposition, allowing him to be only mildly disfluent in the company of fast talkers. The Capacities and Demands Model highlights the importance of lessening demands on the child until he matures enough to be out of danger. The key is to prevent learned anticipatory struggle reactions from forming by reducing experiences of communicative failure. Gottwald and Starkweather (1984; 1985) have used this approach to formulate a sensible and reportedly effective program of stuttering prevention. Figure 3.2 illustrates the ratios of capacities and demands in a child predisposed to stuttering. In one view, the demands are greater than the child's capacities and stuttering appears. In the second, the demands are lessened and, although capacities stay the same, stuttering is diminished.

To illustrate the Capacities and Demands view, we shall take a case from our experience. Lauri was a bright, happy 7 year old. Her mother had been a severe stutterer as a child, but through treatment and her own perseverance she had largely recovered. When Lauri began the second grade she had no history of stuttering nor any problem with school. Some time before Christmas, however, when her class was learning to read, Lauri began to dislike school, and her mother soon discovered that she was having problems academically. After some testing, it was discovered that she had a learning disability; it had been hidden before, but once reading was required it became obvious. As she struggled throughout the rest of the second grade to cope with her reading problem, she began to stutter. Over the course of the next two years, she stuttered in a noticeable way, but did not receive therapy. She was, however, given extra help for her reading disabililty. By the fourth grade, she was making headway with reading, and her stuttering had diminished to an inconsequential level, without treatment.

Although there are many ways to interpret Lauri's onset of stuttering and her recovery, a capacities and demands view would see it this way: Lauri was predisposed to stuttering, but it lay dormant until she was faced with the challenge of reading. Reading, at least when first learned, involves highly conscious control of linguistic processes, in contrast to the more automatic linguistic processing in listening and speaking. As such, learning to read puts a large demand on the pool of available resources for speech and language processing. This demand may result in reduced capacity (fewer available resources) for speech production, which, for a

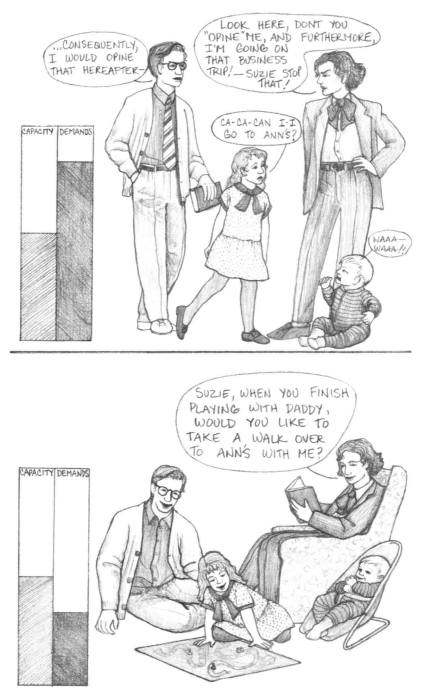

Figure 3.2. Two different ratios of capacities and demands and their hypothesized effect on fluency

vulnerable child, may result in disfluency. In this case, Lauri did not seem to develop a long-lasting fear of speaking as a result of her stuttering. Thus, when she overcame her initial reading difficulty, and reading became more automatic (demanding fewer resources), her available capacity could compensate for the deficit in fluency, and she "outgrew" her stuttering.

Once again, the reader is reminded that the Capacities and Demands view is a metaphor, describing relationships that appear again and again, but are not well understood. As such, its major function is to help the student of stuttering organize these complex inter-relationships into a set of principles that may guide treatment and suggest research hypotheses.

AN INTEGRATION OF CONSTITUTIONAL, DEVELOPMENTAL, AND ENVIRONMENTAL THEORIES

The three theoretical views we have just described are in many ways quite different, but there are points of similarity. In this section, we will highlight these similarities and differences. But in making these comparisons, we will integrate some material from the last chapter into this section to provide a more comprehensive understanding of how constitutional, developmental, and environmental factors may interact to precipitate stuttering.

Constitutional Factors

All three views at least indirectly acknowledge a constitutional factor related to speech, although they differ on what it is. The Diagnosogenic view considers that one factor in the stuttering equation is the child's disfluencies, "ranging from slight and decidedly ordinary to complex and unusual" (Johnson and Associates, 1959). It seems likely that the Diagnosogenic view would attribute at least the more complex and unusual disfluencies to constitutional factors. The Communication Failure view of a constitutional factor is broader, portraying any breakdown in communication as a precipitating influence in stuttering. The breakdown does not have to be explicitly linked to a constitutional deficit, but a glance at Table 3.5 indicates that many of these breakdowns may be constitutionally based. The Capacities and Demands view suggests that there may be a constitutional vulnerability to disfluency (a finite capacity for cognitive and motor processing) that may result in stuttering when demands on any aspect of performance are greater than this capacity can bear.

The Diagnosogenic and Communication Failure views also suggest another factor that may, in some cases, have a constitutional basis. This is the child's sensitivity to his own difficulty and to listener reaction. Recent research in child development has identified a trait in some children that may correspond to this sensitivity. Jerome Kagan and his colleagues (for example, Kagan, Reznick, and Snidman, 1987) have studied two groups of children: those who react "inhibitedly" to the stress of unfamiliar or threatening situations and those who react "uninhibitedly." Inhibited children suppress speech and other activity when confronted with novel stimuli. Kagan also documented high levels of laryngeal tension in inhibited children when they spoke in threatening situations. He attributed this tension to a lower threshold of reactivity in limbic and hypothalamic structures, which would affect laryngeal muscles via the reticular activating system and the nucleus ambiguus, the brainstem way station for laryngeal activation. Kagan corroborated the excess activity in these brain structures by demonstrating that the inhibited children had significantly elevated levels of the neurochemicals known to be associated with hypothalamic activity. Kagan's work suggests that these temperaments are consistent over a number of years, may be biologically based, and are at least partly congenital.

The significance of Kagan's findings for a predisposition to stuttering is this: it has long been suggested that laryngeal disfunction may be a critical element in stuttering; these data suggest a possible mechanism by which the child's constitutional makeup can, in certain situations, affect laryngeal function and thereby contribute to stuttering.[11] Moreover, Kagan's evidence suggests that this makeup may be inherited as well as influenced by the environment.

To summarize, all three views allow the possibility of a constitutional component in the stuttering equation. The Diagnosogenic view acknowledges it least, perhaps because Johnson and Associates (1959) emphasized environmental contributions and minimized physiological explanations, which may have been previously oversold. The Communication Failure view admits a constitutional component to a greater extent, suggesting that some individuals may have a vulnerability to stuttering, either in the form of a speech or language-related problem, a sensitive temperament, or both (Bloodstein, 1987). The Capacities and Demands view is probably the most explicit in attributing part of the problem to some constitutional deficit in most stutterers. This view holds that stutterers lack adequate capacity for the sensorimotor processing demands of rapid, fluent speech (Andrews and Harris, 1964; Andrews et al., 1983; Neilson, 1980; Starkweather, 1987).

Developmental Factors

There is little discussion of developmental factors in either the Diagnosogenic or the Communicative Failure views. It can be inferred from both, however, that the development of speech and language can be a critical factor in the onset of stuttering. Specifically, both views acknowledge that the disfluencies commonly associated with normal development may create negative listener reaction and concern in the child, which in turn may create stuttering. Furthermore, the Communicative Failure hypothesis suggests that delayed development of speech and language (or even normal development in the face of unrealistic parental expectations) may create, in interaction with critical listeners, a conviction that speaking is difficult, which may lead to the anticipatory struggle behaviors of stuttering.

Finally, the Capacities and Demands model clearly acknowledges the role

---

[11] Exactly how laryngeal disfunction could create stuttering is still unclear. However, there is evidence that abnormal laryngeal tension distinguishes stuttering from normal disfluency (Shapiro and DeCicco, 1982) and evidence of laryngeal disfunction even in the fluent speech of young stutterers (Conture, Rothenberg, and Molitor, 1986).

of developmental factors. In this case, the role is broader than in the other two views; most aspects of the child's development are thought to be potential contributors to the overload of capacity. And this overload may give rise to stuttering, in some unspecified way, by interacting with constitutional and environmental factors.

Environmental Factors

The Diagnosogenic view has the simplest hypothesis about environmental factors: they are listeners' reactions to the child's disfluencies. The Communicative Failure view is broader in its depiction of environmental factors. This view includes not only the reactions of all important listeners, but also the atmosphere created in a home or classroom. Both critical listeners and high standards for speaking performance can pressure a child who is vulnerable. The Capacities and Demands view has the broadest hypothesis about these environmental factors. Environmental factors are any influences outside the child that might place a demand on any aspect of his performance. These influences include speech and language models, parental expectations, and stressful life events.

In looking at these three perspectives on environmental factors, it is clear that they form a progression from most specific to most general. It is probably true that advocates of a more general view (e.g., Capacities and Demands) would say that a more specific view (e.g., Diagnosogenic) is correct insofar as it goes, but it doesn't go far enough. To put it another way, Starkweather (1987) would probably agree with Johnson's (1959) hypothesis that the listeners' reactions to normal disfluency can be a precipitant of stuttering, but he would suggest that other things, such as speech and language models in the home, can be equally, and in some cases, more important factors.

STUDY QUESTIONS

1/ The effect of a child's development on fluency has been likened to the effect of multiple tasks for a computer. Explain this analogy.

2/ It has been said that children usually do not learn to walk and talk at the same time. What does this suggest about the way motor development might affect fluency?

3/ There is a high incidence of stuttering among retarded individuals. What might this suggest about the relationship between cognition and fluency?

4/ What aspects of social and emotional development might threaten fluency?

5/ What evidence is there that emotional arousal might increase fluency?

6/ Why would speech and language development be likely to put greater pressure on fluency than physical or congnitive development?

7/ What aspects of parents' behavior might put pressure on a child who is disfluent?

8/ Identify several characteristics of parents' speech that may create a difficult model for a disfluent child to emulate.

9/ Name several life events that have been suggested to increase a child's disfluency.

10/ What is the central hypothesis of the Diagnosogenic view?

11/ The Communication Failure and Anticipatory Struggle view proposes that an experience of communication failure may cause a child to anticipate difficulty speaking and begin to stutter as a result. What characteristic of the child may be another important factor?

12/ How would the Capacities and Demands view account for the fact that some children don't begin to stutter until they are in elementary school?

Suggested Readings

Andrews, G. and Harris, M. (1964). *The syndrome of stuttering.* London: W. Heinemann Medical Books.

These authors present data from longitudinal studies of a thousand families in Newcastle, England. The interpretation of results presents evidence that both genetic and environmental influences are at work to create stuttering. This book gives an early version of the view that stuttering is due to a lack of capacity for some aspect of speech and language processing.

Bloodstein, O. (1987). Inferences and conclusions. In *A handbook on stuttering.* Chicago: National Easter Seal Society.

This chapter presents the Communication Failure and Anticipatory Struggle view of stuttering onset. Bloodstein musters the evidence he has summarized in earlier chapters of this handbook to argue convincingly that stuttering develops from an interaction between the child and his environment.

Crystal, D. (1987). Towards a "bucket" theory of language disability: Taking account of interaction between linguistic levels. *Clinical Linguistics and Phonetics 1,* 7–22.

A theoretical discussion of interaction among levels of speech and language, with an illustrative case of a child whose stuttering increases when language demands are greater. The article makes a clear argument for the influence of speech and language development on stuttering.

Johnson, W. and Associates. (1959). *The onset of stuttering.* Minneapolis: University of Minnesota Press.

This book presents extensive data on parents' perceptions of the onset of their child's stuttering compared with other parents' perceptions of their child's normal disfluency. Johnson eloquently lays out his view of stuttering as the product of an interaction between the child's disfluency, his sensitivity, and the listener's reactions.

Kagan, J., Reznick, J.S., and Snidman, N. (1987). The physiology and psychology of behavioral inhibition in children. *Child Development, 58*, 1459–1473.

This article discusses the findings of Kagan and his colleagues that behaviorally inhibited children show high levels of laryngeal tension. Neurophysiological mechanisms are also discussed, as well as possible genetic and environmental contributions. Recommended for those interested in the hypothesis that behavioral inhibition may be a component in some stuttering.

Lidz, T. (1968). *The person: His development throughout the life cycle.* New York: Basic Books.

This classic text, written by a developmental psychiatrist, traces emotional development from birth to old age. Although heavily psychoanalytic, it gives the reader sensible information about personality and emotion at different ages. With this information, the student interested in the psychology of stuttering can better understand some of the stutterer's responses to his disorder and to treatment.

4

NORMAL DISFLUENCY AND THE DEVELOPMENT OF STUTTERING

To clarify our view of how stuttering develops and why we treat it differently at different stages, we have devised a hierarchy of five levels. The first level is actually normal disfluency, and the last four levels reflect advancing stages of stuttering development. In this chapter, we will explain how these levels differ. In later chapters, we will describe how to treat stuttering at every level. The five levels are shown in Table 4.1, along with the age ranges typically associated with them.

Within each level, you will see that we have divided the characteristics of stuttering into four subcategories. The first three—core behaviors, secondary behaviors, and feelings and attitudes—we described in Chapter 1. The fourth, *under-*

Table 4.1.   Developmental/Treatment Levels of Stuttering

Developmental Level	Typical Age Range
Normal disfluency	1.5-6 years, although a small amount of normal disfluency continues in mature speech
Borderline stuttering	1.5-6 years
Beginning stuttering	2-8 years
Intermediate stuttering	6-13 years
Advanced stuttering	14 years and above

lying processes, we introduce in this chapter to explain why the symptoms change from level to level. Our explanations are hypotheses, based on evidence from animal and human studies of learned behavior, about how stuttering behaviors develop. This subcategory should help you understand the nature of the symptoms, as well as the treatment procedures in Section Two.

These five developmental/treatment levels should become your guide for diagnosing and treating stutterers. Your client's core and secondary behaviors, as well as feelings and attitudes, will indicate a developmental level, and help you develop a plan of treatment for him. Notice that our levels are based somewhat on age. We find that the appropriate treatment for an individual who stutters is determined both by how far the stuttering has advanced and how old the person is. An eight year old may have signs of advanced stuttering, but the stuttering treatment we propose for the advanced level would be inappropriate for this client because it demands considerable self-therapy. We will discuss these sorts of choices in Section Two.

These developmental/treatment levels do not precisely characterize all stutterers. Some stutterers won't fit neatly into any of the levels we've constructed. Some behaviors in the same individual will suggest one level; other behaviors will suggest another level. Generally, this will be rare, and most stutterers can be placed reasonably well within only one level. Moreover, treatment needn't be a problem even though all of a stutterer's behaviors may not reflect a single level, because when some aspects of a person's stuttering seem to be more advanced than others, strategies can be borrowed from other levels to treat them.

Another limitation of our hierarchy of developmental/treatment levels is our implication that all stutterers pass through each stage in sequence. This is generally true, but we have seen exceptions. A very few of our clients have been normal-speaking children one day, according to their parents, and beginning or intermediate stutterers the next. Van Riper (1982) has also described a subgroup of stutterers who show a relatively sudden onset with severe symptoms. He has suggested that many of these children begin to stutter after a traumatic incident, and they stutter with a great deal of tension, even at onset. In these cases, however, the overlay of learned behaviors soon places them in one of the levels we have described. Despite their unusual onsets, many of these clients respond well to our treatment procedures, especially if therapy begins soon after the onset of stuttering.

With these limitations stated, we will begin our description of the levels of stuttering development. We start with a behavior which is really not stuttering at all, but part of normal speech.

NORMAL DISFLUENCY

Children vary a great deal in how easily they learn to talk. Some children pass through the milestones of speech and language development with relatively few disfluencies. Others stumble along, repeating, interjecting, and revising, as they try to master new forms of speech and language, on their way to adult competence. Most children are somewhere in between the extremes of perfect fluency and excessive disfluency, such as the 2 year old shown in Figure 4.1.

Children also swing back and forth in their degree of disfluency. Some days they are more fluent and other days less fluent. The swings in normal disfluency may be associated with language development, motor learning, or another normal process mentioned in the preceding chapter. In the following sections, we will discuss factors that may influence normal disfluency, as well as specific behaviors that we categorize as normal disfluency, and reactions children may have to them. We will also highlight aspects of normal disfluency that distinguish it from early stuttering, since one of our aims in this chapter is to prepare you to make a differential diagnosis.

Core Behaviors

Normal disfluencies have been cataloged by several authors, and there is general agreement among them as to what constitutes a disfluency.[1] Table 4.2 lists eight commonly used categories of disfluency.

Some of the major distinguishing features of normal disfluency—features that differentiate normal disfluency from stuttering—are the amount of disfluency, the number of units in repetitions and interjections, and the type of disfluency, especially in relation to the age of the child.

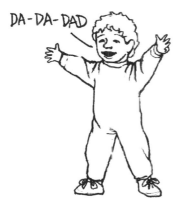

DA-DA-DAD

Figure 4.1.   Child who may be normally disfluent.

---

[1] The following authors discuss categories of nonfluencies: Colburn and Mysak (1982a,b), Yairi (1982), Yairi (1983), Bloodstein (1987).

Table 4.2.   Categories of Normal Disfluencies, with Examples

Type of Normal Disfluency	Example
Part-word repetition	"mi-milk"
Single-syllable word repetition	"I . . . I want that."
Multisyllabic word repetition	"Lassie . . . Lassie is a good dog."
Phrase repetition	"I want a . . . I want a ice-ceem comb."
Interjection	"He went to the . . . uh . . . circus."
Revision-Incomplete phrase	"I lost my . . . Where's Mommy going?"
Prolongation	"I'm Tiiiiiiimmy Thompson."
Tense Pause	"Can I have some more (lips together; no sound coming out) milk?"

Let us first discuss the amount of disfluency. This is usually measured as the number of disfluencies per 100 words, instead of "percent disfluencies." Percent disfluencies implies that the disfluencies are associated with the production of a particular word. If you said, for example, that a child had a disfluency frequency of 10% words disfluent, it would be assumed that 10% of the words spoken were spoken disfluently. However, many disfluencies, such as revisions, interjections, or phrase repetitions, are associated with several words or occur between words. For example, a child may say "Mommie, can you . . . can you . . . um . . . can you buy me dat?" or "I gonna . . . um . . . Dada take me dere." Hence, we calculate the number of disfluencies that occur when the child speaks 100 words.

Some of the earliest research on the amount of disfluency was conducted by Wendell Johnson at the University of Iowa. He assembled a team of researchers in the 1950s to examine the evidence for his "diagnosogenic" theory of stuttering. As we indicated in Chapter 3, Johnson hypothesized that, at the time the child is "diagnosed" a stutterer by his parents, the child's disfluencies are no different from those of nonstuttering children. One of the research team's projects was to record children already identified by their parents as stutterers and compare the amount of disfluency in their speech with that of nonstuttering children (Johnson, 1959). One part of this study compared 68 male stuttering children with 68 male nonstuttering children. The results showed that, although there was some overlap, the stutterers had more than twice the amount of disfluency than did the nonstutterers (an average of 18 disfluencies per 100 words compared to 7 disfluencies per 100 words).[2] Other researchers who have examined disfluencies in nonstuttering children put the amount of disfluencies in normal children at about this level or a little higher (DeJoy & Gregory, 1985; Wexler & Mysak, 1982; Yairi, 1981). Bringing all of these studies together, we can estimate that the average normally disfluent preschool child has about ten disfluencies in every 100 words spoken. This figure may

---

[2] Wendell Johnson's original interpretation was that the two groups were essentially the same, because there was so much overlap in both amount and type of disfluency. Other researchers have reinterpreted the data to suggest that these are two different groups. Johnson's diagnosogenic hypothesis would not be jeopardized by this reinterpretation, however, since he believed that the child's reaction to the parents' labeling of the child as a stutterer caused the child to engage in behavior that would be different from normal disfluency.

be a little high for the whole preschool period, but many children will go through a period of increased disfluency at age two or three that will reach this level.

The range in frequency of normal disfluency is important to note also, especially if frequency of disfluency is used to make a clinical decision. Johnson and Associates (1959) and Yairi (1981) found that at least one normal child in their samples had slightly more than 25 disfluencies per 100 words. Thus, frequency of disfluencies is not, by itself, a very effective clinical measure.

Another distinguishing characteristic of normal disfluency is the number of units that occur in each instance of repetition or interjection. Yairi's (1981) data suggest that, typically, normal repetitions consist of one extra unit: a child might say "That my-my ball." Interjections are likely to be just a single unit, as in "I want some . . . uh . . . juice." Instances of multiple repetitions were occasionally observed in these normal children but this was the exception. The rule was one, and sometimes two, units per repetition or interjection. This agrees with Johnson and Associates' (1959) findings that the average nonstuttering child has one- or two-unit repetitions.

Another major characteristic of normal disfluency is the type of disfluency that is most common. Johnson and Associates (1959) found that interjections, revisions, and word repetitions were the most frequent disfluency types among his 68 nonstuttering males, who ranged in age between two-and-a-half and eight. Yairi (1981) found, in his 33 two-year-old normal subjects that there were two clusters of common disfluency types. One cluster involved repetitions of speech segments of one syllable or less (one-syllable words or parts of words were repeated). The second cluster consisted of interjections and revisions.

The most common disfluency type seems to change as the child grows older. In a follow-up of his original study, Yairi (1982) found that children between two and three-and-a-half showed an increase in revisions and phrase repetitions, but a decrease in part-word repetitions and interjections. Yairi suggests that his data indicate that, as a nonstuttering child matures, part-word repetitions decline, even as other disfluency types might increase. Moreover, if part-word repetitions increase in a child observed longitudinally, this may be a sign that warrants concern.

Although the research is far from complete, we might summarize normal disfluency types as follows: revisions are a common disfluency type in normal children and may continue to account for a major portion of disfluency as the child grows. Interjections are also common, but decline after age three. Repetitions may also be a frequent type of disfluency, especially single-syllable word repetitions of less than two extra units around age 2-3. Repetitions are more likely to involve longer segments (e.g., phrases) as the child grows.

Secondary Behaviors

The normally disfluent child has no secondary behaviors. He has not developed any reactions, such as escape or avoidance, to his disfluencies. Although research suggests that some normal children display "tense pauses," this tension does not appear to be a reaction to the experience of disfluency. If a child shows

Table 4.3. Characteristics of Normal Disfluency in Average Nonstuttering Child

1. No greater than 10 disfluencies per 100 words.
2. Typically one-unit repetitions, occasionally two.
3. Most common disfluency types are interjections, revisions, and word repetitions. As children mature past age 3, they will show a decline in part-word repetitions.

what appear to be normal disfluencies, such as single-word repetitions, yet consistently displays reactions (such as pauses or interjections such as "uh") immediately before or during the disfluencies, he should be carefully evaluated as a possible stutterer.

Feelings and Attitudes

The normally disfluent child does not notice his disfluencies, even though some may be apparent to others. Just as a child may stumble when walking but then regain his balance and keep walking without complaint, a normal child who repeats or interjects or revises will usually continue talking after a disfluency, without evidence of frustration or embarrassment.

Table 4.3 summarizes the major characteristics of normal disfluency.

Underlying Processes

Let us first summarize the behaviors we are trying to account for. Normal disfluency occurs throughout childhood and adulthood. It may begin earlier than 18 months of age[3]; it peaks between ages 2 and 3½. It slowly diminishes thereafter, but also changes in form. Some types of disfluency, such as repetitions, decrease after age 3½, but other types, such as revisions, may increase. Episodic increases and decreases are also common throughout childhood.

What causes these patterns of disfluency? Why are there ups and downs and changes in form? Like most natural phenomena, a multiplicity of forces probably have an impact on fluency at any one moment, but some may be more predominant at certain times. In the last chapter, we talked about the developmental and environmental influences on stuttering and normal disfluency. Let us review them as we discuss studies of normally disfluent children.

The development of language is certainly likely to be one major influence on fluency. As our earlier review showed, children tend to be most disfluent at the beginning of syntactic units (Bernstein, 1981; Silverman, 1974) and when the length and complexity of their utterances increases (DeJoy & Gregory, 1973; Gordon, Luper, & Peterson, 1986; Pearl & Bernthal, 1980). These findings suggest that disfluency is greatest when the child is busy planning a long or complex language structure but must at the same time begin to produce it, putting a heavy load

---

[3] Harris Winitz (1961) studied the vocalizations of infants during the first two years of life and found that repetitions were common throughout that period. During that age span, frequency of repetitions peaked at 12 months. It is not clear whether the repetitions in non-meaningful speech are the result of the same processes that create repetitions in meaningful speech.

on resources. It seems likely that producing newly-learned structures would be hardest of all, resulting in more frequent disfluencies on most recently acquired forms. However, some evidence gathered on four children between 2 and 4 suggests that normal disfluency may be greatest on structures that have been learned, but perhaps not fully automatized, thus requiring more resources than are allocated to their production (Colburn & Mysak, 1982a,b).

Pragmatics may be an important influence on disfluency, too. Studies by Dorothy Davis (1940) and Susan Meyers and Frances Freeman (1985a,b) indicate that disfluency increases under certain pragmatic conditions, such as when interrupting, when directing another's activity, or when asked to change one's own activity. Mastering such pragmatic skills, especially those with more complex social interactions, creates yet another challenge for a developing child. The pressures from developing language, interacting with other factors, can be seen as competition for cerebral resources, which leaves fewer available resources for fluent speech production.

Another likely influence on disfluencies, in addition to language, is speech motor control. Between the ages of 2 and 5, the child must learn to reach all the segmental and supersegmental targets of his native tongue, as well as to increase his speech rate to produce longer and longer utterances. This task must keep the average child fairly busy, although it may not be obvious. He is continually scanning his parents' and older siblings' speech for models of how to sound. He is also continuously correcting his own productions to make them more and more like what he hears. This age, from 2 to 5, also encompasses intensive nonspeech motor learning. Children are mastering a myriad of other motor tasks at the same time they are learning to speak in rapid, complex, fluent sequences. Many children learn to walk, run, ride a tricycle, a bicycle, and a skateboard, to play a dozen sports, to swim, to dance, and to sing, all at about the time they are intensively learning language. These motor activities compete with fluency for use of cortical resources. The view of stuttering, described earlier, that suggests a breakdown may occur when capacity is taken away from a motor control system to be used elsewhere, may fit the normal child as well as the stutterer (Andrews et al., 1983; Starkweather, 1987). Some of the upswings and downswings of disfluency may occur when the normal child is occupied with learning language, speech production, and motor control for other things besides speech fluency.

Besides the continuing demands of normal development, there are also episodic stresses in the child's environment that may temporarily increase normal disfluency. An experiment by Harris Hill (1954) demonstrated that conditioned fear could bring about disfluency in normal speakers' speech. Therefore, it is easy to imagine that there are many psychological stresses in a child's life that would also bring about disfluency. Clinically, we have observed many situations that seem to increase normal disfluency. Among them are stress from moving from one home to another, being part of a family undergoing separation and divorce, the birth of a sibling, and other events which decrease a child's feeling of security. We have also seen increases in normal disfluency during periods of excitement, such as holidays, vacations, and visits by relatives. Disfluency especially increases when excitement combines with competition to be heard, such as dinner table conversations in which everyone tries to talk at once, or after school when several children are competing to tell Mom what happened during the day.

Summary

NORMAL

Between the ages of two and five, most children pass through periods of disfluency. Repetitions, interjections, revisions, prolongations, and pauses are commonly heard during this period. When the average child is between two and three-and-a-half, disfluencies reach 10 per 100 words spoken, and may be even greater in some children. Repetitions are probably most common in younger children, while revisions are more frequent in older children. Despite the fact that children's disfluencies may be evident occasionally to some adults, normally disfluent children seem generally unaware of them in their own speech and consequently have no reactions to them or secondary behaviors to escape or avoid them.

Some factors thought to be associated with increases in normal disfluencies include language development, acquisition of speech motor control, interpersonal stress associated with growing up in a typical family, and threats to security from relocation, family breakup, or hospitalization. Disfluencies may also increase under the daily pressure of competition and excitement while speaking.

BORDERLINE STUTTERING

The borderline stutterer (Figure 4.2) has all the symptoms of the normally disfluent child. However, there are more of these symptoms in the borderline stutterer's speech, and they often differ in several ways. Diagnosis of the borderline stutterer is sometimes difficult, because a child may drift back and forth between normal disfluency and borderline stuttering over a period of weeks or months. Some borderline stutterers gradually lose their stuttering symptoms and grow up without a trace of stuttering. Other borderline stutterers develop more stuttering symptoms and grow up, instead, into beginning, intermediate, and advanced stutterers.

In describing the behaviors of the borderline stutterer, we begin to define

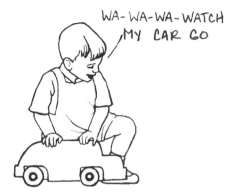

Figure 4.2.   Child who may be a borderline stutterer.

our view of how stuttering differs from normal disfluency. The distinction between stuttering and normal disfluency has been of great interest to theorists for many years. Some theorists (e.g., Wendell Johnson et al., 1942; 1955) suggest, as we have noted previously, that the stuttering child developed his symptoms only after his parents mislabeled his normal disfluencies as stuttering. That is, this child's first "stuttering" symptoms were really the disfluencies of normal speech. An opposing view maintains that there are objective differences between the speech of the normal child and the speech of the child first labeled as a stutterer by his parents or another lay person. We hold the latter view, believing that, when their parents first become concerned, most children who stutter are disfluent in a way that is different from normal. Although the disfluency pattern, considered as a whole, may be different, there are still many behaviors that overlap with normal disfluencies. Moreover, as previously stated, these children often go back and forth between stuttering and normal disfluency over a period of months. For this reason, we use the term "borderline" to indicate that the children are in a gray area, neither entirely normally disfluent, nor definitely stuttering.

Core Behaviors

There is no single behavior that distinguishes the borderline stutterer from the normally disfluent child. However, many researchers and clinicians have suggested a few guidelines. Yairi's (1981) sample of 33 nonstuttering children indicated that their repetitions typically involved only one or two units of repetition (two would be li-li-like this). His data on 22 children whose parents thought they were stuttering (Yairi, 1983) suggested that the parents often reported three to five repetition units at the onset of stuttering. Thus, the appearance of repetitions in which there are more than two units might be one warning sign of borderline stuttering.

Wendell Johnson noted that normally disfluent children and beginning stutterers were not categorically different because all the disfluencies of stuttering children could be found in the speech of nonstuttering children. However, data from his most famous study suggest there may be differences in the *amount* of disfluency. The study (Johnson and Associates, 1959) indicates that the 68 stuttering children had significantly more of the following disfluencies than the 68 normal children: part-word repetitions, word repetitions, phrase repetitions, and prolonged sounds. We believe that high frequency of disfluency is a warning sign of borderline stuttering. We noted in the section on the normally disfluent child that 10 disfluencies per 100 words may be within normal limits. Much more than this would categorize the child as a borderline stutterer, unless other signs indicated the stuttering was even more advanced. From Johnson and his colleagues' study (1959), and from Yairi's work (1981; 1983), we would be more likely to diagnose the child as a stutterer if repetitions and prolongations were more predominant than revisions or incomplete phrases. It should be noted that, even though the borderline stutterer shows a higher frequency of disfluencies, his disfluencies generally sound loose and relaxed. It is only later, when a child crosses over into beginning stuttering, that effort and tension regularly appear in his speech.

Table 4.4.   Characteristics of Borderline Stutterer

1. More than 10 disfluencies per 100 words.
2. Often more than 2 units in repetition.
3. More repetitions and prolongations than revisions or incomplete phrases.
4. Disfluencies loose and relaxed.
5. Child rarely reacts to his disfluencies.

Secondary Behaviors

The borderline stutterer has few if any secondary behaviors. The degree of tension may sometimes seem slightly greater than normal, but repetitions and prolongations will generally look and sound relaxed. The child will not use accessory movements before, during, or after his stutters. In fact, there is usually nothing to indicate he is aware of his stutters.

Feelings and Attitudes

Since the borderline stutterer shows little evidence of awareness of his stutters, he does not show concern or embarrassment. When he repeats a sound or a syllable, even five or six times, he usually goes on talking as though nothing had happened. One exception is that, once in a while, the borderline stutterer might appear to feel surprise or frustration when he is repeating a syllable several times, because he is unable to finish a word. Then he may stop and comment, "Mommy, I can't say that word." But, in general, the borderline stutterer shows no evidence that he has more problems than anyone else.

Table 4.4 summarizes the major characteristics of the borderline stutterer.

Underlying Processes

We hypothesize that the symptoms of borderline stuttering are the result of the constitutional and environmental factors described in Chapters 2 and 3. The constitutional factors—differences in cerebral organization—often first show their effects as an excess of normal disfluencies. As previously stated, environmental and devlopmental pressures may be great between the ages of 2 and $3\frac{1}{2}$, and it is at this time that borderline stuttering typically emerges. This is a time when environmental and developmental pressures may be great. The converging demands of expressive language and motor speech development ordinarily peak between ages two to four, "when an explosive growth in language ability outstrips a still-immature speech motor apparatus (Andrews et al., 1983)." This age is also filled with psychosocial conflicts, as the child struggles with his security needs as an infant and his urge to grow more independent. The child is ready to explore, but he is also afraid. A new brother or sister may be born, triggering the child's insecurity at the threat of being replaced. An older sibling may turn belligerent toward him because of the older child's own need to express aggression as a prelude to puberty. Just as these stresses wax and wane in strength during preschool years, so does stuttering.

After age 4½ or 5, developmental stresses taper off somewhat for most children. Some of the parent-child conflicts are resolved, and the child feels more integrated within himself and within his family.[4] Articulation and language skills, though still not at adult levels, have been mastered to the extent that the child can usually say what's on his mind and be understood. He has mastered other motor skills, such as walking and running, as well as riding a tricycle or a bike with training wheels. He has also adjusted to having a new, younger sibling and may have made at least temporary peace with an older one.

By now, the capacities of a great many children who may have had a modest predisposition to stutter can easily meet demands of the environment. Therefore, many children who were borderline stutterers will have developed normal fluency skills by 4½ or 5. Others who may still have many disfluencies at this age will eventually outgrow them because they are not frustrated by them. They are functioning well in general, feel accepted, and can use their resources to compensate for a little difficulty in speaking.

Some children, however, do not outgrow borderline stuttering. They may continue to stutter and their symptoms may worsen. These may be children who have a substantial predisposition to stutter, which cannot be offset by a "good enough" environment. Their ability to produce speech and language at the rate and level of complexity used by most parents may be inadequate. Their continuing efforts to meet adult speech and language targets may result in excess disfluency, which does not diminish as they pass their third and fourth birthdays. Their frustration tolerance to the multiple repetitions that many 2 and 3 year olds experience may be low. Rather than shrugging it off, they may begin struggling to produce flawless speech, thereby making it worse. Still other children may continue to stutter, because the environmental and developmental stresses do not diminish as described above. They may have continued insecurity from unrelieved sibling rivalry, the breakup of the family by divorce, or a parent's death. They may have language or articulation problems, as well as stuttering, and consequently, may struggle to express themselves throughout their preschool years. Their deficits in processes underlying speech and language, plus the frustration of being unable to communicate easily, may be devastating to fluency. This may lead to the increased tension of beginning stuttering. A child in this situation is unlikely to outgrow stuttering unless parents and professionals can provide extensive support.

Summary
Borderline [handwritten annotation]

The borderline stutterers usually have a greater amount of disfluency than normal children—above 10 nonfluencies per 100 words. They are also likely to have more than 2 units in many of their repetitions, and to have many more repetitions, prolongations, or broken words than revisions or interjections. At the same time, however, their disfluencies, like those of nonstuttering children, are loose and relaxed. Also like nonstuttering children, borderline stutterers show lit-

---

[4] See Theodore Lidz's *The Person* (Basic Books, 1968) for a more detailed description of psychosocial forces throughout an individual's lifetime.

tle or no awareness of their speaking difficulty. Only rarely will they express frustration about it.

Among the underlying processes behind borderline stuttering are probably some of the speech and language processing deficits described in the earlier chapter on constitutional origins of stuttering. These deficits may interact with the high level of demand on communication from speech and language development, the pressure from high rates of speech, complex language, competitive speaking situations, and other attributes of a normal home. In addition, the psychosocial conflicts described earlier, which increase normal disfluency, are likely to be active in creating borderline stuttering.

3. BEGINNING STUTTERING

As stuttering develops, the child who has been a borderline stutterer begins to tense and speed up repetitions, as the child in Figure 4.3 appears to be doing. At first, the child may do this only occasionally, when excited or stressed. Then, gradually, tension and hurry become a regular part of the stuttering. The borderline stutterer is now becoming a beginning stutterer, and he is stuttering more often and is less tolerant of it. The child is impatient with his stuttering and, consequently, uses a variety of escape behaviors. For example, he learns to stop long repetitions by using a quick blink of his eyes or a sudden nod of his head. These signs, and stuttering in general, may still come and go, as in the borderline stutterer. In the beginning stutterer, however, periods of stuttering may last for several months, while the periods of fluency may last only a few weeks.

As the signs progress, tension increases, and struggle is more evident. Instrumental and classical conditioning processes increase the frequency of struggle behaviors, complicate the pattern of stuttering, and spread the symptoms to many more situations.

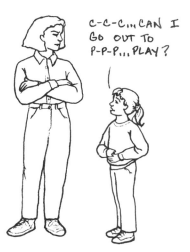

Figure 4.3. Child who may be a beginning stutterer.

Core Behaviors

The core behaviors of the beginning stutterer differ from those of the borderline stutterer in several ways. Repetitions begin to sound rapid and irregular. The final sound of a repeated syllable, if it is a vowel, often sounds abrupt or suddenly cut off. It sounds as though a neutral or schwa vowel ("uh") has been substituted for the appropriate one, as in "luh-luh-luh-like." The repetitions are also produced more rapidly, and with an irregular rhythm. Rather than patiently repeating a syllable as the borderline stutterer does, the beginning stutterer hurries through a repetitive stutter, as though juggling a hot potato.

As the symptom progresses, the beginning stutterer increases tension throughout his speech system. His stuttering will often be accompanied by a rise in vocal pitch, resulting from increased tension in his larynx. Pitch rise may first appear toward the end of a string of repeated syllables, but as time goes on, it appears earlier and earlier in the string.

The beginning stutterer will sometimes prolong sounds he might have previously repeated. Initially, he may prolong the first sound of a syllable, but as stuttering grows more severe, he may prolong the middle sound, and this, too, may be accompanied by an increase in pitch.

As beginning stuttering progresses, the first signs of blockages appear. These are significant landmarks. They indicate that the child is stopping the flow of air and voice at one or more places (Van Riper, 1982). He may inappropriately open or close his vocal folds, interrupting or possibly delaying the onset of phonation (Conture, 1990). This shutting off of the airway, which is usually heard as a momentary stoppage of sound in a child's speech, is sometimes accompanied by a visual cue: the child may seem momentarily unable to move his mouth or may make groping movements as he tries to get air or voice going again. When this stoppage of movement, voice, or airflow first begins, it may be so fleeting that we don't notice it unless we are listening and watching carefully. As these blocks develop, they become so obvious that they overshadow the repetitions and prologations that may remain.

Secondary Behaviors

As the beginning stutterer's symptoms progress, secondary behaviors are added to the stutterer's pattern. They are called secondary because they are responses to the core tension. In addition, although hard evidence is lacking, the core behavior of tension and speeding up seems to be "involuntary," that is, less under the stutterer's control. The secondary behaviors we will be describing seem to be done "voluntarily." They are, at least initially, deliberate. Among the earliest of these are "escape" behaviors, which are maneuvers the stutterer uses to stop the stutter and finish a word. Beginning stutterers often show these escape behaviors after several repetitions of a syllable. They will nod their head or squint their eyes just as they try to push a word out. This extra effort often helps—in the short run. They escape, for the moment, from the punishing repetition or prolongation. Alternately, they may insert a filler such as "uh" or "um" after a string of fruitless repetitions. The "um" releases the word, perhaps by relaxing the tightly squeezed larynx or unlocking the lips. The "um" can always be said fluently. Once the "um" is uttered, phonation and movement associated with the word will often begin. The filler works like sand placed under a car tire stuck in the snow; it gets the child going again when he is stuck in a stutter.

The beginning stutterer will start to use escape behaviors earlier and earlier in the stutter. Their first appearance is usually after the child has repeated a sound several times and is thoroughly frustrated with it. It may sound this way: "Luh-Luh-Luh-Luh-Luh . . . umLet's go!" Soon, however, the child does not want to wait until he has tried to say the sound five times. He will find himself about to say a word and feel convinced it won't come out. Then, he may instinctively employ the escape behavior when he is first starting to stutter, sounding like this: "L-umLet's go!" These "starters" may even appear before the first sound of the word, in this fashion: "umLet's go!" The use of starters is more typical of the intermediate stutterer, but they occasionally appear in the speech of a beginning stutterer.

Feelings and Attitudes

The beginning stutterer has stuttered many times. He is aware of stuttering when it happens. Although he may be conscious that he has some "trouble" when he talks, he has not developed a fear or anticipation of stuttering or a negative picture of himself as a defective speaker. His lack of a negative self-image may be attributed, as Bloodstein (1987) and Van Riper (1982) suggest, to the "episodic" nature of stuttering. Some days it's there; some days it's gone. Sometimes the child feels that he has problems when he talks; other times he forgets about it.

The feelings the beginning stutterer has just before, during, and after a stutter, however, may be strong. He may feel annoyed, frustrated, helpless, and slightly embarrassed. He may stop in the middle of a stutter and say, "Mom, why can't I talk?" This momentary anguish will grow into something more permanent if his stuttering progresses.

The essential characteristics of beginning stutterers are shown in Table 4.5.

Table 4.5.   Characteristics of Beginning Stutterers

1. Signs of muscle tension and hurry appear in stuttering. Repetitions are rapid and irregular, with abrupt terminations of each element.
2. Pitch rise may be present toward the end of a repetition or prolongation.
3. Fixed articulatory postures are sometimes evident when the child is momentarily unable to begin a word, apparently as a result of tension in speech musculature.
4. Escape behaviors are sometimes present in stutters. These include, among other things, eyeblinks, head-nods, and "um's."
5. Awareness of difficulty and feelings of frustration are present, but there are no strong negative feelings about self as speaker.

Underlying Processes

The signs and symptoms of beginning stuttering that we have described above can be observed by any experienced clinician. We have witnessed them in hundreds of stutterers. But the processes underlying these changing symptoms are not so clear. To understand why these symptoms occur, we must rely on hypotheses, or educated guesses, which have been developed in animal behavior laboratories. Although these hypotheses are only tentative and are continually being refined by further research, they will be useful in helping to understand how stuttering may have developed, and how it can be managed. For example, the two types of learning described below—classical and instrumental conditioning—are major influences on the development of stuttering. With an understanding of the principles behind them, the clinician can put them to work to reduce stuttering and increase fluency.

Our first focus is the beginning stutterer's increases in tension and rate. Most clinicians and researchers agree that increased tension is a sign that stuttering is becoming chronic, and several explanations for this increase have been proposed. Oliver Bloodstein (1987) suggests that the appearance of facial tension and hard glottal attacks in the young stutterer's speech may reflect extra muscular effort, which the stutterer uses when he anticipates difficulty. Edward Conture (1990) offers a related view. He conceptualizes the increased laryngeal and articulatory muscle tension as the stutterer's attempt to control the sound-syllable repetitions, which are so distressing to the child and his parents. Increased rate is cited by a number of authors as a sign that stuttering is worsening. Van Riper (1982), in describing the developmental course of the majority of stutterers, suggests, " . . . the tempo changes as the disorder develops. The repetitive syllables become irregular and are often spoken more rapidly than other fluent syllables." Starkweather (1987) explains this increase in speed of repetitions as the product of pressure the child feels as he becomes more aware of the extra time it takes him to produce an utterance.

We agree with the views expressed in these comments about increased muscle tension and speech rate during repetitive disfluencies, but we would add a further speculation. We think that increased muscle tension and repetition rate begin as natural or "reflexive" responses, which the child makes when he is affected, first by frustration and then, later, by fear. These responses, we feel, are further shaped through the processes of conditioning. Before we describe our view of how this takes place, we will first review the elements of classical conditioning.

CLASSICAL CONDITIONING

The famous Russian physiologist Ivan Pavlov offered the first scientific description of classical conditioning. At the time, Pavlov was studying the reflexive secretion of fluids in dogs' mouths and stomachs when they were fed. After several days, Pavlov found that the dogs were starting to drool when he walked into his laboratory in the morning, thereby delaying his assessment of food-elicited salivation. As he pondered the problem, he grew curious and began to experiment with the dogs' anticipatory drooling. He realized that the dogs were associating his presence with being fed, and this association produced premature salivation. Would they make the same association to anything that was present when they were fed? Pavlov tried a tuning fork. He sounded the fork several times just before a dog was fed and looked for the response. Initially, no response was forthcoming; the dog salivated only when it was fed. But Pavlov persisted, again and again sounding the tuning fork just before feeding the dog. After many such pairings, Pavlov found that the dog would respond to the tuning fork just as it had been responding to Pavlov as he walked through the door. The dog now salivated in response to the sound of the tuning fork, although the food was nowhere in sight.

Pavlov's observation provided the first insight into classical conditioning. Since then, classical conditioning has been studied intensively, and scientists have been able to describe how it takes place. Figure 4.4 depicts the "paradigm" (a model or diagram of how a process takes place) for classical conditioning.

The first stage of this process is the presentation of an unconditioned stimulus (UCS) which elicits an unconditioned response (UCR). These are often reflexive or "hardwired" responses, such as flinching to a loud noise. For Pavlov's dog, the UCS is the food and the UCR is salivation.

The second stage is the repeated presentation of a neutral stimulus just before the UCS. Pavlov sounded the tuning fork immediately before he fed the dog.

The last stage is presentation of the neutral stimulus (now that learning has occurred, the neutral stimulus is called the conditioned stimulus or CS). The CS now elicits the UCR (now called the conditioned response or CR). Pavlov sounded the tuning fork without presenting food, and the dog salivated.

Note that for conditioning to take place, the pairing of the neutral stimulus and the UCS must take place repeatedly. Moreover, the pairing between the CS and the UCS must occur intermittently; otherwise, extinction occurs. If Pavlov didn't occasionally feed the dog in the presence of the tuning fork, the tuning fork would eventually no longer elicit the salivation response.

Classical Conditioning and Stuttering

Let us now turn to the early stages of stuttering and examine the role that classical conditioning may play. An excellent theoretical account of classical conditioning and the onset of stuttering was provided by Eugene Brutten and Donald Shoemaker, a speech pathologist and a psychologist at the University of Southern Illinois (Brutten & Shoemaker, 1967).[5] These authors suggested that stuttering symptoms (repetitions and prolongations) are the result of the cognitive and motor disorganization that occurs when the child experiences learned negative emotion (autonomic arousal) as a response to various stimuli in speaking situations. That is, the child first has a fluency breakdown under real stress when he is speaking in a particularly difficult situation, such as with an angry parent or after a traumatic event. At that time, various neutral stimuli, such as the words spoken or the room in which the child is speaking, are associated in the child's mind with the

---

[5] Brutten and Shoemaker postulate a "two factor" theory of stuttering. Instrumental conditioning is the second factor. It shapes the pattern of stuttering when tension, escape behaviors, and avoidances are rewarded. We will be discussing the role of instrumental conditioning in the next section.

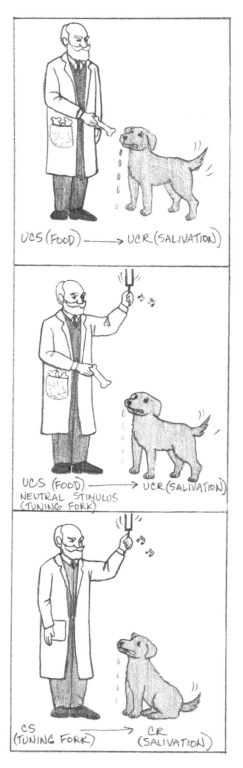

Figure 4.4. Classical conditioning paradigm. Dog salivates naturally when given food. Food is paired frequently with sound of tuning fork. Tuning fork without food then elicits salivation.

stimulus that elicits negative emotion. When these neutral stimuli appear again, without the unconditioned stimulus, they elicit negative emotion through learned association, and they cause the child's speech to disintegrate into the repetitions and prolongations of borderline stuttering.

Although our account owes much to Brutten and Shoemaker's pioneering work, we don't believe classical conditioning is usually responsible for the earliest signs of stuttering. Instead, we believe, along with Starkweather (1987, p. 372) that, " . . . it seems likely that physiological sources play more of a role in stuttering onset, whereas conditioning processes play more of a role in stuttering development." And we agree with a very similar assessment by Van Riper (1982) that, " . . . the real contribution of classical conditioning theory as it is applied to stuttering lies in its ability to explain the development of the disorder." Our view is that most borderline stutterers develop their excessive repetitions and prolongations as a result of the interactions of constitutional, developmental, and environmental factors. We believe these excessive repetitions and prolongations then create considerable frustration, which triggers reflexive responses of increased muscle tension and rate of repetitions. These reactions to frustration form the unconditioned responses, which are classically conditioned to speech. But before discussing the conditioning process, we will first elaborate on the reflexive responses of increased muscle tension and speech rate during disfluencies.

Our speculation about the child's responses has been influenced by studies of animal conditioning and human phobias, particularly those reviewed by Jeffrey Gray in his book *The Psychology of Fear and Stress* (1987). Gray argues that frustration and fear are essentially similar emotions, affecting and affected by the same brain mechanisms. Fear responses are, however, more intense—further along on the continuum of negative emotion. As will be evident in our discussion of the intermediate stutterer, fear plays an increasingly important role as stuttering develops. Studies of fear and frustration in animals suggest that biological inheritance and early environment play an important role in determining an individual's vulnerability to threat, and hence the likelihood that the frustration and fear response will be elicited easily. The innate reaction of the frightened animal, including Man, Gray suggests, is "one of the three Fs—freezing (keeping absolutely still and silent), flight, or fight—when he is faced with a punishment or threat of a punishment." These responses are mediated by the autonomic nervous system and are not under voluntary control. We suggest that the increased muscle tension is, at first, the direct result of this unconditioned frustration/fear response ("keeping absolutely still and silent"). And increased rate of repetitive stutters is the flight component of the response ("a great increase in activity . . . frantic scampering and jumping"). Both will later form the basis for instrumentally conditioned escape responses.

Let us examine the stutterer's responses again, to see if they might fit the pattern of these reflexive reactions. Many of the descriptions of excessive muscle tension can be seen as analogous to the freeze response; that is, they have the effect of "freezing" by silencing or immobilizing the repetitive disfluencies, which are the source of the stutterer's frustration. For example, Freeman and Ushijima's (1978) and Shapiro and DeCicco's (1982) research suggests that stuttering is associated with abnormal muscle cocontraction in the larynx. Such cocontraction would be a means of stiffening the structures and silencing vocal output. Other studies have demonstrated cocontraction in the articulatory structures (Fibiger, 1971; Guitar et al., 1988; Platt & Basili, 1973), which would also produce immobility and silence.

There is, however, little research which would directly support the notion that the increased rate of repetitions has its basis in the flight response. We have some tentative evidence that stutterers do have more rapid productions during repetitions than do nonstutterers. An unpublished study carried out in our clinic (Allen, 1988) indicated that the durations of stutterers' repeated segments and the silences between them were shorter than similar durations in the disfluencies of nonstuttering children matched for age. This increased rate may derive from the "great increase in activity" seen in the flight response, although these particular data do not exclude the possibility that the stuttering children were more rapid speakers to begin with. Thus the possibility that increased muscle tension and speech rate during disfluencies are a result of an innate freezing, flight, or fight response is highly speculative at this time.[6] It is, however, a potentially powerful explanation of why some children develop stuttering so rapidly, and why the tension response is so difficult to change.

We have suggested in this chapter that borderline stutterers develop into beginning stutterers because of an innate reaction to the frustration created by excess repetitions and prolongations. This reaction would increase muscle tension and speech rate during disfluencies. But we also believe that there are many individual differences in this response, and that these differences may explain why many borderline stutterers outgrow their stuttering and why other stutterers who continue to stutter develop at different rates and reach different levels of severity. Gray (1987) reviews a large body of literature which suggests that genetics and early environment create wide, individual differences in vulnerability to stress and in conditionability. Brutten and Shoemaker (1967) cite this literature to suggest that individuals who stutter may be especially vulnerable to autonomic arousal and thus to conditioned negative emotion. Individual differences in response to stress and autonomic arousal were the major focus of the research of Kagan and his collegues, reviewed in Chapter 3 (Kagan, et al., 1987). Although they studied nonstuttering children, their results may have application to borderline and beginning stutterers. They found several indicators of physiological arousal under stress that were much higher in inhibited children than in uninhibited children. One of the most reliable differences between the groups, and one of particular interest to us, is an increase in laryngeal tension (assessed acoustically) in stressful situations. If Kagan and his colleagues' findings are reliable and apply to the general population, a tendency to increase laryngeal tension under stress might be another predisposing factor for stuttering. We might then theorize that there are three factors that put children at risk for stuttering: (a) a constitutional predisposition for speech

---

[6] Research to support this speculation could make use of the supposition that the responses are mediated by the autonomic nervous system. Correlates of autonomic activity, such as EEG (Morrell, 1961) or the use of drugs that decrease autonomic arousal, may someday provide evidence that the increases in tension and rate are a result of unconditioned responses triggered by autonomic arousal. Research on children in the early stages of stuttering would be crucial, because autonomic arousal may decrease once the responses are conditioned (Morrell, 1961).

motor discoordination (discussed in Chapter 2), (*b*) developmental and environmental pressures (Chapter 3), and (*c*) a constitutional or environmental predisposition to develop excess laryngeal tension in conditions of frustration or fear. These three factors might combine in a variety of ways to produce the individual differences we see in the acquisition of fluent speech.[7]

We now turn to our view of the role of classical conditioning in the development of stuttering. For ease of explanation, we will refer to the hypothesized increase in muscle tension and speech rate during disfluencies under conditions of frustration and fear as "the tension response." The basic paradigm for this conditioning is shown in Figure 4.5.

To illustrate how this paradigm applies to an individual stutterer, we will use a young client from our clinic, a beginning stutterer named Richard. The actual changes in Richard's stuttering were neither as sudden nor as absolute as we describe them below. We have taken some liberties with Richard's stuttering to make the process more easily understood.

The Previously Neutral Stimulus. The neutral stimulus is the child's borderline stuttering, relatively free of tension and hurry. In our example, Richard's disfluencies consisted of frequent instances of part-word repetitions, which were neither tense nor hurried.

Pairing the Neutral Stimulus with the UCS. As stuttering develops, a child's relaxed disfluencies (NS), which have previously not bothered him, become paired with an event (UCS) which elicits the tension response (UCR). This event might be a parent's correction of the child's repetitive disfluency, the child's own experience of being unable to communicate quickly, or both.

In Richard's case, at about age 4, he began to become more disfluent than ever, possibly in response to having a new baby in the family and to moving into a new house. His parents tried to help him by suggesting that he stop and try again if he seemed to be caught up in a particularly long and frustrating stutter. Whenever he was corrected or felt frustrated, his repetitive stuttering became tense and hurried.

The Formerly Neutral Stimulus (Now the CS) Now Elicits the UCR (Now the CR). In this third stage of classical conditioning, the formerly neutral stimulus, now the CS (a disfluency), occurs without the threatening experience and yet elicits the CR (tension response).

Richard showed this effect of conditioning in the increased muscle tension and speech rate associated with his disfluencies in situations where he previously stuttered without tension or hurry, such as talking to playmates. Richard's stuttering then gradually became more and more widespread, through processes we will discuss below.[8]

We should add here that our treatment for Richard taught him a slower style of speaking which was free from disfluencies and, therefore, free from the CS that elicited the tension response. In fact, slow speech may be incompatible with

---

[7] Vulnerability to developing laryngeal tension under stress may also explain why some children and adults develop hyperfunctional voice disorders and others do not.

[8] Such rapid learning and widespread generalization as we sometimes see in stuttering children has a parallel in "prepared classical conditioning," wherein animals can be rapidly and deeply conditioned to such potentially dangerous stimuli as snakes (Mineka, 1985). Children who are inherently sensitive may likewise rapidly condition to such possibly threatening stimuli as a critical parent.

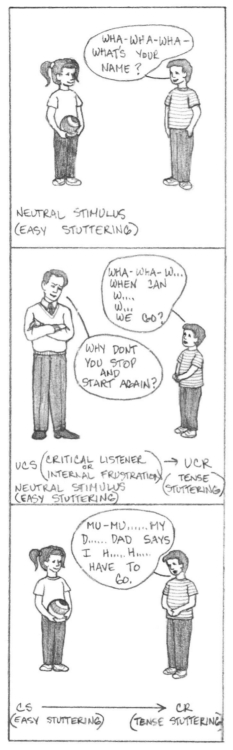

Figure 4.5. An example of classical conditioning of tension in a beginning stutterer. The repeated pairing of easy stuttering with a critical listener or internal frustration, which elicits tension, makes the easy stuttering a conditioned stimulus for tension. Consequently, tense stuttering occurs in more and more situations.

tense and hurried disfuencies. Richard only needs to speak slower when stress threatens to bring out his disfluencies. As his system matures, this may be less frequently necessary.

Spread of Conditioning

Conditioning is a continuing and active process. Whenever the conditioned stimulus elicits the conditioned response (the child is disfluent [CS] and experiences the tension response [CR]), a host of other stimuli are incidentally present. When the child stutters, he is talking to someone, uttering a particular word or sound, speaking in a particular room, and talking about a particular topic. Because of the power of classical conditioning, the pairing of these other stimuli with the conditioned stimulus gives them the potency to elicit the tension response. They become conditioned stimuli. Thus, as conditioning takes place again and again, the stimulus becomes a complex of many things, including words and sounds, listeners, and physical surroundings or situations. This chaining of stimuli is called "higher-order conditioning."[9] Figure 4.6 illustrates the process.

The spread of conditioning to other conditioned stimuli results in changes in the stuttering response as well. Initially, a child might emit several repetitive disfluencies, or a long prolongation, before the tension response appears. Soon, however, muscle tension occurs earlier and earlier in the stuttering. When other conditioned stimuli, such as words, elicit the tension response, the easy repetitive disfluencies may not occur at all. Instead, a child will increase muscle tension on the very first sound he tries to utter, resulting in the "fixed articulatory postures" that are a sign of beginning stuttering.

As a child's stuttering frequency increases as a result of the spread of conditioning to more and more stimuli, the duration of the child's stuttering may also increase. This may be explained by the fact that the tension response soon becomes a stimulus that itself elicits more tension. After all, the tension response makes it harder to utter a word, and the experience of "squeezing hard" without being able to speak for a second or two is undoubtedly frustrating, leading to another tension response.

In Richard's case, his slow speech treatment included a carefully constructed hierarchy of people and situations where he was previously disfluent. By associating fluent speech with many situations, we were able to counteract the previous conditioning and prevent these stimuli from triggering disfluency, frustration, and the tension response. This is counter-conditioning, a major element in the treatment of beginning, intermediate, and advanced stutterers. Counter-conditioning is part of well-constructed fluency shaping programs for beginning stutterers and is the essence of the desensitization phase of stuttering modification for intermediate and advanced stutterers.

Conditioning as Patterns of Connectivity

The above description of the spread of conditioning may seem confusing. For years, clinicians and researchers have been trying to figure out why, for exam-

---

[9] Higher-order conditioning and related aspects of learned behavior are described with clarity and detail in Zimbardo's *Psychology and Life* (1985).

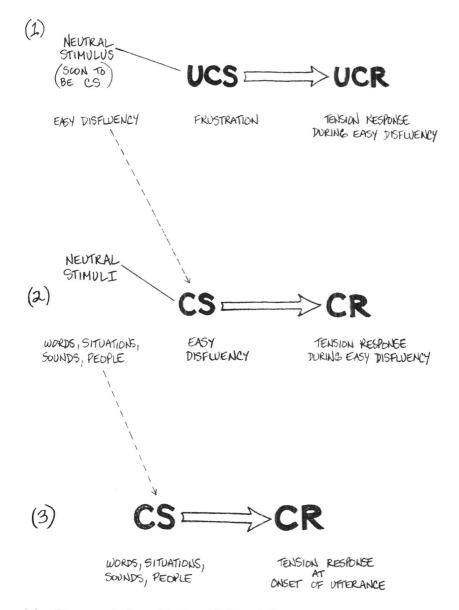

Figure 4.6. The spread of conditioning. (1) Easy disfluency repeatedly elicits the tension response, producing tense stuttering. (2) Easy disfluency, which occurs with various words, situations, sounds, and people, is then a conditioned stimulus that elicits the tension response and tense stuttering. (3) Words, situations, sounds, and people become the conditioned stimuli, which elicit the tension response at the onset of an utterance, producing fixed articulatory postures (or blocks) when the child begins an utterance.

ple, a child will stutter at home but not at school, or will stutter more severely during the summer than during the winter. They were also baffled by the wide individual differences that occur in stutterers. Why do some stutterers have a great deal of stuttering on the telephone while others have little or none? Why do some stutterers stutter more with women or with older men?

Some recent cognitive models of how we learn and how we store knowledge may be appropriate descriptions of this process (Rumelhart, McClelland, and the PDP Research Group, 1986). In these models, learning is viewed as the storing of patterns of connections in memory. Since nothing is learned in isolation, all the stimuli associated with an event that is learned is also stored as part of the pattern which encodes the event. When events are experienced again and again with similar stimuli, the patterns of connectivity are strengthened. Undoubtedly, when events are associated with strong emotions, the learned patterns are particularly strong. Applying this model to language, utterances are learned and stored in patterns that reflect all their past uses and all their emotional and cognitive contexts.

The application to stuttering is this: A child stutters in a variety of places, on various words, with various listeners. Memories of these experiences are interconnected patterns which encode much of the context in which the stuttering occurred. As stuttering develops, certain connections are strengthened more than others because they occur more frequently or occur with stronger emotion. In the ongoing process of evaluation, the clinician must discover which stimuli have the strongest connections to trigger stuttering. In treatment, the clinician, whether she is a behaviorist or a cognitivist, must strengthen connections associated with fluency and weaken those associated with stuttering.

Classical Conditioning and the Onset of Stuttering

In the preceding sections, we have suggested that classical conditioning comes into play only after the child has developed the first signs of stuttering—an excess of normal-sounding disfluencies. There may be, however, a subgroup of stutterers for whom classical conditioning is a major element in the onset of the disorder. These individuals may have experienced other difficulties in communication that, like disfluency, are conditioned to frustration, fear, and increased tension. Articulation disorders, cluttering, or a traumatic experience reading aloud are examples of such difficulties. These communicative frustrations may, like disfluencies, have become associated with caustic or critical remarks by listeners or with the speaker's own sense of inadequacy. This resulted in high levels of emotion, triggering increased tension in speech. Bloodstein's (1987) view of stuttering as the result of communicative failure and anticipatory struggle is largely responsible for our thinking in this regard. Our only addition to his view is the intervening variable of the fight, flight, or freeze response, elicited by the communicative failure and causing increases in tension, which may then create beginning stuttering without a preceding stage of borderline stuttering.

INSTRUMENTAL CONDITIONING

Instrumental conditioning is a fact of daily life. It creates in us such quirks as pushing an elevator button over and over when the elevator is already on its way. It is a major force in the development of stuttering and an important therapy tool.

Instrumental conditioning occurs when, for example, a behavior is followed immediately by a reward. This is *positive reinforcement*, and it causes the behavior to increase. Instrumental conditioning also includes *punishment*, when behavior is followed by a negative consequence. Punishment decreases the frequency of a behavior. A third kind of instrumental conditioning occurs when, for example, a behavior reduces negative stimulation. This is *escape* (sometimes called negative reinforcement). It makes a bad situation better, so the behavior occurs more often.

Instrumental conditioning can work rapidly in the young stutterer, in conjunction with classical conditioning, to increase the secondary behaviors called escape devices. Consider how this escalation may begin in a beginning stutterer, such as Richard. At some point, he may be caught up in an experience of seemingly endless repetitions that produce frustration in the child and impatience in his parents. These in turn increase the tension and rate of disfluencies. The increased tension may result in lip squeezing, which is followed by release of the word. The increased rate of activity related to speech may produce head nods or eye blinks that are followed by release of the word. When these behaviors are successful in releasing the word, the child's frustration and his parents' impatience are relieved, and the escape behavior is thus negatively reinforced. This makes it more likely that the child will use this escape behavior again the next time he stutters. In addition, the child may sense completed communication with his parents. This is positive reinforcement for the escape behavior that he used to get the word out, and this also increases the likelihood that the behavior will be used again.

Unfortunately, like most of the behaviors that stutterers use to relieve their stuttering, an escape behavior is only temporarily helpful. For reasons we don't entirely understand, when a child uses an escape behavior more and more, it becomes less and less effective in releasing the word. The young stutterer then turns to additional escape devices to terminate his stutters.

Classical conditioning also plays a major role in the escalation of escape behaviors. As you will remember, classical conditioning works by generalizing responses from an original stimulus with which it is associated to other stimuli that happen to occur when the response occurs. When an escape behavior is used in a particular context, such as a word, a listener, a situation, or even a feeling, it may generalize to other times when that word, listener, situation or feeling occurs. As Starkweather (1983) has pointed out, the joint occurrence of classical and instrumental conditioning in treatment is beneficial. The clinician who reinforces the stutterer's changes becomes, by association, a reinforcement in and of herself. Likewise, the therapeutic setting (for example, the treatment room) and, in general, all stimuli associated with it (e.g., parents, peers, and others) become reinforcers for change, and can be used as such to encourage the therapeutic response.

Summary

In summary, the principal differences between the borderline and beginning stutterer are these:

The beginning stutterer shows more tension and "hurry" in his stuttering. This is often manifested in abruptly ended syllable repetitions, irregular rhythms of repetitions, evident stoppages of phonation, and momentarily fixated articulatory postures. The beginning stutterer uses secondary behaviors such as escape devices and starters. In addition, the beginning stutterer sees himself as someone who has trouble talking.

We speculate that one major factor underlying beginning stuttering is the child's inherent sensitivity to stress, which may easily result in the emotion of frustration, triggering a tension response. Classical conditioning then links this unconditioned response to disfluency (when the child is disfluent and feels threatened, frustrated, or afraid), creating the rapid, tense disfluencies that begin to appear in the beginning stutterer. After repeated pairing, the disfluency itself elicits the increased tension and rate. Classical conditioning also links the disfluency to more and more people and places. A third factor in beginning stuttering is instrumental conditioning, which increases the frequency of escape devices. These behaviors are negatively reinforced when the frustration of a stutter is terminated by an escape behavior. They are positively reinforced when the stutterer completes his communication after using an escape behavior.

INTERMEDIATE STUTTERING

The intermediate level stutterer, typically a youngster between the ages of 6 and 13 (Figure 4.7), has two major characteristics that distinguish him from the beginning stutterer. First, he is starting to *fear* his stuttering, whereas the beginning stutterer is only frustrated, surprised, or annoyed by it. Second, he reacts to his fear of stuttering by *avoiding* it, something the beginning stutterer doesn't do.

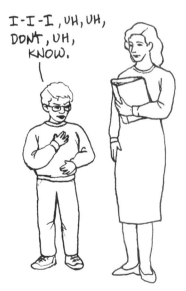

Figure 4.7. A child who may be an intermediate stutterer.

These new symptoms emerge gradually as the young stutterer more frequently experiences negative emotion during stuttering. For example, he blocks and feels helpless. His listeners respond with discomfort or pity. After this has happened frequently, he becomes afraid.

His fear may be first attached to the sounds and words on which he has stuttered most. He starts to believe that these sounds are harder for him. Then he begins to scan ahead to see if he might have to say them. When he anticipates them, he tries to avoid them. For example, he may say, "I don't know" to questions, or he may substitute "my sister" for his sister's name when talking about her. He may start a sentence, realize a feared word is coming up, and then switch the sentence around to avoid it, producing a maze of half-finished sentences.

The intermediate stutterer's fear of stuttering may be attached to situations as well as words. The youngster may find that he stutters more in some situations than in others. At first, he approaches these situations with dread. Then, later, he may go to great lengths to avoid them. Van Riper (1982) suggests that the development of these situational fears and avoidances depends on listener reactions. Interventions with key listeners in the stutterer's environment can prevent them.

Core Behaviors

What are the intermediate stutterer's moments of stuttering like, when he doesn't avoid them? What are his core behaviors? He will still repeat and prolong, but his most frequent core behaviors are now blocks. The intermediate stutterer's blocks seem to grow out of the increasing tension we saw in the beginning stutterer. The child at the intermediate level usually stutters by stopping airflow, voicing or movement (or all three) and then struggling to get it going again. His stutters seem to surprise him less than they did when he was a beginning stutterer. Instead, as evidenced by his voice and manner in certain situations, he anticipates them. We have the impression that the intermediate stutterer's blocks are frequently characterized by excessive laryngeal tension, but he often blocks elsewhere as well. He may squeeze his lips together, jam his tongue against the roof of his mouth, or even hold his breath. In general, he is not highly conscious of just what he's doing during a block, but he has a vivid awareness that he is stuck, that he is helpless, and that the word he wants to say seemingly won't come out.

Secondary Behaviors

The blocks described above can be devastating to a young stutterer. He is not only frustrated with his own inability to make a sound, but he is often faced with a surprised and uncomfortable listener, as well. Even patient listeners may not know what to do. They may interrupt, look away, or fidget. The stutterer then concludes that he is doing something wrong and tries to escape or avoid these painful moments.

The escape behaviors, which the stutterer uses to break out of his stutters, are present in the beginning stutterer, but they are far more frequent in the intermediate stutterer. They are often more complex, too. The intermediate stutterer may blink his eyes and nod his head to get out of a block. Sometimes, he may do both, and if the word still hasn't come out, he may resort to yet another device, such as slapping his leg. As these patterns grow more complex, they also may become more disguised to look like natural movements, and they are performed more rapidly.

In addition to escape behaviors, the intermediate stutterer uses both word and situation avoidances, as mentioned above. Word avoidances develop after a child has had repeated difficulty with a particular word or sound and then learns to take evasive action before he has to say it. For example, a young stutterer in our clinic was once asked his name by a particularly stern nun. He blocked severely on it and, subsequently, developed a fear of saying his name, as well as other words with the same sound. He could usually think up synonyms for other words, but he found it awkward to substitute for his name. He then learned to get a running start on his name by beginning with "My name is . . . " whenever he was asked his name. This worked to avoid the stuttering about half of the time. This is a subtle form of avoidance which many clinicians would call a "starter." More obvious examples of avoidances are given below.

Van Riper (1982) has cataloged many word avoidance techniques used by stutterers. His list includes *substitutions* (substituting one word or phrase for another when stuttering is expected, as in "he my u-u-u . . . my father's brother"), *circumlocutions* (talking all around a word or phrase when stuttering is expected, as in "well, I went to . . . yes, I really had a good time there, I saw the Empire State Building."), *postponements* (waiting for a few beats or putting in filler words before starting a word on which stuttering is expected, as in "My name is . . . . Bill") and *anti-expectancy devices* (using an odd manner or funny voice to avoid stuttering when it is anticipated). Like escape behaviors, these word avoidance techniques often become more rapid and more subtle with time. A clever stutterer can disguise his word avoidances to look like normal behavior. He can put on a pensive expression and appear to search for a word while he postpones the attempt to say a feared sound. Experienced clinicians learn to pick up subtle cues in the rate and manner of speaking that tip them off to the use of avoidances.

Situation fears and situation avoidances are also beginning to appear in the intermediate stutterer. Past stuttering in specific places or with specific people are the seeds from which situation fears grow. In school, for example, stutterers usually have more trouble in situations like reading aloud or giving oral reports. Most stutterers (and many nonstutterers) have dreaded those classes in which the teacher calls on students by going up and down the rows. As in our earlier example, a stutterer's fear steadily mounts as his teacher goes down the row, getting closer and closer to him. Then, if he's called on, he may take a failing grade rather than give his oral report. In contrast, other situations in school, especially casual ones like gym class or lunch period, hold little fear and expectation of stuttering for him.

Situation fears quickly generate situation avoidance. The student who fears giving answers in class will learn to slouch low in his seat in hopes of being overlooked. The stutterer who is afraid of making introductions will contrive to let other people handle them. One of the authors coped with his fear of ordering in restaurants by ducking into the bathroom when the waitress came, leaving his friends to order for him. Every stutterer will have his own pattern of situation avoidances. They provide an important focus for therapy in many cases.

Feelings and Attitudes

The intermediate stutterer has gone well beyond the momentary frustration and mild embarrassment of the beginning stutterer. He has felt the helplessness of being caught in many blocks and runaway repetitions. The anticipation of stuttering and subsequent listener penalty have been fulfilled many times. These experiences pile up like cars in a demolition derby to create the entanglement of fear, embarrassment, and shame that accompanies moments of stuttering. These feelings may not be pervasive yet; they do not dog the stutterer all the time. But now stuttering has changed from an annoyance to a serious problem.

The intermediate stutterer shows his increasingly negative feelings about stuttering in numerous ways. He looks away from his listener during a stutter and flushes with embarrassment afterwards. He becomes stiff and uneasy at the prospect of speaking. His stuttering pattern shows an increasing number of avoidance devices, and he is beginning to evade situations in which he may stutter. These are all signs that his feelings and attitudes are pervaded by fear.

Table 4.6 give the characteristics of intermediate stutterers.

Underlying Processes

Many of the intermediate stutterer's symptoms result from the same processes that underlie those of the beginning stutterer. There are, however, major differences. In the intermediate stutterer, the classically conditioned tension response is more evident, conditioned frustration changes toward the more intense reaction of fear, and avoidance conditioning emerges as a factor in shaping stuttering behaviors.

AVOIDANCE CONDITIONING

The word and situation avoidances of the intermediate stutterer arise from the combined effect of instrumental and classical conditioning. These two factors join forces to produce avoidance conditioning, one of the most potent of learning mechanisms. Unfortunately, behaviors that are avoidance conditioned are so well learned that they are hard to unlearn. This may be one of the reasons that stutterers often relapse after therapy.

To understand avoidance conditioning in stutterers, it may helpful to see how animals can be avoidance conditioned. One of the best examples comes from the work of two early experimenters in avoidance conditioning, Richard Solomon

Table 4.6. Characteristics of Intermediate Stutterers

1. Most frequent core behaviors are blocks in which the stutterer shuts off sound or voice. He may also have repetitions and prolongations
2. Stutterer uses escape behaviors to terminate blocks.
3. Stutterer appears to anticipate blocks, often uses avoidance behaviors prior to feared words. He also anticipates difficult situations and sometimes avoids them.
4. Fear before stuttering, embarrassment during stuttering, and shame after stuttering characterize this level, especially fear.

and L.C. Wynne (1953). These experimenters first trained dogs to escape an electric shock by placing them in a box with a low door on one side and administering a shock until they learned to jump over the door to safety. Once the dogs learned to escape the shock promptly, the experimenters then gave them a warning signal before the shock began. After only a few trials in which the warning signal was paired with the shock, the dogs learned to jump over the door at the warning signal, before the shock. This was avoidance learning.

The analogous behavior in stutterers is this: a stutterer first learns to escape from a stutter by, for example, saying another word when he is blocked, as in "I went to New Y-Y-Y . . . the Big Apple." After many pairings of anticipating a particular word and stuttering on it, he learns to use his escape behavior (to substitute "The Big Apple" for "New York," for example) before he stutters on "New York," and the stutter is avoided. Figure 4.8 depicts this transformation of an escape behavior into an avoidance behavior.

Word avoidances often become less and less effective, but they continue to be used despite this intermittency. The fact that they sometimes work and sometimes don't makes them all the more resistant to treatment. The stutterer has a strong urge to use an avoidance device if he thinks there is a chance that he might

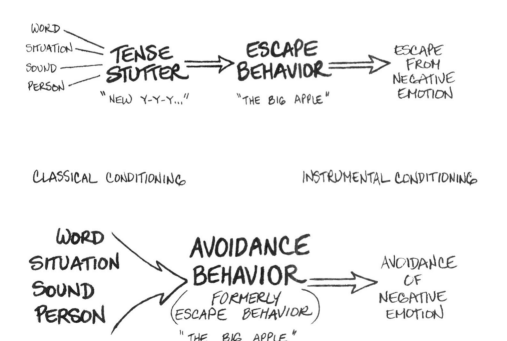

Figure 4.8.   The creation of an avoidance response from an escape behavior. At first, in the presence of various words, situations, sounds, and people, a tense stutter is followed by an escape behavior, which terminates a negative emotion. Then, the words, situations, sounds, and people elicit the avoidance response (formerly the escape behavior). This is rewarded by the successful avoidance of stuttering and its negative emotion.

stutter. Treatment must deal with this tendency of word avoidances to recur when stuttering is expected.

The intermediate stutterer has learned to fear and avoid situations, as well as words. This is a phenomenon well-known in the animal conditioning literature (Bouton & Bolles, 1985; Mineka, 1985). The experimental psychologist would say that when a stimulus has been conditioned to produce a response in a particular context, the context itself becomes part of the stimulus that elicits the response. Other similar contexts can, by associative learning, become eliciting contexts. Thus, if a stutterer stutters badly in a classroom at school, that classroom and similar classrooms become feared situations for the stutterer. He will do his best to avoid talking in these classes. If he has terrible blocks on the telephone, he begins to fear talking on the telephone, and eventually avoids using the dreaded instrument. This contextual learning, as we shall see, is an important consideration in the treatment of the advanced stutterer.

Experimental treatment with animals has taught us much about deconditioning the avoidance learning in stutterers. Our primary method is to bring the stutterer into contact with the feared object without the level of arousal he has experienced before. For many intermediate stutterers, this often consists of teaching him ways of speaking that produce fluency and then gradually teaching him to use more and more words and sounds of which he was previously afraid and to speak in more and more situations he feared. Some intermediate stutterers (as well as most advanced stutterers) also fear stuttering itself. For them, treatment consists of teaching them to decrease their fear during stuttering. This decreases tension and rate and provides an opportunity to change their stuttering behavior toward fluency.

Summary

Intermediate

The intermediate level of stuttering is characterized by increasingly tense blocks, repetitions, and prolongations. This increased tension results from feelings of frustration, fear, and helplessness. These feelings trigger the tension response, which, because increased tension interferes with fluency, in turn produces more frustration, fear, and feelings of helplessness. As tension mounts, this vicious cycle continues: blocks are longer and more noticeable, listeners react with surprise and impatience, and the stutterer's fear increases in response to this punishment.

These negative feelings spur the stutterer to use various devices to escape from blocks. Instrumental conditioning increases the frequency of escape behaviors. Classical conditioning generalizes the conditioned anticipation of stuttering to specific sounds, words, and situations. These anticipations give rise to word and situation avoidance behaviors.

5. ADVANCED STUTTERING

The last developmental/treatment level, advanced stuttering, is characterized more by the age of the stutterer than by differences in the stuttering pattern or underlying processes. The advanced level deals with older adolescents and adults (Figure 4.9). Treatment is unique at this level because the client can take much of the responsibility for therapy, including substantial work outside the clinic.

The advanced stutterer's increased capability in therapy compensates for another characteristic of this level, the individual's long history of stuttering. The advanced stutterer's pattern is highly overlearned because of this history and, therefore, may be hard to change. The advanced stutterer's self image is also a consideration. After many years, the stutterer increasingly thinks of himself as a stutterer, rather than as someone who occasionally has difficulty speaking. Except for a few safe situations, in which the advanced stutterer is relatively fluent, most speaking situations hold some fear for him, and he shapes his life accordingly. His friends, his social activities, and his job are often influenced by the fact that he thinks of himself as a stutterer. He believes that his stuttering is as noticeable to other people as his having two heads would be, and is just as unacceptable.

Core Behaviors

Core behaviors in the advanced stutterer are typically blocks—stoppages of airflow and/or phonation. These may be longer and more struggled in the advanced stutterer than in the intermediate stutterer, but they are essentially the same behavior. Because the blocks are longer, tremors of lips, jaw, or tongue may be more evident.

There are, however, some advanced stutterers whose blocks are hardly evident at all. These stutterers have honed their avoidance behaviors to such a fine edge that core behaviors are practically invisible. When their stuttering does escape this suppression, it usually devastates them. Consequently, much of their energy is spent anticipating blocks that don't occur and mustering avoidances to keep anxiety at bay.

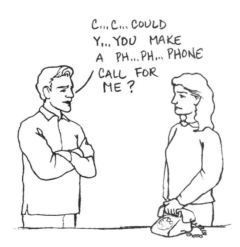

Figure 4.9.   An individual who may be an advanced stutterer.

Secondary Behaviors

The advanced stutterer has many of the same word and situation avoidances that the intermediate stutterer has, but they are likely to be more extensive. Some show these behaviors more obviously than others. They may have a pattern of several attempted word-avoidance devices (such as "uh . . . well . . . you see," and a gasp of air) followed by a block, which is long in duration, filled with unsuccessful escape attempts, and finally released with great effort. Others approach feared words cautiously and use subtle mannerisms, such as appearing to think just before saying them, so that most listeners wouldn't realize they were stuttering.[10] These stutterers usually have to be on guard much of the time, scanning ahead with their verbal early-warning systems. Many advanced stutterers also control their environments carefully so that they can avoid situations in which they may stutter. They may feign sickness when they would have to give a speech, use answering machines to avoid answering the telephone, or arrange to have their spouses or children deal with store clerks.

Often, with careful questioning of these stutterers who use avoidance a great deal, we can learn what occurs when his avoidances don't work. Even the most skillful avoiders are sometimes caught with their defenses down, and become stuck in block. Core behaviors may also be elicited by asking a stutterer to stutter openly, without using secondary behaviors. Stutterers who can do this, especially those who can do this without excessive discomfort, are more amenable to change.

Feelings and Attitudes

The feelings and attitudes of the advanced stutterer, like his stuttering pattern, are shaped by years of conditioning. Over and over, the stutterer has learned that much of his stuttering is unpredictable. When it is predictable, it comes when he wants it least—when he wants more than anything to be fluent. As a result, he often feels out of control. These uncomfortable internal feelings are confirmed by the stutterer's view of how others see him. Listeners' reactions look overwhelmingly negative to him. Even when listeners say nothing, the looks on their faces say everything. It is as though the stutterer drove a rattletrap car that always stalled in heavy traffic amid honking drivers. These experiences gradually shape the advanced stutterer's attitudes toward feelings of helplessness, frustration, anger, and hopelessness.

Of course, individual responses to stuttering vary greatly. If the stutterer is handsome, rich, and talented, as well as assertive, he may be less devastated by his stuttering. But if he has many other problems and has learned to be dependent, his feelings and attitudes may be an important component of his problem.

The point is, that by the time the stutterer is an adult, he has had years of experiencing stuttering, feeling frustrated and helpless, and developing techniques to minimize his pain. Unless he has strong attributes to compensate, he will feel

---

[10] Several well-known television and radio personalities fit into this pattern, using bizarre speaking styles to avoid stuttering. The next time you see or hear someone in the media with an odd manner of speaking, consider whether they might be a successful avoider.

that stuttering is a big part of the self that he presents to other people. It is a part that he hates, a part on which he hangs many other troubles, and a part he wants to eliminate.

On the other hand, some stutterers who have reached the advanced level have become reconciled to their handicap. If they are in their twenties or thirties or beyond, there may be some natural resistance to treatment, because stuttering has become part of their identity. After years of doubt and turmoil, they've grown accustomed to themselves as stutterers. To contemplate treatment is to reject themselves, to open old wounds. Those who succeed in treatment may find this worthwhile. But for those who relapse to their former level of stuttering after treatment, there may be a difficult battle inside to regain ground that had been won before and was given up.

Table 4.7 lists the major characteristics of advanced stutterers.

Underlying Processes

In advanced stuttering, unlike in the lower levels, constitutional, developmental, and environmental factors are no longer so directly influential. The effects of home environment, developmental pressures of speech and language, and perhaps even some differences in the stutterer's central nervous system have been diminished by maturation and learning. However, conditioned habits that are learned in response to these early factors are stronger than ever. Their effects have been magnified by years of experience. Moreover, the stutterer's characteristic patterns of tension, escape behaviors, and word and situation avoidance have become almost automatic through years of practice. For example, he may have a string of avoidance and escape behaviors, but he only remembers that "the word got stuck."

The advanced stutterer's disorder is affected by cognitive learning, as well. He has developed a self-concept as an impaired speaker, and for most, this carries highly negative connotations. Self-concept for any individual begins to be formed in preschool years and is initially a picture of what one can do, rather than of what one is (Clarke-Stewart & Friedman, 1987). More enduring traits are added as a result of social interactions in later childhood, adolescence and beyond

---

Table 4.7. Characteristics of Advanced Stutterers

---

1. Most frequent core behaviors are longer, tense blocks, often with tremors of lips, tongue, or jaw. Individual will also probably have repetitions and prolongations, as well.
2. Stuttering may be suppressed in some individuals through extensive avoidance behaviors.
3. Complex patterns of avoidance and escape behaviors characterize the stutterer. These may be very rapid and so well habituated that the stutterer may not be aware of what he does.
4. Emotions of fear, embarrassment, and shame are very strong. Stutterer has negative feelings about himself as a person who is helpless and inept when he stutters. This self-concept may be pervasive.

(Roessler & Bolton, 1978). The stutterer's self-concept at the earliest levels of development is then determined in part by his perception of how he talks. It is a fleeting notion, not necessarily negative, that sometimes he has difficulty talking. At later levels of development, the reactions of significant listeners—his parents, his peer group, or other adults—have a major impact. Now his self-concept may become filled with enduring and negative features as a result of listener impatience and rejection. The negative self-concept is not only formed by perceptions of listener reactions, it also, in turn, affects those perceptions. Researchers in the psychology of disability suggest that "one's perception of self influences one's perception of others' views of oneself, rendering social interaction more difficult" (Roessler & Bolton, 1978). Applied to the advanced stutterer, it suggests that he projects his own rejection of his stuttering onto his listeners, inhibiting his interactions with them. This vicious cycle can only be stopped when an outsider helps the stutterer test the reality of his perceptions.

In addition to working on cognitive aspects of the problem, therapy for the advanced stutterer also deals directly with the avoidances he has learned so well. As mentioned in the discussion of the intermediate stutterer, as avoidance conditioning advances, the stutterer fears not only the words and situations, but the stuttering itself. To decondition this fear and change these responses, treatment enables the stutterer to stutter with less fear by associating the clinician's approval with a calmer, more relaxed form of stuttering. Gradually, the tension and hurry fade away from the stutterer's disfluencies, and he feels more in control. Consequently, his fear further diminishes.

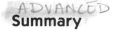

Summary

Advanced stuttering characterizes a treatment orientation as well as a developmental level. Treatment may be easier because the stutterer can assume much of the responsibility for generalization beyond the clinic. On the other hand, treatment may be difficult because the stutterer's patterns are more thoroughly learned than at earlier levels. The advanced stutterer's core behaviors are often long blocks with considerable tension and sometimes with visible tremors. Secondary behaviors can consist of long chains of word avoidance and escape behaviors. Situation avoidance is common. Advanced stutterers may hide and disguise their stuttering well enough to avoid detection by many listeners, but this is at a cost of constant vigilance. Feelings of frustration and helplessness accumulate over the years, leading to coping behaviors and a lifestyle that can often be highly constraining. These responses create a self-concept of an inept speaker whose stuttering is unacceptable to listeners. This, in turn, affects the stutterer's perceptions of the listener's reactions.

STUDY QUESTIONS

1/   Name the five developmental and treatment levels of stuttering and give their associated age ranges.

2/   What is the difference between core behaviors and secondary behaviors?

3/   Name five types of normal disfluency and give an example of each.

4/   At what ages is normal disfluency likely to be most frequent?

5/   Name 3 influences that may cause normal disfluency to increase.

6/   What are 3 ways in which core behaviors of normal disfluency are different from those of borderline stuttering?

7/   Describe the core behaviors of the beginning stutterer.

8/   What causes the beginning stutterer's increase in tension in his disfluencies?

9/   Describe why an escape behavior is used by a stutterer. Give examples.

10/   How does instrumental conditioning work to increase the frequency of escape behaviors?

11/   Give an example of a stutterer's (a) word avoidance, (b) situation avoidance.

12/   How does classical conditioning work to generalize stuttering from a specific word or situation to many other words and situations?

13/   What is the major secondary behavior that differentiates the intermediate from the beginning stutterer?

14/   Compare the feelings and attitudes of the borderline, beginning, and intermediate stutterer.

15/   Why might the treatment of the advanced stutterer be different from that of the intermediate stutterer?

16/   Describe the role of the listener in the development of the advanced stutterer's self-concept.

Suggested Readings

Bloodstein O. (1987). Symptomatology. In *A handbook on stuttering*. Chicago: National Easter Seal Society.

The subsection titled, "Developmental changes in stuttering" in this chapter describe four stages similar to our levels of stuttering development. Other schemas of developmental changes are also discussed in a clear and logical style.

Gray, J.A. (1987). *The psychology of fear and stress*. Cambridge, J K.: Cambridge University Press.

This is a very readable exposition of relatively recent findings about innate fears, conditioning, and brain processes involved with escape and avoidance learning. Gray also describes his concept of the "behavioral inhibition system," a model of the role of conditioning, language, the limbic system, and anxiety on behavior.

Luper, H.L., & Mulder, R.L. (1964). *Stuttering: Therapy for children*. Englewood Cliffs, New Jersey: Prentice Hall.

An excellent treatment text that describes four developmental levels of stuttering similar to our own. Although out of print, this book is available at most university libraries.

Starkweather, C.W. (1983). *Speech and language: Principles and processes of behavior change*. Englewood Cliffs, New Jersey: Prentice Hall.

This book describes the principles of instrumental, classical, and avoidance conditioning that underlie much of stuttering behavior. It gives a clear account of how these principles create stuttering behavior, and how conditioning is used in treatment.

Van Riper, C. (1982). *The development of stuttering*. In *The nature of stuttering*. Englewood Cliffs, New Jersey: Prentice Hall.

In this chapter, Van Riper describes four developmental tracks of stuttering, three of which depart substantially from our stages of stuttering development. This chapter will give the reader a good sense of individual variability in stuttering.

Section II

ASSESSMENT AND TREATMENT OF STUTTERING

5

TREATMENT CONSIDERATIONS

We believe there are a number of clinically relevant issues the clinician needs to consider and resolve for herself before initiating an assessment or treatment program with a stutterer. This is important because the position she takes on these matters will guide her clinical judgment and behavior. In other words, what she believes about these issues will determine not only her assessment procedures, but also her long-term treatment goals and daily clinical procedures with her client.

The first issue the clinician needs to consider is her beliefs regarding the causes and development of stuttering. Her assessment strategies and therapy goals and procedures should be compatible with her beliefs about the nature of stuttering.

Secondly, we believe there are a number of important questions that are related to therapy goals that she will need to consider. These are as follows: (*a*) What are the appropriate speech behaviors to target in therapy? (*b*) What are realistic fluency goals to have for the client? (*c*) How much attention should be given to her client's feelings and attitudes about his speech? (*d*) What procedures or strategies are needed to help the client maintain his improvement? (*e*) What should be done about any concomitant speech and language problems her client may have?

Finally, the clinician needs to consider the methods she will employ with her client. For example, will her therapy be characterized by behavior modification with its emphasis upon instrumental or operant conditioning and programmed instruction principles, or will it be more loosely structured?

Quite obviously, these issues are related. The clinician's view on one of them could influence her position on another one. Nevertheless, it seems important to us to discuss each of these issues separately. These issues will be outlined in this chapter, and our point of view will be given. In the next seven chapters, these issues will be expanded upon in the discussion of assessment and treatment procedures.

CLINICIAN'S BELIEFS

We believe it is important for the clinician to weigh her beliefs about the nature of stuttering against the available data and then develop clinical procedures compatible with her beliefs. Our beliefs about the nature of stuttering, that is, the etiology and development of stuttering, were presented in Section I of this book. Our position will be reviewed in only enough detail here to illustrate how the clinician's theoretical views will affect clinical decisions. As you will recall, we believe that predisposing physiological factors interact with developmental and environmental influences to produce or exacerbate the core behaviors or easy repetitions. The child also responds to these early disfluencies with increased tension in an effort to inhibit them. Then, through a series of developmental levels, various secondary or coping behaviors and negative feelings and attitudes are learned. Escape and starting behaviors are learned through instrumental conditioning. Speech fears are classically conditioned. Word and situation avoidances are acquired through avoidance conditioning.

How does holding this point of view about the etiology and development of stuttering affect our clinical behavior? Three examples regarding the treatment of school-age children who stutter should clarify this point. First and foremost, we believe the development/treatment level of the child's stuttering will determine the nature of his therapy program. The therapy for each level is different. For example, we believe a second grade, beginning stutterer who is not embarrassed or afraid to talk and who is not avoiding talking should be managed quite differently from a fifth grade intermediate stutterer who is beginning to develop fear and avoidance behaviors relative to his speech. Thus, we believe that knowing the child's development/treatment level is essential to making appropriate therapy decisions.

At this time, we should point out to the reader that we will be discussing therapy for the development/treatment levels in the following order: advanced, beginning, and intermediate. We will begin with the treatment of the advanced stutterer because we believe stuttering modification and fluency shaping therapies are the most dissimilar at this level. Consequently, the reader will be able to clearly see the differences between these two major therapy approaches. We will then discuss the treatment of the beginning stutterer. We will discuss the treatment of the intermediate stutterer last because the therapy procedures for the intermediate stutterer are often a combination or modification of procedures for the advanced and the beginning stutterer. Thus, understanding the treatment of the intermediate stutterer is easier if one first understands the treatment of the other two levels.

The second example of how our belief regarding the etiology and development of stuttering affects our clinical behavior involves our assessment procedures. Since knowing the child's development/treatment level is important, it is necessary that the clinician employ assessment procedures that will provide her with the essential information to determine the child's treatment level. For example, with the above two children it would be necessary for the clinician to evaluate each child's feelings and attitudes about his speech, as well as his use of word and situation avoidances, to accurately diagnose each child's treatment level.

The third, and last, example of how our theoretical position on the nature of stuttering influences our clinical behavior is the counseling of the parents of these two school-age stutterers. We would discuss with each set of parents the importance of factors in their child's environment that could be contributing to his stuttering problem, and we would discuss possible ways of modifying these factors. However, we would also discuss with these parents possible predisposing constitutional or physiological factors that could be contributing to their child's stuttering. In other words, it is not all the parents' responsibility. Their children brought something to the problem, too.

These, then, are some of the ways our beliefs about the nature of stuttering influence our work with stutterers and their families. There are many others, and we will discuss them in subsequent chapters. In addition, we will also point out how other clinicians' beliefs influence their therapies. However, the above examples should be enough to illustrate to the clinician that her views on stuttering will influence her work with her clients.

SPEECH BEHAVIORS TARGETED FOR THERAPY

Which speech behaviors should be targeted for therapy? Should the clinician work directly on the client's stuttering in an effort to modify or reduce its severity, or should the clinician target some other aspect of the stutterer's speech behavior, such as reducing his rate of speech? Recently, there has been considerable controversy relative to this topic. For example, Hugo Gregory (1979) in his book, *Controversies about Stuttering Therapy*, grouped therapies for the advanced stutterer into two general approaches, namely, the "stutter more fluently" approach and the "speak more fluently" approach. The stutter more fluently approach is based on the premise that the stutterer should first study and become familiar with his stuttering and then learn to modify it by stuttering more easily. The stutterer should also reduce his avoidance behavior. The speak more fluently approach involves replacing stuttering with fluent speech. To do this, various procedures are used to establish a form of fluency, and then features of this initial fluency are gradually modified to obtain speech that sounds normal.

More recently, Richard Curlee and William Perkins (1984) also grouped current therapies into two approaches similar to Gregory's. They referred to the two approaches as "those that manage stuttering" and "those that manage fluency." The former group focuses on techniques to help the stutterer stutter more fluently and with less effort, while the latter group emphasizes teaching the stutterer how to talk more fluently. Curlee and Perkins also observed that there are some other philosophical differences between these two approaches. Many clinicians who favor managing fluency also advocate applying behavior modification principles in their therapy. Generally, this has not been true for those clinicians who support managing stuttering.

In an earlier publication (Guitar & Peters, 1980), we attempted to resolve the above controversies. We discussed the similarities and differences between these two approaches to stuttering therapy and attempted to integrate them. We referred to the two approaches as "stuttering modification therapy" and "fluency shaping therapy." We stated that, in addition to differing with regard to the speech behaviors targeted in therapy, these two approaches often, but not always, differ with regard to fluency goals, attention given to feelings and attitudes, maintenance procedures, and clinical methods. In the following pages, we will outline how stuttering modification therapy and fluency shaping therapy often differ on these five clinical issues, and we will give our point of view on each of the issues.

Stuttering Modification Therapy

We described stuttering modification therapy as helping the stutterer learn to modify his moments of stuttering (Fig. 5.1). This can be done in a variety of ways. For example, the clinician can teach the stutterer to reduce his struggle behavior and smooth out the form of his stuttering. The clinician can also help the stutterer learn to reduce the tension and rapidity of his stuttering and learn to stutter in a more relaxed, easy, and open manner. A good example of this type of therapy is Charles Van Riper's (1973) therapy for the advanced stutterer. In this therapy, Van Riper teaches the stutterer to stutter more fluently by using the techniques of cancellations, pull-outs, and preparatory sets. By using these techniques, the advanced stutterer is not taught to speak normally; rather he is taught to stutter in a more fluent, less abnormal manner. In our opinion, other proponents of stut-

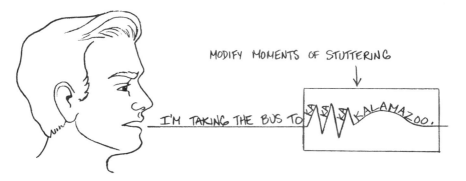

Figure 5.1.   Stuttering modification therapy.

tering modification therapy include Oliver Bloodstein, Edward Conture, Carl Dell, Harold Luper and Robert Mulder, David Prins, and Joseph Sheehan. This list is not exhaustive, but we believe these clinicians' therapies are clearly representative of stuttering modification therapy.[1] We will be referring to the writings of these clinicians in subsequent chapters.

Fluency Shaping Therapy

Whereas the goal of stuttering modification therapy is to modify the moments of stuttering, the goal of fluency shaping therapy is to systematically increase fluent responses until they replace the moments of stuttering. This fluency is first established in the clinical setting, and then it is generalized to the person's daily speaking environment. Fluency shaping clinicians usually use one of two approaches, or a combination of these two approaches, to establish fluency in the clinic. In one, a basal level of fluency is first established by having the stutterer produce short fluent responses, such as single words or simple phrases. These fluent responses are reinforced, and any stuttering may be punished. The length and spontaneity of these responses are then systematically increased until the client achieves fluent conversational speech in the clinical environment. In the second approach, the clinician helps the stutterer establish fluency by altering his speech pattern (Fig. 5.2). For example, this may involve the stutterer's speaking fluently at a substantially slower speech rate. This slow, fluent pattern is then gradually modified to approximate normal sounding speech. Regardless of which approach is used to establish fluency in the clinic, once it has been established, it is then generalized to the stutterer's daily speaking environment.

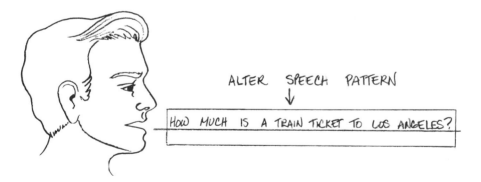

Figure 5.2. Fluency shaping therapy.

---

[1] In choosing these clinicians to illustrate stuttering modification therapy, we attempted to select clinicians whose therapies are clear examples of this approach. We also attempted to do this in selecting clinicians to illustrate fluency shaping therapy and the integration of the two approaches. In doing this, we regrettably excluded some well-known clinicians whose therapies do not fit perfectly within any of the above three approaches to treatment. Examples of this latter situation include Gene Brutten's two-factor behavior therapy (1970, 1975) and Dean Williams' normal talking therapy (1957, 1971, 1979).

A writer whose therapy is representative of fluency shaping therapy is Bruce Ryan (1974). Ryan has a number of programs to increase or to establish fluent speech in the clinical setting. One of these is the Delayed Auditory Feedback (DAF) Program. In a DAF program, a delayed auditory feedback machine is used to help the client speak in a slow, prolonged, fluent manner. The delay times on the delayed auditory feedback machine are systematically changed to allow the client to gradually increase his speaking rate by reducing his prolongation of speech sounds until his rate approaches normal. He is then taken off the machine, and this new fluency is gradually transferred to everyday speaking situations. In this DAF program, the stutterer is not taught to stutter more easily; rather fluency is first established in the therapy session, and then it is transferred to the client's daily speaking environment. In our opinion, other advocates of fluency shaping therapy include Martin Adams, Einer Boberg, Janis Costello, William Perkins, George Shames and Cheri Florance, Richard Shine, and Ronald Webster. Again, this list is not exhaustive, but we believe these clinicians' therapies are clear examples of fluency shaping therapy. In the following chapters, we will be referring to the therapies of these clinicians, as well.

Integration of Approaches

In the following chapters, the terms stuttering modification therapy and fluency shaping therapy will be used, and more detailed descriptions of both approaches will be presented for the different development/treatment levels of stuttering. Many clinicians believe they need to decide to use one approach or the other in working with their clients. They believe that either they need to modify their clients' moments of stuttering or they need to target their overall speaking patterns. The two approaches appear to them to be incompatible. To many clinicians, this can be a difficult and confusing choice. Fortunately, however, the two approaches are not necessarily antagonistic. On the contrary, techniques based on one approach can be helpful to the clinician employing the other approach. In fact, one of our prime goals in writing this book is to demonstrate how stuttering modification therapy and fluency shaping therapy can be integrated. Consequently, in the following chapters, we will give many examples of ways the clinician can combine aspects of both approaches into an integrated approach. To do this, we will discuss our clinical procedures in detail. We will also review the therapies of the following clinicians: Hugo Gregory and his colleagues Diane Hill and June Campbell, C. Woodruff Starkweather, and Meryl Wall and Florence Myers. These are not the only clinicians who are integrating the two major approaches, but we believe these are clear examples. For now, we will only outline our position with regard to the speech behaviors that we feel should be targeted for therapy.

We believe it can be beneficial for the advanced stutterer to learn to stutter more easily on given moments of stuttering, as well as to learn to modify certain aspects of his overall speaking pattern, such as his rate of speech, to enhance his fluency. We believe these two skills are not incompatible; in fact, we believe they can complement one another. We also believe this is true for most intermediate stutterers. For beginning stutterers, however, we believe the issue of which speech behaviors to target in therapy becomes less critical. The reason is that the differences between stuttering modification and fluency shaping therapies generally are less pronounced at this level.

What we have said above regarding the speech behaviors targeted for therapy is also true for many of the other clinical issues we will be discussing. We believe that, for the advanced stutterer, the two approaches are the most dissimilar. As one moves toward the lower development/treatment levels of stuttering, the differences between stuttering modification and fluency shaping therapies usually become less, and their similarities become greater. Applications and in-depth discussions of the above points of view will be presented in the following chapters on treatment.

FLUENCY GOALS

Dimensions of Fluency

What are realistic therapy goals to have when working with stutterers? Before responding to this question, it is first necessary to take a closer look at fluency. Starkweather (1985, 1987) suggests that speech fluency has four basic dimensions: (*a*) the continuity of speech, (*b*) the rate of speech, (*c*) the rhythm of speech, and (*d*) the effort with which speech is produced (Fig. 5.3). These four dimensions of fluency, that is, continuity, rate, rhythm, and effort, will now be examined more closely from a clinical management point of view.

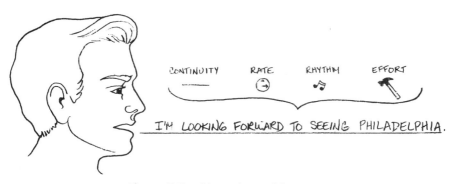

Figure 5.3.   Dimensions of fluency.

CONTINUITY

By continuity, Starkweather means the smoothness of speech or the extent to which speech is broken up by disfluencies. In terms of clinical management, we are interested in the number of part-word and monosyllabic word repetitions, prolongations, and blocks that occur in our client's speech. In terms of therapy goals, we are interested in the frequency of stutterings remaining in our client's speech at the end of therapy. This seems self-evident. After all, our clients come to us to rid themselves of these disfluencies.

RATE

Fluency consists of more than just the absence of disfluencies; fluent speech is also rapid. Thus, we need to be concerned about our client's speech rate. This is particularly true when rate control strategies are used in therapy to eliminate or significantly reduce the number of disfluencies. For example, one very common technique used in fluency shaping therapy is to teach the stutterer to slow his speech rate by prolonging each syllable as he talks. This will, indeed, reduce the number of disfluencies. However, unless the stutterer is also taught how to use this technique and still approximate a normal speaking rate, our experience suggests that he will not use it in everyday speaking situations. Our clients want to sound normal in this regard, too.

RHYTHM

Rhythm is the third dimension of fluency. Rhythm has to do with the stress patterns of speech. For a client's speech to sound normal at the end of therapy, it is important that he use normal stress patterns. He should not sound monotonous. He should not be giving each syllable equal stress. Monotonous sounding speech can be a by-product of fluency shaping programs in which the client is instructed to slow his speech by prolonging each syllable. We have also heard this quality in the speech of stutterers who have been treated in stuttering modification programs. It is important that this monotonous quality not remain in the client's speech at the end of therapy. Both the stutterer and his listener will object to it. Furthermore, many stutterers will not use this monotonous fluency in everyday speaking situations. They would rather stutter and be spontaneous.

EFFORT

The last dimension of fluency is effort. Starkweather observes that effort could be either physical effort or mental effort. We think that mental effort is the most clinically significant. Normal fluent speech is spontaneous; it does not require the constant monitoring of the act of speaking in order to sound normal. The speaker pays attention to his ideas; he does not pay attention to his mouth. When speech is closely monitored, it is not normal. Normal speakers do not constantly monitor their speech, and stutterers do not like to constantly monitor their speech either. It requires too much effort. In our experience, stutterers will not be happy in the long run with speech that has to be constantly monitored. We believe this is true whether the stutterer is using stuttering modification techniques to modify his moments of stuttering or using fluency shaping strategies to enhance his fluency.

Types of Fluency

With this background, let us consider possible fluency goals for stutterers. We observe that clinicians, depending upon their particular beliefs, subscribe to three possible successful outcomes to therapy. These are spontaneous fluency, controlled fluency, and acceptable stuttering.

Spontaneous Fluency

By spontaneous fluency, we are referring to the fluency of the normal speaker. In terms of continuity, spontaneous fluency contains neither tension nor struggle behaviors, that is, no abnormal monosyllabic repetitions or blocks. Neither does spontaneous fluency contain more than an occasional number of easy repetitions and prolongations. The rate and the rhythm are normal. With regard to the effort of speaking, spontaneous fluency is not maintained by paying attention to speech; rather, the person just talks and pays attention to his ideas.

Controlled Fluency

Controlled fluency, in terms of continuity, is somewhat similar to spontaneous fluency except that the stutterer must monitor and change his manner of stuttering and/or speaking to maintain relatively normal sounding speech. He may do this in a variety of ways. For example, he may use preparatory sets to modify his moments of stuttering, or he may slightly reduce his speaking rate by prolonging syllables to enhance his fluency. In other words, the listener, especially the experienced listener, may often hear small differences in the stutterer's speech. The stutterer, however, in terms of continuity, will not be exhibiting noticeable moments of stuttering. It is apparent, then, that in controlled fluency, rate and/or rhythm may be modified at times. On the other hand, effort of speaking is definitely adversely affected all the time in controlled fluency. The stutterer exhibits this relatively normal sounding speech only by paying attention to and modifying how he talks.

Acceptable Stuttering

The third possible outcome of therapy is acceptable stuttering. Acceptable stuttering occurs when the speaker exhibits noticeable but not severe disfluency and feels comfortable speaking despite this disfluency. In other words, the stutterer is not embarrassed by or fearful of his stuttering. As with controlled fluency, the stutterer may be monitoring his speech to maintain this acceptable stuttering. In this case, all dimensions of fluency; continuity, rate, rhythm, and effort, may be adversely affected. In other cases, it is quite possible that the stutterer is not monitoring his speech to maintain this acceptable stuttering. He is just talking spontaneously. In this case, the effort with which speech is produced is not significantly affected.

Stuttering Modification Therapy

We believe that advocates of stuttering modification therapy see spontaneous fluency as the ultimate goal for treatment. This is especially true for beginning stutterers. It is less true for intermediate stutterers and much less true for advanced stutterers. If spontaneous fluency is unobtainable with these latter two groups, then most stuttering modification clinicians work for controlled fluency. If this is unobtainable, then they try for acceptable stuttering.

Fluency Shaping Therapy

Adherents of fluency shaping therapy also have as their ultimate goal for their clients the attainment of spontaneous fluency. If this were not obtainable, then controlled fluency would become the goal. We believe, however, that most fluency shaping clinicians would not have acceptable stuttering as one of their goals for their clients. This is regarded as non-success.

Integration of Approaches

We believe these three possible therapy goals, spontaneous fluency, controlled fluency, and acceptable stuttering, vary with the treatment level of the client's stuttering. We believe the ultimate goal for the advanced stutterer should be spontaneous fluency. In our opinion, though, most advanced stutterers do not reach this goal on a consistent basis. They may have periods when they are spontaneously fluent; however, at other times, they will need to monitor their speech in order to use their controlled fluency, or they will need to be tolerant of acceptable stuttering. Thus, we believe, a realistic goal for most advanced stutterers is the development of the ability to use, and a feeling of comfort with, both controlled fluency and acceptable stuttering. In other words, there will be times with friends or family when the advanced stutterer is spontaneously fluent; but at other times in more stressful situations, he may need to use his controlled fluency or be willing to exhibit acceptable stuttering.

With the intermediate stutterer, that is, the child who is beginning to avoid talking, the goal should still be spontaneous fluency. However, in some cases, it is more realistic to expect the outcome of therapy to be controlled fluency or, more frequently, acceptable stuttering. This is especially true for children as they approach adolescence.

We believe, along with many others, that a realistic goal to have when working with many beginning stutterers is spontaneous fluency or normal speech. These children often regain spontaneous fluency with a minimum of therapy. It is indeed fortunate, both for the child and the clinician, that these young stutterers gain or regain spontaneous fluency relatively easily. Our experience would suggest that it is usually unrealistic to expect children this young to carefully monitor their speech to use controlled fluency or acceptable stuttering.

FEELINGS AND ATTITUDES

How much attention in therapy should be given to the stutterer's feelings and attitudes about his speech (Fig. 5.4)? Stuttering modification therapy and fluency shaping therapy differ to a considerable degree on this issue. This is particularly true in dealing with the advanced stutterer. It is less true when dealing with younger stutterers or stutterers whose stuttering is less developed.

Stuttering Modification Therapy

Stuttering modification therapy for the advanced stutterer places a great deal of emphasis upon reducing the fear of stuttering. Much of the therapy is con-

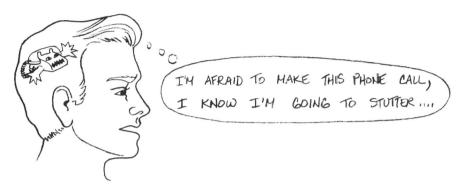

Figure 5.4. How much attention should be given to feelings and attitudes?

cerned with reducing the fear of stuttering and eliminating the avoidance behavior associated with this fear. In addition, stuttering modification clinicians are also interested in developing positive attitudes toward speaking. They encourage the stutterer to develop an approach attitude toward speaking situations, rather than an avoidance attitude. Stutterers are encouraged to seek out speaking situations that they formerly avoided.

With younger stutterers, stuttering modification clinicians put less emphasis upon modifying the child's feelings and attitudes than they do with the older stutterer. As a general rule, the younger the child and the less developed his stuttering, the less attention is given in therapy to dealing with feelings and attitudes. This is because most stuttering modification clinicians believe that stuttering goes through stages in its development. They believe that fears, avoidances, and negative attitudes develop only after the child has been stuttering for a period of time and that these fears, avoidances, and negative attitudes increase in severity as the child matures. Thus, it makes sense to target these feelings and attitudes only when they become part of the stuttering problem.

Fluency Shaping Therapy

As a general rule, we believe that fluency shaping clinicians do not directly attempt to reduce the stutterer's fear and avoidance of words and speaking situations. This would be true for the advanced stutterer, as well as for the lower level stutterer. Thus, with regard to working on feelings and attitudes with the advanced stutterer, fluency shaping clinicians would differ substantially from stuttering modification clinicians. The difference, however, would be much less pronounced in working with the beginning stutterer. This is because neither clinician would be focusing on feelings and attitudes with this younger stutterer.

Integration of Approaches

We have been strongly influenced by proponents of stuttering modification therapy on this issue of targeting feelings and attitudes in treatment. Our position on this issue varies with the treatment level of the stuttering problem. For example, advanced stutterers exhibit chronic frustration, embarrassment, and fear associated with their stuttering. They are avoiding feared words in their speech, and they are avoiding fearful speaking situations. The disorder has become a severe handicap. Based upon our experience, these negative emotions and avoidance behaviors should receive considerable attention in therapy. These speech fears need to be reduced if the stutterer is going to have success in applying either stuttering modification techniques to reduce the severity of his stuttering or fluency shaping techniques to enhance his fluency. If the stutterer is too fearful in a speaking situation, the result will be excessive muscular tension in his speech mechanism. Under these conditions, his motor control will break down, and he will not be able to alter his speech production. These fears and avoidance behaviors also need to be substantially reduced if the advanced stutterer is to maintain the improvement in fluency he made during therapy. If these fears and avoidance behaviors are not significantly reduced, we believe they will become the seeds for relapse, which is so common among advanced stutterers.

The intermediate stutterer, on the other hand, is just beginning to develop some embarrassment and fear relative to his speech. He is just beginning to use some word and situation avoidances. We believe the clinician will need to spend some therapy time, though considerably less than with the advanced stutterer, helping the child reduce his fears and avoidances. The intermediate stutterer will need help in becoming more comfortable with his speech.

As was pointed out earlier, beginning stutterers have little or no concern about their speech. They do not exhibit word or situation fears and avoidances. Accordingly, these children's feelings and attitudes about their speech will require little, if any, attention during the course of their therapy. The focus of treatment will be on speech behaviors. We believe the primary goal of treatment is to increase the child's fluency.

MAINTENANCE PROCEDURES

What strategies or procedures, if any, does the clinician need to employ to help the stutterer maintain the progress he has made during therapy? In other words, do clients, once we get them fluent, automatically maintain their fluency forever, or do they perpetually need to work at being fluent? Stuttering is different from most other speech and language disorders in this regard. Most clients with other speech and language disorders, once they have generalized their new target behaviors to their everyday speaking environment, maintain these new behaviors with very little effort. This is not true with many stutterers, especially advanced stutterers. They are notorious for relapsing. Beginning stutterers, on the other hand, tend to maintain their fluency much better and with much less effort. Let us take a look at what stuttering modification and fluency shaping clinicians do with regard to this matter of maintenance.

Stuttering Modification Therapy

Since beginning stutterers tend to regain spontaneous or normal fluency as a result of therapy, they also tend to maintain this fluency rather easily. They may have an occasional mild relapse, but this is often short-lived. At these times, the stuttering modification clinician will bring the child back into therapy for a booster session or two. This is usually all that is needed.

With some intermediate stutterers and with almost all advanced stutterers, the problem of relapse is a significant one. Stuttering modification clinicians tend to do the following things to combat relapse. They urge their clients not to avoid words or situations. They stress the importance of keeping speech fears at a minimum level. They also help their clients thoroughly master their stuttering modification skills. Finally, they help the stutterer become his own speech clinician so that he can assume responsibility for his own therapy.

Fluency Shaping Therapy

Like stuttering modification clinicians, fluency shaping clinicians have few problems with their young or beginning stutterers relapsing after they have generalized their fluency to their everyday speaking environment. If they do relapse, they will be recycled through part of the fluency shaping program they completed earlier.

Also like stuttering modification clinicians, fluency shaping clinicians find relapse to be a significant problem in their work with older stutterers. To help their clients maintain fluency, fluency shaping clinicians will stress the importance of their clients' mastery of the fluency enhancing skills, for example, using a slower speech rate, which they learned in their treatment program. The assumption is that, if they thoroughly master and use these skills, they will have the ability to use controlled fluency. However, if the stuttering does recur, they will be recycled through the fluency shaping program again.

Integration of Approaches

We believe that the treatment level of the client's stuttering will determine the procedures to be used to maintain his fluency. For maintaining improvement with the advanced stutterer, we rely a great deal upon stuttering modification strategies. It is important for the stutterer to keep his speech fears and avoidances at a very low level. We need to help him become comfortable with both controlled fluency and acceptable stuttering. We also need to encourage him to thoroughly master stuttering modification and fluency shaping techniques so that he can both modify his moments of stuttering and enhance his fluency. Finally, we need to help him become his own speech clinician.

We believe the intermediate stutterer, the stutterer who is beginning to avoid talking, will need help in maintaining his improvement, whether it is spontaneous fluency, controlled fluency, or acceptable stuttering. This stutterer will need to be impressed with the importance of not avoiding talking. He may need continued work on desensitization to his speech fears. He may also need to develop skill and confidence in his ability to use stuttering modification and/or fluency shaping techniques.

We have found that beginning stutterers generalize and maintain their fluency much more readily than do the older or more developed stutterers. Thus, we believe all the clinician needs to do is to provide a setting in which the beginning stutterer can develop spontaneous fluency and then provide the conditions that will allow this fluency to generalize. Maintenance will usually take care of itself. If it does not, a brief return to therapy may be needed.

CLINICAL METHODS

With the term clinical methods, we are referring to two dimensions of the therapy process. The first is the structure of therapy; the second is data collection. Stuttering modification therapy and fluency shaping therapy differ substantially with regard to these two aspects of therapy.

Stuttering Modification Therapy

With regard to the structure of therapy, we observe that in stuttering modification therapy, the stutterer and the clinician typically interact in a loosely structured manner. With the adult and older child, the structure of therapy is characterized by a teaching/counseling interaction. With the younger child, the nature of the interaction may be more of a play situation.

The second dimension mentioned above was data collection. Traditionally, stuttering modification clinicians do not put a great deal of emphasis upon the collecting and reporting of objective data, for example, the frequency of stuttering before and after therapy. This is apparent from their writings. It is not that stuttering modification clinicians are not interested in their client's progress; rather, they consider their own and their client's global descriptions and impressions of progress as more valid than frequency counts of stuttering made in the treatment environment.

Fluency Shaping Therapy

In terms of the structure of therapy, fluency shaping therapy is usually performed in a highly structured situation. With their roots in operant conditioning and programmed instruction, fluency shaping clinicians put a great deal of emphasis upon preparing behavioral objectives and sequencing antecedent events, responses, and consequent events in a series of steps. Specific instructions and materials are prescribed. Specific responses are called for from the stutterer with specific reactions to these responses required from the clinician.

As might be anticipated from their theoretical orientation, fluency shaping clinicians put a great deal of emphasis upon the collection and reporting of objective and reliable data. They regard this as extremely important in documenting their client's progress.

Integration of Approaches

What should the clinician do about these issues? There are strong advocates of both approaches. With regard to the structure of therapy, we have used both approaches and today find ourselves borrowing from both sides. Sometimes we use one approach, and at other times we use the other approach. Quite often our therapy is characterized by the loose application of programming principles. The clinician, however, will need to make up her own mind on this matter.

On the issue of data collection, however, we are less ambivalent. We have been strongly influenced by the fluency shaping advocates. We believe it is important for the clinician to routinely collect data on her client so that she knows if her therapy procedures are having an effect upon her client's problem. This is a critical ingredient to effective therapy. In addition, with today's emphasis upon accountability, record keeping has become more and more important for the public school clinician who must write an Individual Education Program (IEP) for each child.

We routinely obtain data before treatment, during treatment, and after treatment. As a minimum, we measure our client's frequency of stuttering and rate of speech. These data are always obtained from samples of our client's speech before and at the termination of treatment and are sometimes obtained in a probe during a therapy session. Furthermore, we attempt to assess our client's speech at home and at school. We also attempt to assess our client's feelings and attitudes towards his problem. More will be said about these matters when we discuss our assessment procedures in the next chapter and when we discuss our clinical methods in the treatment chapters.

TREATMENT OF CONCOMITANT SPEECH AND LANGUAGE PROBLEMS

As noted in our review of the research in Chapter 2, children who stutter, or a subgroup of these children, tend to be delayed in their speech and language development. In particular, they are likely to be delayed in their articulation development. Thus, it seems reasonable to conclude that a number of young stutterers whom the clinician will encounter will have concomitant speech and language problems. Despite the above conclusion, until very recently little has been written regarding the clinical management of these concomitant speech and language problems. For example, we reported in 1980 (Guitar & Peters) that we were unable to find, either in the stuttering modification or in the fluency shaping literature much discussion dealing with treatment considerations for children who have articulation and language problems accompanied by stuttering. Very recently, however, a number of clinicians, particularly Hugo Gregory and Diane Hill, Glyndon and Jeanna Riley, and Meryl Wall and Florence Myers, have responded to this issue. In different ways, these writers integrate the work on the child's stuttering or fluency with treatment of other aspects of his speech and language system. We strongly support this clinical approach and will cite examples from the above clinicians' and from our own clinical experience to illustrate how this can be accomplished.

It should be noted, however, that there are some clinicians who express concern in regard to working on a young stutterer's articulation or language. They believe that, by working on the child's articulation or language, the child will come to believe that he needs to work hard at speaking correctly. This extra effort the exacerbates the stuttering. Yet, on the basis of our clinical experience, we believe that work on both fluency and articulation or language can be integrated. We believe the clinician can approach this task without making the child believe that talking is difficult.

SUMMARY

We have suggested that the clinician's beliefs on treatment issues will not only affect her goals for her client, but they will also affect her daily clinical behaviors. Thus, it is incumbent upon her to give serious thought to seven treatment issues.

The first issue is the clinician's beliefs about the onset and development of stuttering. We stress the fact that her beliefs regarding the nature of stuttering will influence her clinical decisions. To illustrate this point, we described how our belief in developmental levels of stuttering significantly influences our clinical goals and procedures.

The second issue involves the speech behaviors targeted for therapy. With the advanced stutterer, we believe it is important to integrate aspects of both stuttering modification therapy and fluency shaping therapy. In other words, the stutterer can learn to stutter with less struggle on given moments of stuttering, as well as learn to change certain aspects of his overall speech pattern to increase his fluency. This integration is less critical with beginning stutterers because the differences between stuttering modification and fluency shaping therapies become less pronounced with these children.

The next issue is the type of fluency to be expected as a result of therapy. The three possible outcomes are spontaneous fluency, controlled fluency, and acceptable stuttering. We believe the type of fluency to be expected varies with the treatment level. For the advanced stutterer, we believe the most realistic goal is the development of the capacity to use both controlled fluency and acceptable stuttering. With the intermediate stutterer, the goal should be spontaneous fluency, but controlled fluency or especially acceptable stuttering is the most realistic outcome to expect. Spontaneous fluency is a realistic expectation with the beginning stutterer.

The fourth issue is the attention given to feelings and attitudes in therapy. Again, we believe this varies with the treatment level. With the advanced stutterer, we believe this dimension of therapy needs to receive considerable attention. With the intermediate stutterer, some attention will need to be focused on the client's feelings and attitudes. With the beginning stutterer, very little attention will need to be given to this aspect of therapy.

The next issue is the choice of procedures or strategies, if any, needed to help the client maintain his improvement. Older stutterers, that is, intermediate and advanced stutterers, require considerable help to keep avoidances and speech fears at a minimum and to master the stuttering modification and fluency shaping skills that allow them to modify their moments of stuttering and/or enhance their fluency. Beginning stutterers need little help in maintaining the fluency they acquire in therapy.

The sixth issue is clinical methods. Some prefer loosely structured therapy characterized by a teaching/counseling interaction. Others prefer a highly structured approach with behavioral objectives and antecedent events, responses, and consequent events carefully sequenced in a series of steps. Regardless of the approach, we especially encourage the use of data collection to document the effects of therapy.

The last issue involves the treatment of concomitant speech and language problems in young stutterers. Several recently developed programs successfully meet these needs. We strongly support these new developments.

We will return to these clinical issues again and again in subsequent chapters. Our goal is to impress upon the clinician the impact of one's clinical beliefs upon one's clinical practice.

STUDY QUESTIONS

1/ List the seven clinically relevant issues that were discussed in this chapter.

2/ Give an example of how a clinician's beliefs about the nature of stuttering could influence her approach to therapy.

3/ What are the speech behaviors targeted for therapy in stuttering modification therapy? in fluency shaping therapy?

4/ Define the following dimensions of fluency: continuity, rate, rhythm, and effort.

5/ Define the following terms: spontaneous fluency, controlled fluency, and acceptable stuttering. Be sure to include all four dimensions of fluency in your definitions.

6/ Should a clinician have the same fluency goals for a beginning stutterer as for an advanced stutterer? If not, why not?

7/ How does the approach of stuttering modification clinicians and fluency shaping clinicians differ with regard to targeting feelings and attitudes in treatment? How are they similar?

8/ Why is it important for the clinician to be concerned about maintenance of fluency following treatment, especially with the intermediate or advanced stutterer?

9/ As a general rule, how do stuttering modification clinicians and fluency shaping clinicians differ with regard to clinical methods?

10/ Why is it important for a clinician to have a position with regard to the treatment of concomitant speech and language disorders in stutterers?

Suggested Readings

Gregory, H. H. (1979). Controversial issues: statement and review of the literature. In H. H. Gregory (Ed.), *Controversies about stuttering therapy* (pp. 1–62). Baltimore: University Park Press.

In this chapter, Gregory defines the "stutter more fluently" and the "speak more fluently" approaches to treatment. He also raises many excellent questions relevant to the evaluation and treatment of stuttering.

Guitar, B. & Peters, T. J. (1980). Comparison of stuttering modification and fluency shaping therapies. In B. Guitar & T. J. Peters, *Stuttering: An integration of contemporary therapies* (pp. 13–23). Memphis: Speech Foundation of America.

The similarities and differences, as well as the pros and cons, of stuttering modification and fluency shaping therapies are discussed.

6

ASSESSMENT AND DIAGNOSIS

This chapter is a bridge between our description of the nature of stuttering (Chapters 1–4) and our recommendations for treatment (Chapters 7–12). It is written to help clinicians develop an effective treatment program for their clients by showing them (*a*) how to assess the predisposing, precipitating, and learning factors currently influencing their client's stuttering, and then describing (*b*) how to use this information to select the appropriate developmental/treatment level.

Figure 6.1 illustrates the components of assessment and diagnosis and the sequence in which we employ them.

We will describe assessment procedures for three age levels: the adolescent/adult, the preschool child, and the elementary school child. Age levels are used because we are aware of a client's age before the evaluation but know little else about him. Our sequence of age levels reflects that, as in treatment, very different procedures are used for the assessment of adult and adolescent clients compared to those of preschool age. Procedures for elementary school students borrow from both of the other age levels; therefore, evaluation of these students is best understood after learning about evaluation of older and younger clients first.

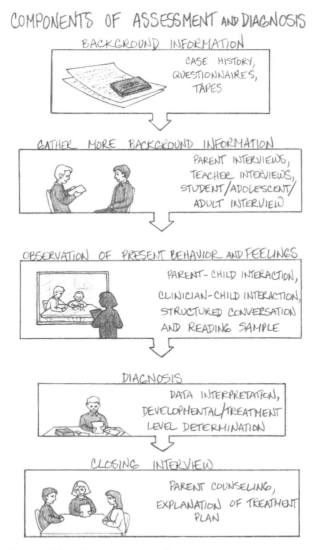

Figure 6.1.   The sequence of assessment and diagnosis.

We will use the terms "assessment" and "diagnosis" to specify two different stages of our evaluation procedures. Our initial data-gathering will be termed "assessment," and our steps to pull this information together to decide if the client is indeed a stutterer and to specify the level of treatment appropriate for him will be termed "diagnosis."

SOME CONSIDERATIONS

Before getting into the techniques of assessment, we will describe a few things to keep in mind when seeing a new client.

1. Every client is different. We have found that, the more experienced you become, the more you need to resist the tendency to jump to conclusions. A warning bell should go off in your head if you find yourself thinking, "Ah, yes, I understand this client. Just like that child I saw last year." Be cautious about letting referral information, past experience, and other sources cloud your ability to see all aspects of the client and his problem. Also be wary of simple explanations and quick judgements about the critical factors for a client. If, for instance, a child's parents tell you they often ask their child to stop and start again when he stutters, and that they both work long hours outside the home, and dinner time is noisy and confusing, try not to assume that pressures at home are the major problem for the child. They may be, but other things may be critical also. Ask more questions. Explore how the child responds to these situations and others before you decide where to begin the process of change.

2. Consider the person as well as the problem. The client, no matter what age, will sense quickly whether you are seeing him as an individual or only seeing his stuttering. An effective clinician is genuinely interested and empathetic; she accepts failures and backsliding as well as victories and progress. The evaluation is your first opportunity to show the client that you accept him just as he is and do not reject or fear his stuttering. In this atmosphere, the client can start to accept himself and his stuttering and make the first critical steps toward fluency.

3. Diagnosis is an ongoing process. As treatment progresses (or doesn't), try to keep asking, "Am I using the best approach with this person? Is there something else or something different I should be doing?" Decide what measures of progress are important for your clients, and apply these measures at regular intervals. Our own approach is to assess stuttering behavior at the beginning and the end of each semester. In other settings, we often assess a client after every ten hours of treatment. In our periodic assessments, we try, although we don't always succeed, to obtain samples of our clients' speech in a non-clinical situation, such as in their classrooms or on their jobs. We also assess our clients' stuttering when we bring them in for maintenance checks at increasingly wider intervals after formal treatment is over. In addition, we assess our clients' feelings and attitudes at the beginning and end of treatment, and we may assess

them at other times if we are concerned about progress. If we are working on changing attitudes and feelings, change should be reflected in our measures, or we should try a different approach. Decreases in negative attitudes and feelings should be accompanied by decreases in stuttering severity, and our measures should show this. The tools for making these various assessments are described in the section for each age level in this chapter.

ADOLESCENT AND ADULT

Pre-Assessment

CASE HISTORY FORM

We usually send a case history form to adult clients—those over age 18 and beyond high school—several weeks before their appointment. A sample of this form can be seen in Figure 6.2. Because adolescents are usually seen in a school, we encourage them to fill out the form themselves but suggest they may want to get their parents' help for parts of it.

This form requests information that would be appropriate for most speech or language disorders. Consequently, it can be used with all adult clients referred for speech or language problems. It also allows the clinician to learn ahead of time if the client who was referred for stuttering appears to have a different or an additional disorder. The form will give the clinician information about the extent to which the stuttering, if that is the problem, affects the client's life.

ATTITUDE QUESTIONNAIRES

We assess clients' communication attitudes through observations, direct questions, and questionnaires. Because we want to be able to review the completed questionnaires before we interview a client, we may send them to the client and ask that they be returned before the interview. Alternately, we may ask clients to complete them when they arrive for the evaluation, before we interview them. After we have scored the questionnaires, we have preliminary information about the clients' attitudes, and we can prepare to explore them further through follow-up questions.

Assessment

INTERVIEW

We begin by welcoming the client and explaining what procedures we will use to evaluate his problem—videotaping and audiotaping of his speech, questions about his past and current difficulties, and questions about his feelings and attitudes regarding his speech. This, we explain, will be followed by our analysis of the information and a concluding interview in which we will share our diagnosis with him and discuss the things that can be done about his problem. We also must remember to have the client complete any questionnaires we haven't obtained previously. We then begin our interview with an open-ended question such as, "What is the problem that brings you here today?"

<u>Adult Case History Form</u>

Date: _____

A. <u>Personal Information</u>

1. Name:_____
           First   Middle   Last

2. Address: _____

              _____

              _____

3. Telephone Home:_____ Work: _____

4. Date of Birth: _____ Sex: ____ Marital Status: _____

5. Social Security Number: _____
      Medicaid/Medicare Number: _____

6. Referred by: _____

7. Education Level: _____ Occupation: _____

8. Employed by: _____

9. Name of spouse or nearest relative: _____

10. Address of above person: _____

11. List and describe all members of your present family and indicate whether they live in your home. Indicate any speech, hearing or language problems present in other members of the household.

Name   Relationship   Sex   Communication Problem

Name	Relationship	Sex	Communication Problem

Figure 6.2. Case history form for adults and adolescents.

Once the client has had a chance to describe his speech problem, we then ask further questions to try to get a deeper understanding. Below are typical questions we ask and a brief commentary about each one. In some cases, we have grouped two questions together—a question to start the client talking about a particular topic, and a follow-up question to be asked if the first question doesn't elicit some related information.

B. Present Speech, Language, or Hearing Problem

How long have you had this problem? _____

Have you ever received treatment for this problem?_____

If so, where? _____ How long?_____

Does any member of your family have a similar problem? (Specify)

_____ _____

What do you think caused the problem? _____

_____

How do you feel about the problem?_____

_____

What are significant other people's feelings about the problem?

_____ _____

Do you avoid speaking situations (If so, please explain)?

_____

Does the problem affect your job/school performance? _____

_____

Are there times when the problem is better or worse? _____

_____

Why are you seeking help at this time? _____

_____

Please provide in the space below any additional information which
may be useful in evaluating your communication and in planning a
treatment program.

_____

_____

_____

Figure 6.2.—Continued

C. <u>Current Health Status</u>: Answer yes or no and explain more fully where appropriate.

Are you in good health at the present time?

Is your hearing good?

Is your vision good?

Are you ambulatory?

Are you taking any medications at the present time (specify)?

Is there any associated medical pathology (i.e., cleft palate, cerebral palsy, post-CVA, accident or injury) which may be contributing to your communicative problem (specify)?

Have you been hospitalized within the last year?
If yes, give name and address of hospital.

May we contact this hospital for your discharge summary?

If, in order to help you, it is appropriate to send reports to other agencies or to contact other agencies or professional persons for information, please indicate your permission by signing below.

I authorize and request ___(clinic name and address)_____
to obtain and/or exchange pertinent medical/educational information. It is understood that all information will be kept confidential.

Signed: _____   Date: _____

If signed by a person other than the client, please state name and capacity of that person:

_____

Please provide in the space below any additional information that may be useful in evaluating your communication and in planning a treatment program.

_____

Figure 6.2.—Continued

1. When did you begin to stutter? How has the way you stutter changed over the years?

We realize that, by answering the first part of this question, the client may be just reporting what his parents told him. The accuracy of this may be questionable, but at least we will learn of his perception of the onset. The second part of the question—about recent changes—may reveal what kinds of things affect the way the client stutters. Does he stutter more severely because of a recent job change or because of a threat to self-esteem such as a divorce or loss of employment? Less frequently, we may find out that the client began to stutter in late adolescence or adulthood. If so, we would want to consider the possibility of neurogenic or psychogenic stuttering, which we discuss briefly below, in the section on diagnosis.

2. What do you believe caused you to stutter?

This may give us some insights that may affect motivation. For example, one client reported that her mother and several of her brothers stuttered and that, therefore, it was a genetic problem and could not be helped. This led us to confront the issue, early in treatment, of whether she could change or not.

We also find that sometimes clients have misinformation about the possible cause of their stuttering and we can correct this, thereby changing some of our clients' attitudes about their problem. We have met clients who come to therapy believing that their problem is entirely psychological. As they learn our view of stuttering, they are relieved to know that we believe they can modify their speech behaviors without longterm psychotherapy.

3. Does anyone else in your family stutter?

Here we might find that a parent stutters. This is of interest because the parent's attitudes about his or her own stuttering may have a profound effect on the client. Moreover, knowing about other family members who stutter may help us develop a better understanding of factors related to this client's stuttering. This may be useful in treatment, especially in helping the client understand the nature of the problem.

4. Have you ever had therapy? What did the therapy consist of? How effective do you think it was?

This information is important in planning therapy. For example, if a client had a type of therapy previously that he felt did not help, it would be unwise to put the client back into the same type of therapy. But if the client has had success with therapy, but regressed slightly or moved before the treatment was finished, using this type of therapy again may be most appropriate. It is important that the clinician be familiar with various types of therapy that clients may have undergone. Most current therapies will emphasize either a stuttering modification or a fluency shaping approach.

5. Has your stuttering changed or caused you more problems recently? Why did you come in for help at the present time?

The responses to these questions make it possible to see the current problems faced by the client. We also can usually get some inkling of the client's motivation. For example, the client may have been offered a promotion if he can improve his speech, or the client may just have recently learned of the treatment program and hoped for some relief of a long-standing problem.

The following four questions about the client's pattern of stuttering are closely related to one another:

6. Are there times or situations when you stutter more? Less? What are they?

7. Do you avoid certain speaking situations in which you expect to stutter? If so, which ones?

8. Do you avoid certain words that you expect to stutter on? Do you substitute one word for another if you expect to stutter? Circumlocute?

9. Do you use any "tricks" to get words out? Escape behaviors?

These four questions will provide information useful in therapy planning. They tell us something about the client's most difficult situations, how he feels about them, and how he deals with them. This information may also corroborate what we learn from the questionnaires we give him. It will also give us an impression of how aware he is of his stuttering behaviors.

10. Have your academic/vocational choices and/or performance been affected because you stutter? How?

The client's answers will be incorporated into therapy, to help plan later stages of treatment in which new behaviors and new challenges are attempted. The answers may also prompt us to refer clients, in the later stages of treatment, to an academic or vocational counselor to help them choose a more appropriate option for themselves.

11. Have your relationships with people been affected because you stutter? How?

As in the question above, we can use this information to plan a hierarchy of generalization for our clients, moving from easy to difficult social situations gradually if the client finds social interactions difficult. We also need to know how much a client blames any difficulties he has in social interactions on the fact that he stutters. A client may be socially inhibited because he is sensitive and vulnerable to expected listener reactions. Such sensitivity can be assessed by observing the client's affect when he is stuttering. If he appears to be relatively unaffected emotionally by his stuttering, but professes to have difficulty relating to people, he may benefit from counseling or psychotherapy focused on resolving this interpersonal difficulty.

12. What are your feelings or attitudes toward your stuttering? What do you think other people think about your stuttering?

The responses will be used to help determine some of the foci of treatment, such as procedures in desensitization to decrease the stutterer's shame and guilt about stuttering. Perceptions about others' views of his stuttering may need to be confronted via various "reality-testing" tasks to find out what people really think.

13. What are your family's (parents, spouse, children) feelings, attitudes, and reactions toward your stuttering and toward the prospect of your being in therapy?

This information could affect, positively or negatively, the client's motivation. It may be an important consideration in planning therapy.

14. Are there any additional things that you think we ought to know about your stuttering?

This gives the client a chance to get anything off his chest that he may be holding back, or it may be an opportunity for him to speak about things that have only occurred to him after the other questions were asked.

SPEECH SAMPLE

Pattern of Disfluencies.   Throughout our evaluation of the adult or adolescent stutterer, we observe the pattern with which the client stutters. We would try to determine, for example, roughly what proportion of the core behaviors are repetitions, prolongations, and blocks. During blocks, where and how does the stutterer shut off airflow or voicing? What are the client's escape and avoidance behaviors? Is this client able to tolerate being in a block, or does he speak in an unusual or vague way to avoid stuttering? More detail on various escape and avoidance patterns can be found in Chapter 4. This information will be useful when we help the client learn more about his stuttering and help him decrease his fear of it.

Stuttering Severity Instrument.   Another way in which we assess disfluency is to employ the Stuttering Severity Instrument (Riley, 1972), illustrated in Figure 6.3.

This instrument measures the following components of stuttering: frequency, duration, and physical concomitants. In addition, we assess speech rate from this sample for reasons we explain in the section on rate below. Although Riley suggests using a 100-word sample of oral reading and conversation, we prefer to use a larger sample to increase reliability. We ask the client to read aloud for 5 minutes, using material believed to be at an appropriate level. Then we ask him to converse about his job or school for 5 minutes. It is important to measure these samples accurately with a stopwatch. In measuring the amount of speaking time in the conversational sample, we stop the watch whenever the client is not talking, but allow it to run during moments of stuttering. Short pauses (less than 2 seconds) are incorporated into the 5 minutes, but long pauses, for formulation, are excluded. We usually videotape these samples and score them later. If they are audiotaped, the clinician must score the physical concomitants on line, since these are not accurately scored from an audio recording.

The total overall score for the SSI is the sum of the three subcomponents measured. (*a*) Frequency is assessed as percentage of stuttering in reading and conversation. Riley uses percent of words stuttered; this is converted to a Task Score, found on the form. (*b*) Duration is assessed by estimating the length of the three longest blocks, calculating the mean duration, and finding the appropriate Task Score on the form. (*c*) Physical concomitants are assessed by adding the scale values from each subcomponent and deriving a total score. Percentiles and Severity ratings (e.g., mild, moderate, severe) for various total overall scores are given on the form. The clinician should read Riley's directions on administering this measure in the *Journal of Speech and Hearing Disorders* (1972) before using it.

When counting frequency of stuttering we count as stutters: part-word

STUTTERING SEVERITY INSTRUMENT (SSI)

Name _____   Date_____

I. FREQUENCY

1. JOB TASK		2. READING TASK		3. PICTURE TASK		
PERCENT	TASK SCORE	PERCENT	TASK SCORE	PERCENT	TASK SCORE	
1	2	1	2	1	2	
2-3	3	2-3	3	2-3	6	
4	4	4-5	4	4	8	FREQUENCY
5-6	5	6-9	5	5-6	10	TASK SCORE
7-9	6	10-16	7	7-9	12	
10-14	7	17-26	8	10-14	14	(1 + 2, OR 3)
15-28	8	27+	9	15-28	16	
29+	9			29+	18	I._____

II. DURATION

ESTIMATED LENGTH OF THREE LONGEST BLOCKS COMBINED   SCORE

```
FLEETING..................................... ......................1
ONE-HALF SECOND...................................................2
ONE FULL SECOND...................................................3
2 TO 9 SECONDS....................................................4
10 TO 13 SECONDS..................................................5
30 TO 60 SECONDS..................................................6
MORE THAN 60 SECONDS..............................................7
```

DURATION
SCORE

(SCORE FOR MEAN
DURATION OF THREE
LONGEST BLOCKS)

II. _____

III. PHYSICAL CONCOMITANTS

EVALUATING SCALE: 0 = NONE; 1 = NOT NOTICEABLE UNLESS LOOKING FOR IT; 2 = BARELY NOTICEABLE
TO CASUAL OBSERVER; 3 = DISTRACTING; 4 = VERY DISTRACTING; 5 = SEVERE AND PAINFUL LOOKING.

DISTRACTING SOUNDS: NOISY BREATHING, WHISTLING, SNIFFING, BLOWING,
CLICKING SOUNDS...........0 1 2 3 4 5

PHYSICAL
CONCOMITANTS

FACIAL GRIMACES: JAW JERKING, TONGUE PROTRUDING, LIP PRESSING,
JAW MUSCLES TENSE.........0 1 2 3 4 5

(TOTAL OF FOUR
CATEGORIES)

HEAD MOVEMENTS: BACK, FORWARD, TURNING AWAY, POOR EYE CONTACT,
CONSTANT LOOKING AROUND...0 1 2 3 4 5

III. _____

MOVEMENTS OF EXTREMITIES: ARM AND HAND MOVEMENTS, HANDS ABOUT
FACE, TOSO MOVEMENTS, LEG MOVEMENTS, FOOT TAPPING
OR SWINGING...............0 1 2 3 4 5

TOTAL OVERALL SCORE (TOS): I + II + III = _____

CHILDREN'S SEVERITY			ADULTS' SEVERITY		
TOS	PERCENT	SEVERITY	TOS	PERCENT	SEVERITY
0-5	0-4	VERY MILD	0-16	0-4	VERY MILD
6-8	5-11	MILD	17-19	5-11	MILD
9-13	12-23	MILD	20-21	12-23	MILD
14-15	24-40	MILD	22-24	24-40	MODERATE
16-19	41-60	MODERATE	25-27	41-60	MODERATE
20-23	61-77	MODERATE	28-30	61-77	MODERATE
24-27	78-89	SEVERE	31-33	78-89	SEVERE
28-30	90-96	SEVERE	34-36	90-96	SEVERE
31-45	97-100	VERY SEVERE	37-45	97-100	VERY SEVERE

Figure 6.3. The Stuttering Severity Instrument. (From Riley, G. (1972). A stuttering severity instrument for children and adults. *J Speech Hear Disord, 37,* 314–322. Copyright 1972, American Speech-Language-Hearing Association. Reprinted with permission.)

repetitions, single syllable or whole word repetitions, prolongations, blockages of sound or airflow, as well as successful avoidance behaviors. One of the present authors counts frequency as percent of words stuttered; the other author uses percent of syllables stuttered. Because frequency is assessed as percentage of syllables (or words) stuttered, we make the assumption that a syllable (or word) can be stuttered only once. Thus, "Where is my ba-ba-ba-ba-ba-basketball?" is one stutter. "Where is my uh well my my ba-ba-ba-ba-basketball?" is also one stutter, since we would assume that the repetition of the word "my" and the use of "uh" as a postponement are part of the same stutter as the repeated first syllable, "ba". There are rare occasions when a word might have more than one stutter (for instance, "ba-ba-basketba-ba-ball). This presents no problem for counting frequency as percentage of stuttered syllables, since there is, in this case, one stutter on the first syllable and one stutter on the third syllable. When counting frequency as percentage of words stuttered, both stutters are counted and "percentage of words stuttered" become a slightly inaccurate description of the procedure.

We also compare the client's stuttering during reading with that during conversation. It is often true that, if stuttering is markedly worse during reading, the stutterer may be avoiding words he thinks he may stutter on during conversational speech. It is important that the clinician select appropriate reading material for the particular client. Some stutterers may have reading problems; if the reading material is above their level, their stuttering may increase as their resources are stressed on the reading task.

Speech Rate.   In addition to the above measures, we assess the client's speech rate. Rate often reflects the severity of stuttering and the effect it is having on his communication. If the client's speech rate is markedly below normal, communication may be difficult for him.

Rate can be measured as either words per minute or syllables per minute, depending on the clinician's preference. Some clinicians find it easier to calculate rate using words per minute, because words are easily observable units. Others note that syllables per minute can be calculated more rapidly than words, because the clinician can use the "beat" of the syllable to count "on-line" (i.e., while the speaker is talking). The syllables per minute approach also allows for the fact that some speakers will use more multisyllable words than others. Speakers who use many polysyllabic words might otherwise be penalized because their words may take longer to produce than those who speak using mostly one-syllable words. No matter which method is used, the following rules can be used for counting words or syllables: Count only the words/syllables that would have been said if the person had not stuttered. Thus if the person says, "My-my-my, uh, well my name is Peter," this should be counted as 4 words or 5 syllables, because it would be assumed that the extra "my's" and the "uh" are part of the stuttering. If the person says, "When I went to Boston, I mean when I went to New York . . . " and it does not appear that the person was postponing or using any other "trick" to avoid stuttering, this would be counted as 13 words or 14 syllables, because the person's stuttering did not interfere with the utterance. Only words (or syllables in words) are counted: "uh" or "um" are not counted. "Oh" or "well" are counted, unless they are used as a postponement, starter, or other component of stuttering.

When words per minute are calculated, a transcript is made of the client's 5-minute sample of conversational speech, and his 5-minute reading sample is marked to indicate where he finished. Total number of words are counted, and this figure is divided by 5 to give a per-minute conversation or reading rate.

The normal speaking rate has a range of about 115 to 165 words per minute (Andrews & Ingham, 1971).[1] Normal reading rate has a range of about 150 to 190 words per minute (Darley & Spriestersbach, 1978).

When syllables per minute are calculated, it is often easiest to use an inexpensive calculator to count syllables cumulatively, as they are being spoken (although this takes some practice). Before the speaker begins, push the "1" key, then the "+". When the speaker starts speaking, depress the "=" key for each syllable spoken or read. The cumulative total appears in the readout window.[2] We find it easiest to count by reading a transcript of the conversational sample aloud slowly and pushing the "=" key for each syllable spoken. The inexperienced rater should learn to count first from a transcript. The experienced rater can, as we suggested above, assess conversational speech rate directly from the tape recording, pressing the "=" key for each syllable spoken. If this latter procedure is used, it is wise to recheck your figures to ensure accuracy.

Normal speech rate has a range of from 162 to 230 syllables per minute, with a mean of 196 (Andrews & Ingham, 1971). Normal reading rate is about 210 to 265 syllables per minute.

FEELINGS AND ATTITUDES

A variety of questionnaires are available to assess various aspects of the stutterer's feelings and attitudes about communication and about stuttering. We obtain information about the client's communication attitudes via the Modified Erickson Scale (Andrews & Cutler, 1974). This questionnaire, illustrated in Figure 6.4, has been normed on both stutterers and nonstutterers. Moreover, research has suggested that changes in attitude during treatment may be related to long term outcome (Guitar & Bass, 1978), although there is debate in the literature about the interpretation of this finding (Ingham, 1979; Guitar, 1979; Young, 1981).

We also use questionnaires to assess the client's tendency to avoid stuttering. We use the Avoidance scales of the Stutterer's Self Ratings of Reactions to Speech Situations (Johnson, Darley, and Spriestersbach, 1952)—which will be referred to as SSR—to assess the tendency to avoid specific speaking situations. This form is shown in Figure 6.5.

Our research suggests that clients with Avoidance scores higher than 2.56 prior to treatment may be more likely to have an appreciable level of stuttering a year after treatment with fluency shaping therapy than clients with lower scores (Guitar, 1976).

---

[1] All rate figures given in this section are for adults.

[2] Although many calculators require pressing the "1", then "+", then "=" button repeatedly to count cumulatively, others will count cumulatively when the "1" is pressed, followed by repeated pressing of the "+" button. Some experimentation may be necessary to find the appropriate sequence on your calculator. Some of the more expensive calculators cannot be used to count cumulatively because of the types of microchips used in them.

<u>MODIFIED ERICKSON SCALE OF COMMUNICATION ATTITUDES (S-24)</u>

Name: _____   Date: _____   Score:_____

<u>Directions</u>: Mark the "true" column with a check (✔) for each statement that is true or mostly true for you and mark the "false" column with a check (✔) for each statement which is false or not usually true for you.

                                                                                    TRUE   FALSE

1. I usually feel that I am making a favorable impression when I talk. _____ _____

2. I find it easy to talk with almost anyone........................   _____ _____

3. I find it very easy to look at my audience while speaking
   to a group..   _____ _____

4. A person who is my teacher or my boss is hard to talk to.........   _____ _____

5. Even the idea of giving a talk in public makes me afraid...........   _____ _____

6. Some words are harder than others for me to say.................   _____ _____

7. I forget all about myself shortly after I begin a speech...........   _____ _____

8. I am a good mixer....................................   _____ _____

9. People sometimes seem uncomfortable when I am talking to them..   _____ _____

10. I dislike introducing one person to another.......................   _____ _____

11. I often ask questions in group discussions........................   _____ _____

12. I find it easy to keep control of my voice when speaking..........   _____ _____

13. I do not mind speaking before a group.............................   _____ _____

14. I do not talk well enough to do the kind of work I'd
    really like to do....................................   _____ _____

15. My speaking voice is rather pleasant and easy to listen to........   _____ _____

16. I am sometimes embarrassed by the way I talk......................   _____ _____

17. I face most speaking situations with complete confidence.........   _____ _____

18. There are few people I can talk with easily.......................   _____ _____

19. I talk better than I write...   _____ _____

20. I often feel nervous while talking................................   _____ _____

21. I find it hard to make talk when I meet new people...............   _____ _____

22. I feel pretty confident about my speaking ability.................   _____ _____

Figure 6.4.   The Erickson S-24 Scale of Communication Attitudes. (From Andrews, G. & Cutler, J. (1974). Stuttering therapy: The relation between changes in symptom level and attitudes. *J Speech Hear Disord*, 39, 312–319. Copyright 1974, American Speech-Language-Hearing Association. Reprinted with permission.)

23. I wish that I could say things as clearly as others do............   ____ ____

24. Even though I knew the right answer, I have often failed
to give it because I was afraid to speak out.....................   ____ ____

Data on the "Modified Erickson Scale of Communication Attitudes"

I. Answers (Andrews and Cutler, 1974)

Score one point for each answer that matches this:

1. False	7. False	13. False	19. False
2. False	8. False	14. True	20. True
3. False	9. True	15. False	21. True
4. True	10. True	16. True	22. False
5. True	11. False	17. False	23. True
6. True	12. False	18. True	24. True

II. Adult Norms (Andrews and Cutler, 1974)

	Mean	Range
Stutterers	19.22	9-24
Non-Stutterers	9.14	1-21

Figure 6.4—Continued

We may also use Perceptions of Stuttering Inventory (PSI) (Woolf, 1967), shown in Figure 6.6, which examines the stutterer's perception of the presence of struggle, avoidance, and expectancy of stuttering in his communication. Woolf suggests the PSI can be used to help the stutterer view his problem more objectively, to develop treatment goals, and to assess progress. We find that the avoidance section of the PSI complements the Avoidance scale on the SSR because the SSR focuses more on situations and the PSI deals more with the stuttering behaviors.

OTHER SPEECH AND LANGUAGE BEHAVIORS

As we interact with the client during the interview, we informally assess his comprehension and production of language, his articulation, and his voice. We also screen his hearing. If we suspect that there is an articulation, language, or voice problem, we follow up with further evaluation in the potential deficit areas. Adolescent language assessment procedures can be found in McLoughlin and Lewis (1990) and articulation assessment procedures in Hoffman, Schuckers, and Daniloff (1989). We find that the client's concern about other disorders guides us in treatment. If, as we have found upon occasion, the stuttering client also lisps, we will discuss it with him. If he is not concerned about it, we don't feel it is necessary to treat the problem. If, however, he feels an articulation or language (or other) problem handicaps him communicatively, we will treat that problem also.

STUTTERERS' SELF RATING OF REACTIONS TO SPEECH SITUATIONS

Name_____ Age _____ Sex_____
Examiner _____ Date_____

After each item put a number from 1–5 in each of the four columns.

Start with the right hand–column headed Frequency. Study the five possible answers to be made in responding to each item, and write the number of the answer that best fits the situation for you in each case. Thus, if you habitually take your meals at home and seldom eat in a restaurant, certainly not as often as once a week, write number 5 in the Frequency column opposite item No. 1, "Ordering in a restaurant". In like manner respond to each of the other 39 items by writing the most appropriate number in the Frequency column.

Now, write the number of the response that best indicates how much you stutter in each situation. For example, if in ordering meals in a restaurant you stutter mildly (for you), write the number 2 in the Stuttering column.

Following the same procedure, write your responses in the Reaction column, and, finally write your responses in the Avoidance column.

Numbers for each of the columns are to be interpreted as follows:

A. Avoidance
1. I never try to avoid this situation and have no desire to avoid it.
2. I don't try to avoid this situation, but sometimes I would like to.
3. More often than not I do not try to avoid this situation, but sometimes I do try to avoid it.
4. More often than not I do try to avoid this situation.
5. I avoid this situation every time I possibly can.

B. Reaction
1. I definately enjoy speaking in this situation.
2. I would rather speak in this situation than not.
3. It's hard to say whether I'd rather speak in this situation or not.
4. I would rather not speak in this situation.
5. I very much dislike speaking in this situation.

C. Stuttering
1. I don't stutter at all (or only very rarely) in this situation.
2. I stutter mildly (for me) in this situation.
3. I stutter with average severity (for me) in this situation.
4. I stutter more than average (for me) in this situation.
5. I stutter severely (for me) in this situation.

D. Frequency
1. This is a situation I meet very often, two or three times a day, or even more, on the average.
2. I meet this situation at least once a day with rare exceptions (except Sunday perhaps).
3. I meet this situation from three to five times a week on the average.
4. I meet this situation once a week, with few exceptions, and occasionally I meet it twice a week.
5. I rarely meet this situation--certainly not as often as once a week.

Figure 6.5. Stutterers' Self-Rating of Reactions to Speech Situations. (From Johnson, W., Darley, F., & Spriestersbach, D.C. (1952). *Diagnostic Manual in Speech Correction.* New York: Harper & Row. Copyright 1952 by Harper & Row. Copyright renewed 1980 by Edna B. Johnson, Frederick L. Darley and Duane C. Spriestersbach. Reprinted with permission of the publisher.)

	Avoidance	Reaction	Stuttering	Frequency
1. Ordering in a restaurant.	_____	_____	_____	_____
2. Introducing myself (face to face).	_____	_____	_____	_____
3. Telephoning to ask price, train fare, etc.	_____	_____	_____	_____
4. Buying plane, train or bus ticket.	_____	_____	_____	_____
5. Short class recitation (10 words or less).	_____	_____	_____	_____
6. Telephoning for taxi.	_____	_____	_____	_____
7. Introducing one person to another.	_____	_____	_____	_____
8. Buying something from store clerk.	_____	_____	_____	_____
9. Conversation with a good friend.	_____	_____	_____	_____
10. Talking with an instructor after class or in his/her office.	_____	_____	_____	_____
11. Long distance call to someone I know.	_____	_____	_____	_____
12. Conversation with father.	_____	_____	_____	_____
13. Asking girl for date (or talking to man who asks me for date.	_____	_____	_____	_____
14. Making short speech (1–2 minutes).	_____	_____	_____	_____
15. Giving my name over telephone.	_____	_____	_____	_____
16. Conversation with my mother.	_____	_____	_____	_____
17. Asking a secretary if I can see the employer.	_____	_____	_____	_____
18. Going to house and asking for someone.	_____	_____	_____	_____
19. Making a speech to unfamiliar audience.	_____	_____	_____	_____
20. Participating in committee meeting.	_____	_____	_____	_____
21. Asking instructor question in class.	_____	_____	_____	_____
22. Saying hello to friend going by.	_____	_____	_____	_____
23. Asking for a job.	_____	_____	_____	_____
24. Telling a person a message from someone else.	_____	_____	_____	_____
25. Telling a funny story with one stranger in a crowd.	_____	_____	_____	_____
26. Parlor game requiring speech.	_____	_____	_____	_____
27. Reading aloud to friends.	_____	_____	_____	_____
28. Participating in a bull session.	_____	_____	_____	_____
29. Dinner conversation with strangers.	_____	_____	_____	_____
30. Talking with my barber/hairdresser.	_____	_____	_____	_____
31. Telephoning to make appointment or to arrange to meet someone.	_____	_____	_____	_____
32. Answering roll call in class.	_____	_____	_____	_____
33. Asking at a desk for book or card to be filled out, etc.	_____	_____	_____	_____
34. Taking with someone I don't know well while waiting for bus, class, etc.	_____	_____	_____	_____
35. Talking with other players during game.	_____	_____	_____	_____
36. Taking leave of a host or hostess.	_____	_____	_____	_____
37. Conversation with friend while walking.	_____	_____	_____	_____
38. Buying stamps at post office.	_____	_____	_____	_____
39. Giving directions to stranger.	_____	_____	_____	_____
40. Taking leave of a girl/boy after date.	_____	_____	_____	_____
TOTALS	_____	_____	_____	_____
AVERAGES (divide total by # of answers)	_____	_____	_____	_____

Figure 6.5.—Continued

PERCEPTIONS OF STUTTERING INVENTORY (PSI)

The symbols S, A, and E after each item denote struggle (S), avoidance (A), and expectancy (E). In practice, these symbols are not included in the Inventory, but are listed on a separate scoring key.

$$\underline{S} \quad \underline{A} \quad \underline{E}$$

Name _____ Age _____   # _____

Examiner _____ Date _____   % _____

Directions

Here are sixty statements about stuttering. Some of these may be characteristic of your stuttering. Read each item carefully and respond as in the examples below.

Characteristic
of me

_____   Repeating sounds

Put a check mark (x) under "characteristic of me" if repeating sounds is part of your stuttering; if it is not characteristic, leave the space blank.

"Characteristic of me" refers only to what you do now, not to what was true of your stuttering in the past and which you no longer do; and not what you think you should or should not be doing. Even if the behavior described occurs only occasionally or only in some speaking situations, if you regard it as characteristic of your stuttering, check the space under "characteristic of me."

Characteristic
of me

_____   1. Avoiding talking to people in authority (e.g.,
                       a teacher, employer or clergyman). (A).

_____   2. Feeling that interruptions in your speech (e.g.,
                       pauses, hesitations, or repetitions) will lead
                       to stuttering. (E).

_____   3. Making the pitch of your voice higher or lower
                       when you expect to get "stuck" on words. (E).

Figure 6.6. Perceptions of Stuttering Inventory. (From Woolf, G. (1967). The assessment of stuttering as struggle, avoidance, and expectancy. Br J Disord Commun, 2, 158–171. Reprinted with permission of the publisher.)

_____   4. Having extra and unnecessary facial movement (e.g., flaring your nostrils during speech attempts). (S).

_____   5. Using gestures as a substitute for speaking (e.g., nodding your head instead of saying "yes" or smiling to acknowledge a greeting). (A).

_____   6. Avoiding asking for information (e.g., asking for directions or inquiring about a train schedule). (A).

_____   7. Whispering words to yourself before saying them or practicing what you are planning to say long before you speak. (E).

_____   8. Choosing a job or hobby because little speaking would be required. (A).

_____   9. Adding an extra or unnecessary sound, word or phrase to your speech (e.g., "uh," "well," or "let me see") to help yourself get started. (E).

_____   10. Replying briefly using the fewest words possible. (A).

_____   11. Making sudden, jerky, or forceful movements with your head, arms or body during speech attempts (e.g., clenching your fist, jerking your head to one side). (S).

_____   12. Repeating a sound or word with effort. (S).

_____   13. Acting in a manner intended to keep you out of a conversation or discussion (e.g., being a good listener, pretending not to hear what was said, acting bored, or pretending to be in deep thought). (A).

_____   14. Avoiding making a purchase (e.g., avoiding going into a store or buying stamps in the post office). (A).

_____   15. Breathing noisily or with great effort while trying to speak. (S).

_____   16. Making your voice louder or softer when stuttering is expected. (E).

_____   17. Prolonging a sound or word (e.g., m-m-m-m-my) while trying to push it out. (S).

Figure 6.6.—Continued

_____ 18. Helping yourself to get started talking by laughing, coughing, clearing your throat, gesturing, or some other body activity movement. (E).

_____ 19. Having general body tension during speech attempts (e.g., shaking, trembling, or feeling "knotted up" inside). (S).

_____ 20. Paying particular attention to what you are going to say (e.g., the length of a word, or the position of a word in a sentence). (E).

_____ 21. Feeling your face getting warm and red (as if you are blushing) as you are struggling to speak. (S).

_____ 22. Saying words or phrases with force or effort. (S).

_____ 23. Repeating a word or phrase preceding the word on which stuttering is expected. (E).

_____ 24. Speaking so that no word or sound stands out (e.g., speaking in a singsong voice or in a monotone). (E).

_____ 25. Avoiding making new acquaintances (e.g., not visiting with friends, not dating, or not joining social, civic, or church groups). (A).

_____ 26. Making unusual noises with your teeth during speech attempts (e.g., grinding or clicking your teeth). (S).

_____ 27. Avoiding introducing yourself, giving your name, or making introductions. (A).

_____ 28. Expecting that certain sounds, letters or words are going to be particularly "hard" to say (e.g., words beginning with the letter "s"). (E).

_____ 29. Giving excuses to avoid talking (e.g., pretending to be tired or pretending lack of interest in a topic). (A).

_____ 30. "Running out of breath" while speaking. (S).

_____ 31. Forcing out sounds. (S).

Figure 6.6.—Continued

Perhaps we should place a voice problem in a separate category. We sometimes find that stutterers may be hoarse. We feel that many times this may be the result of laryngeal tension related to stuttering. If stuttering treatment is successful, the hoarseness may disappear. Once again, we take our cue from the client. If the problem bothers the client, and isn't remediated by treatment, we address it in therapy. If the hoarseness is of recent origin, we may refer the client for an otolaryngological exam to rule out a serious laryngeal pathology.

_____ 32. Feeling that your fluent periods are unusual, that they cannot last, and that sooner or later you will stutter. (E).

_____ 33. Concentrating on relaxing or not being tense before speaking. (E).

_____ 34. Substituting a different word or phrase for the one you had intended to say. (A).

_____ 35. Prolonging or emphasizing the sound preceding the one on which stuttering is expected. (E).

_____ 36. Avoiding speaking before an audience. (A).

_____ 37. Straining to talk without being able to make a sound. (S).

_____ 38. Coordinating or timing your speech with a rhythmic movement (e.g., tapping your foot or swinging your arm). (E).

_____ 39. Rearranging what you had planned to say to avoid a "hard" sound or word. (A).

_____ 40. "Putting on an act' when speaking (e.g., adopting an attitude of confidence or pretending to be angry). (E).

_____ 41. Avoiding the use of the telephone. (A).

_____ 42. Making forceful and strained movements with your lips, tongue, jaw or throat (e.g., moving your jaw in an uncoordinated manner). (S).

_____ 43. Omitting a word, part of a word, or a phrase which you had planned to say (e.g., words with certain sounds or letters). (A).

_____ 44. Making "uncontrollable" sounds while struggling to say a word. (S).

_____ 45. Adopting a foreign accent, assuming a regional dialect, or imitating another person's speech. (E).

_____ 46. Perspiring much more than usual while speaking (e.g., feeling the palms of your hands getting clammy). (S).

_____ 47. Postponing speaking for a short time until certain you can be fluent (e.g., pausing before "hard" words). (E).

Figure 6.6.—Continued

_____ 48. Having extra and unnecessary eye movements while speaking (e.g., blinking your eyes or shutting your eyes tightly). (S).

_____ 49. Breathing forcefully while struggling to speak. (S).

_____ 50. Avoiding talking to others of your own age group (your own or opposite sex). (A).

_____ 51. Giving up the speech attempt completely after getting "stuck" or if stuttering is anticipated. (A).

_____ 52. Straining the muscles of your chest or abdomen during speech attempts. (S).

_____ 53. Wondering whether your will stutter or how you will speak if you do stutter. (E).

_____ 54. Holding your lips, tongue, or jaw in a rigid position before speaking or when getting "stuck" on a word. (S).

_____ 55. Avoiding talking to one or both of your parents. (A).

_____ 56. Having another person speak for you in a difficult situation (e.g., having someone make a telephonecall for you or order for you in a restaurant). (A).

_____ 57. Holding your breath before speaking. (S).

_____ 58. Saying words slowly or rapidly preceding the word on which stuttering is expected. (E).

_____ 59. Concentrating on how you are going to speak (e.g., thinking about where to put your tongue or how to breath). (E).

_____ 60. Using your stuttering as the reason to avoid a speaking activity. (A).

Figure 6.6.—Continued

OTHER FACTORS

In this section, we will be discussing evaluation of the following factors: intelligence, academic adjustment, psychological adjustment, and vocational adjustment. Each of these factors can affect the treatment of the adult or adolescent stutterer and, therefore, must be considered in planning therapy.

If a stutterer has below normal intelligence, he may have difficulty following the regimen of a typical therapy program. Usually, the clinician will know beforehand if the stutterer she is to evaluate has below normal intelligence. Adolescent stutterers in the schools will usually be identified as mentally handicapped if they are, and they are likely to be, in a special class. Adults, too, are usually previously identified as mentally handicapped if such is the case, because either the referral source will indicate this or it will be evident that a guardian has filled out the case history form.

Problems of academic adjustment in the adolescent stutterer usually become apparent either through the original referral or when the clinician interviews the child's teachers in the evaluation process. These interviews with the child's teachers are described in more detail in the next section, the Elementary School Child. An example of poor academic adjustment relevant to stuttering is a student's being in conflict with a teacher who insists he should present orally when the student is unwilling to do so.

In Chapter 3, we indicated that there are no group differences between stutterers and nonstutterers in their degree of psychological health. However, we sometimes see stutterers who do not function well in their environments. They may be unable to achieve a satisfying marriage. They may be unable to hold a job, or they may be socially withdrawn. The clinician should be alert to the effect these adjustment problems may have on treatment. If she suspects, as treatment progresses (or doesn't), that psychological problems are interfering with treatment, she may wish to refer these clients for psychological help. The clinician should take care, in this case, to ask professional colleagues for recommendations as to who are the most effective psychotherapists in the area.

Psychological problems relevant to stuttering may also become apparent in the interview when the onset of stuttering is explored. Sudden onset after a psychological trauma, particularly if the onset is in late adolescence or adulthood, may indicate psychogenic stuttering. We have found that, if the psychological effects of the trauma have subsided, the adolescent or adult client may respond well to our treatment approach, which is described in Chapter 8. If it is clear that psychological factors are still affecting the client's speech and behavior, or if there is doubt, refer the client for a psychological evaluation. Unless the disorder is psychosis, in which case stuttering therapy is not recommended, a client with a psychological problem may respond well to a combination of psychotherapy and stuttering therapy.

INTERVIEW WITH PARENTS OF ADOLESCENT

When we evaluate an adolescent stutterer, we want to talk with his parents to obtain more background information about the client, to give them an opportunity to express their concerns and feelings privately, and to let them know what we will be doing with their child.

We begin the initial interview with the parents of the adolescent stutterer by asking them to describe the problem as they see it. We encourage them to express their fears, concerns and frustrations, and we listen carefully. We try to get an understanding of how the young client functions within his family. We usually ask questions such as these: What is their child's stuttering like at home? How does he seem to feel about it—is he embarrassed or does he show fear of talking or anger? How do the parents feel about it? What are family members' reactions to it—what do they do when he stutters? Has their child been seen anywhere else for therapy? If so, what were the results? Although parents may ask what can be done with their child and what they should do, we prefer to wait until after we've seen the youngster before answering these questions.

Adolescents strive to become more and more independent from their parents. Therefore, we find that therapy works best if the adolescent is treated as an adult. We begin fostering this independence by first talking to the teenaged client separately from his parents so that he can give us his own view of the situation and how he views the prospect of treatment. Following this, and following our meeting with the parents, described above, we meet with the parents and the teenaged client together to find mutual agreement about the parents' and the teenager's role in treatment. This is often an important time. It serves to let the youngster know that we respect his ability to work independently from his parents; it serves to let the parents know that they can be most helpful by being supportive but not directive.

Diagnosis

After we gather the information described above, we need to integrate this material to determine if the client stutters, and if so, what treatment level would be appropriate. Typically, clients in this age range will be advanced stutterers. However, some of the adolescent stutterers may be in the intermediate stage. Let us first consider the possibility that our client turns out not to be a stutterer.

In rare cases, individuals who are normally disfluent, though perhaps highly normally disfluent, may be referred by teachers, employers, or friends. These individuals will have phrase repetitions, circumlocutions, revisions, and hesitations—the types of disfluencies we descibed in Chapter 4 as characteristic of normal disfluency. These types of disfluencies are relatively infrequent in children after their elementary school years. However, some adolescents and adults may simply be on the disfluent end of the continuum of normal fluency. In addition to differences in the unit-size of their disfluencies, they will be clearly distinguishable from stutterers because they will have neither secondary behaviors nor negative feelings and attitudes. Our role in this case is to explain to the individual and to the referring person, when there is one, that these disfluencies are normal and need not be of concern. It might be emphasized to the referring source, particularly in the case of the adolescent, that excessive attention to these disfluencies is probably more harmful than helpful.

Another need for differential diagnosis, besides instances of normal disfluency, is in cases where cluttering, neurogenic disfluency, and psychogenic disfluency must be distinguished from stuttering.

Some of the salient features of cluttering in the adult or adolescent are rapid, somewhat unintelligible speech, frequent repetitions of syllables, lack of awareness or concern about speech, disorganized thought processes, and language problems. Cluttering sometimes coexists with stuttering and both disorders may respond to a highly structured fluency-shaping approach for treatment. The book *Cluttering* by Deso Weiss (1964) is a prime source for diagnostic and treatment information. In addition, an excellent chapter by David Daly (1986), "The Clutterer," in the book *The Atypical Stutterer* describes assessment and therapy procedures.

Neurogenic disfluency in the adolescent or adult may appear as the result of stroke, head trauma, or neurological disease. Symptoms are likely to be repetitive disfluencies, but may include blockages as well. Since stuttering commonly begins in childhood, if a client reports onset after age 12, neurogenic disfluency is a possibility. A chapter by Nancy Helm-Estabrooks (1986), "Neurogenic Stuttering in Adults," in *The Atypical Stutterer*, discusses diagnostic signs and treatment possibilities.

Disfluency that begins in adolescence or adulthood may also result from psychological trauma. A recent article by Carole Roth, Arnold Aronson, and Leo Davis (1989) suggests that psychogenic disfluency may be caused by "environmental stress or interpersonal conflict." They found that disfluencies were often accompanied by what appear to be neurological signs such as weakness, numbness, tingling, and seizure-like activity. Disfluencies included repetitions, prolongations, blocks, secondary behaviors, and feelings and attitudes similar to those of stutterers. Psychogenic disfluency was generally found to be amenable to traditional therapy approaches both during the diagnostic interview and during treatment. In our own experience, however, not all psychogenic disfluency responds to treatment. In one case of a man who had been mute for several years before beginning to show symptoms of severe stuttering, we were unable to make any change in his disfluencies whatsoever using slow speech, singing, and delayed auditory feedback. Further information about psychogenic disfluency can be obtained from another recent article about this disorder, by Mahr and Leith (1990). In summary, when late onset disfluencies are seen and they are associated with psychological stress and conflict, psychogenic disfluency should be suspected. Traditional treatments such as those described in Chapter 8 may be helpful. The patient should be referred for both psychological and neurological assessment, in case underlying factors in these areas require treatment.

When the clinician determines that stuttering treatment would be appropriate for the client, whether the client's stuttering is of the "garden variety" type or has another etiology, the focus turns to consideration of what level of treatment to select for the client. As we said earlier, adult and adolescent stutterers are most likely to be at the advanced developmental/treatment level. Signs of this level include core behaviors—repetitions, prolongations, and blocks—all with tension, secondary behaviors of escape and avoidance, and negative feelings and attitudes about communication in general and about stuttering in particular.

DETERMINING DEVELOPMENTAL/TREATMENT LEVEL

The determination of developmental/treatment level for the adolescent or adult stutterer is based to a large extent on the client's age. The intermediate and advanced treatment approaches are both suited for stutterers' whose core behaviors are blocks, who have escape and avoidance as secondary symptoms, and whose attitudes about speech are relatively negative. The stutterer suited to the advanced level will usually have more entrenched negative attitudes about speech and about himself as a speaker simply because he has been stuttering longer. The major difference beween the intermediate and advanced treatment levels is that the advanced level demands more independence and responsibility from the client.

Consequently, the clinician will place adult clients at the advanced level, but will determine the adolescent's placement by how much he can take responsibility for a certain amount of self-therapy.

Intermediate Stuttering.   The stutterer who is at the intermediate level will probably be younger than 14. His stuttering pattern will be characterized by escape and avoidance behaviors and considerable tension on his blocks, prolongations, and repetitions. He will, as well, be avoiding some speaking situations. Moreover, his feelings and attitudes revealed by our interview, by his parents and teachers, and by the questionnaires we have used will suggest fairly negative speech attitudes.

Advanced Stuttering.   The stutterer who fits into the advanced developmental/treatment level will usually be 14 or older, and be sufficiently mature to handle the assignments which are involved in advanced treatment. His stuttering pattern will be similar to the intermediate stutterer's, but he may have even more habituated patterns of avoidance and escape (i.e., patterns that appear to be highly automatized and rapidly performed). He will probably avoid difficult speaking situations as well. We also often find in the advanced stutterer strong negative concepts of himself and his impression of his listeners' view of him. He may feel, for example, "I must be awfully incompetent to talk like this" or "People think I'm dumb because I stutter."

Closing Interview

We will make the assumption here that our client is a stutterer. By this point in the evaluation, we have a pretty good picture of our client's stuttering and where we will start therapy. We begin by summarizing to the client our impression of his stuttering pattern (core and secondary behaviors) and his attitudes and feelings. One of our aims here is to let him know we understand him and understand why he does what he does. We feel it is important to let him know that, given the stuttering that he has, it is no surprise that he would use the various secondary behaviors and avoidance tactics that he does. We accept his behaviors rather than criticize them. We then let him know that we feel we can work with him to help him discover other ways to respond. Here we ensure that he feels that he will not be alone, but we will be working alongside him, and that we will gradually give him more and more responsibility to work on his own.

We then outline the particular type of therapy we have chosen for this client. Afterward, we may give an adult client an assignment to begin the process of his taking part of the responsibility for treatment. This will also take advantage of the fact that many adult clients are highly motivated to change at the time they come in for an evaluation. We don't generally do this with adolescent clients, but there are exceptions. Some adolescent clients may be highly reluctant, rather than highly motivated at this time. With them, we often end our evaluation session by striking a bargain to try at least four sessions of therapy before they make a decision about treatment. We may also give them the booklet *Do You Stutter: A Guide for Teens* (Fraser & Perkins, 1987), so they can read about the process of therapy on their own and develop realistic (and motivating) expectations about its potential outcome.

PRESCHOOL CHILD

Preassessment

CASE HISTORY FORM

This form, shown in Figure 6.7, is sent out to the parents several weeks prior to the assessment. The information in it informs the clinician about the parents' perception of the problem at present, as well as background on the onset and

<u>Case History for Children</u>

Date:_____

Child's Name:_____
            (First)   (Middle)   (Last)

Address: _____

             _____ Tel:_____

Date of Birth:_____ Place of Birth:_____

Medicaid #:_____ Referring Physician:_____

Child lives with: Own parent/s:_____ Other relative:_____
                  Foster parent/s:_____ Institution:_____
(If other than own parents, give name/s):
_____

Name of person completing this form:_____

Relationship to child:_____

FAMILY:
<u>Father:</u>
  Name:_____ Age:_____
  Is he living with family?_____ Occupation:_____
  Employed by:_____
  Educational level: _____
  Telephone (Home): _____ (Work): _____
  Social Security #:_____

<u>Mother:</u>
  Name:_____ Age:_____
  Is she living with family?_____ Occupation:_____
  Employed by: _____
  Educational level:_____
  Telephone (Home): _____ (Work):_____
  Social Security #:_____

Brothers and sisters:
  (Name)   (Age)   (Name)   (Age)

  _____ _____ _____ _____
  _____ _____ _____ _____
  _____ _____ _____ _____

Figure 6.7. Case history form for children.

PROGRESSION OF SPEECH/LANGUAGE PROBLEM:

1. Describe your child's problem: _____

   _____

   _____

   _____

2. How has your child's problem changed since you first noticed
   it? _____

   _____

   _____

3. How does this problem affect your child? (In family interactions, social interactions, school, etc.) _____

   _____

   _____

4. Check items you feel apply to your child:

   ___Talks very little   ___Has limited vocabulary
   ___Talks excessively   ___Speech cannot be understood
   ___Talks too fast   ___Has nasal-sounding speech
   ___Uses poor grammar   ___Stutters
   ___Has poor memory   ___Cleft Palate
   ___Has hearing loss

5. Do any other members of your family have speech or hearing
   problems? Please describe:_____

   _____

6. Have you ever questioned your child's ability to hear
   normally? Yes_____ No_____ Why?:_____

   _____

7. Has your child had ear infections? Yes_____   No_____
   Which ear?:_____   Describe:_____

   _____

8. Has your child received medical attention for his/her
   earaches/infections?:_____   Name of Physician:_____

Figure 6.7.—Continued

development. This information is used as a starting place for further questions during the parent interview.

TAPE RECORDING

We ask the parents of a preschool child to send us an audiotape of their child's speech, along with the case history form. When they are able to do so, we

9. Is child's hearing the same from day to day? Yes____   No____
    Please describe:_____

    _____

10. Does your child have difficulty determining which direction
    sound comes from? Yes____   No____   Describe:_____

    _____

11. Does your child seem to favor one ear over the other when
    listening? Yes____   No____   When? _____

12. Has your child ever had his/her hearing tested? Yes___
    No___   By Whom?_____   When?_____

13. What doctors, clinics or diagnostic centers have seen your
    child? _____

    _____

14. Is your child receiving help now? Yes___   No___
    Where?_____

MEDICAL HISTORY
Prenatal:
  Did mother have any of the following during pregnancy?
  When? (Check appropriate column.)

  Condition_____0-3 months_____3-9 months
   German measles_____
   Hepatitis_____
   Toxemia_____
   Bleeding_____
   Anemia_____
   Extreme nausea_____
   Rh incompatibility_____
   High blood pressure_____
   Unusual fatigue_____
   Emotional upset_____

   Were drugs or medications given to mother? _____
   If so, what?_____

Postnatal: (Fill in with information you remember.)
   Was delivery in a hospital?_____   Birth weight:_____
   Length of pregnancy (weeks): _____   Length of labor:_____
   Was labor induced? _____   Caesarian delivery?_____
   Was baby premature?_____   Postmature?_____
   Did baby require oxygen?_____   Incubator?_____
   Did baby leave hospital with mother?_____
     If not, why?_____

Figure 6.7.—Continued

find this helpful because we can preview the child's speech soon after the parents
have contacted us. In cases where several weeks go by between the parents' contact
and our evaluation, the child's stuttering may have diminished substantially and we
may witness only the most fluent cycle of the child's speech. In addition to pre-
viewing the child's stuttering, the tape often gives us a chance to learn a little about
the parent-child interactions.

HEALTH:
Child has had: (Check appropriate items.)

___ German measles	___ Mumps	___ Bronchitis
___ High fever	___ Measles	___ Convulsions
___ Chicken pox	___ Allergies	___ Myringotomy
___ Scarlet fever	___ Influenza	___ Adenoidectomy
___ Tonsillitis	___ Earaches	___ Tonsillectomy
___ Frequent colds	___ Asthma	

Other serious conditions or accidents? (Please describe.)

Is child taking any medication at present? (Please specify.)

DEVELOPMENTAL HISTORY: (Check appropriate items.)

___ Development appears to be usual in every way
___ Development unusual (as compared to other children in family)
___ Sleeps excessively
___ Sleeps little   ___ Toilet trained (age___)
___ Behavior no problem   ___ Dresses self
___ Behavior difficult   ___ Child is aggressive
___ Child is sociable   ___ Child is explosive
___ Child is withdrawn   ___ Fearful of new situations
___ Coordination poor   ___ Family upset
___ Difficulty swallowing   ___ Child is impulsive

At what age did child: Sit up alone?___   Walk alone?___
   Say single words?____   Use sentences?____

EDUCATIONAL HISTORY:

Child's present school:_____ Grade:_____

Kindergarten/Nursery School experiences? Yes____   No____
   Where?_____

His/her schoolwork is: Good___   Average___   Poor___

Grades failed (if any): _____

History of school problems? Yes____   No_____ (Describe:)
_____

Describe behavior in school:_____
_____

Has difficulty with: Reading____   Math____   Writing____

Figure 6.7.—Continued

Assessment

PARENT-CHILD INTERACTION

When possible, we observe one or both parents interacting with their child. We prefer to do this at the beginning of the evaluation for several reasons. First, parents may be less affected by our orientation toward stuttering and may thereby give us a more natural sample. Second, this interaction gives us a chance to

What specific questions do you have about your child that you
   would like us to try to answer? (Use back of sheet if
   necessary.)

If, in order to help your child, it is appropriate to send
reports to other agencies or professional persons, or to contact
other agencies or professional persons, please indicate your
permission by signing below.

I authorize and request _(clinic name and address)__ to obtain
and/or exchange pertinent medical/educational information. It is
understood that all information will be kept confidential.

Name:_____

Relationship to child:_____

Date:_____

Figure 6.7.—Continued

see the child's stuttering first-hand. We can see, for example, how much the child
seems aware of the stuttering, how much accessory behavior there is, and whether
or not the child appears embarrassed. These are all things that may not be evident
from an audiotape. Third, we can observe the ways in which the parents interact
with their child. Do they interrupt? Do they correct? Do they talk at a high rate,
with complex vocabulary and syntax? These observations add to what we may have
learned from an audiotape, and they provide a good information base from which
we can plan our parent interview and our recommendations for treatment.

The parent-child interaction can be done formally or informally. Some
clinicians observe the interaction in the waiting room and make only mental notes
about it. Others who work in preschool programs may visit the child's home and
arrange to observe a parent-child interaction while they sit quietly in the same
room. Still others, ourselves included, videotape the parents and the child in a play-
style interaction in a treatment room supplied with toys and games. In cases where
audio or videotaping can be done, this sample of the child's speech may be assessed
as described below, in the section on analysis of speech and related behavior.

PARENT INTERVIEW

We begin by letting the parents know the kinds of things we will be doing
with them and their child during the evaluation, and assure them there will be a
time at the end when we will share our opinions and recommendations. Sometimes
in the initial interview, parents will ask direct questions about whether the things
they are doing are wrong. We let them know that, in our view, stuttering is often
the result of many things acting together and that parents do not cause it. We try

not to give advice about what they should change or what they should do until we have interviewed the parents and assessed the child directly. In our experience, we are more accurate and parents are more receptive to recommendations if we delay the discussion of what to do until after the available information can be pulled together, in the closing interview.

We begin the initial interview by asking the parents to describe the problem their child is having. We ask an open-ended question such as "Tell me about Billy's speech" or "Please describe Billy's speech and tell me what concerns you." When they have had a chance to share their concerns, we then gather information about the child's birth and development. It should be noted that we rarely ask all of the nineteen questions listed below. Instead, we find out what we want to know in a long discussion punctuated by both their questions and ours. We list these questions because we have found information in these areas to be helpful.

1. Were there any problems with your pregnancy or the birth of this child?

Although there is little indication that stutterers as a group have difficult birth histories, there is an increased incidence of stuttering in brain-damaged individuals. Thus, with this question, we are seeking to rule out the possibility of congenital brain damage. If a difficult pregnancy or birth is noted, we might be prepared to examine the child's motor and cognitive development more closely.

2. What was the child's speech and language development like? How did it compare to his siblings' development and to your expectations?

Because we believe that the first appearance of stuttering may be influenced by the "processing load" that language development may put on speech production, we think it is important to understand the course of a child's overall speech and language development. We explore the possibility that the child's language is developing so rapidly that his motor system cannot contend with it. We also examine the possibility that the child is delayed in language development and is frustrated and finding it hard to talk.

3. What was the child's motor development like, compared to his brothers and sisters or to other children?

Here, we are interested in the parents' general impressions. Did this child seem to develop motor skills at an average pace, or do they think he might have been delayed? Some indications of the normal range of gross and fine motor development, as well as personal-social and speech-language development, can be found in the Denver Developmental Screening Test (Frankenburg & Dodds, 1967).

In our experience, many children who stutter appear to be slightly advanced in language development and, to a lesser extent, slightly delayed in motor skills. They may benefit from reduced language stimulation and from models of speech produced at a slow rate. Other children who stutter may be delayed in several areas; they may need treatment for language and articulation, integrated with therapy for stuttering.

4. Have any other members of your family had speech or language disorders?

We ask this general question and then ask, more specifically, if family members or any relatives have ever stuttered, had articulation or language disorders, or have been clutterers. To confirm that the disorder may have been a problem, we ask if the person ever received treatment. We use this knowledge when we describe our view of stuttering as a disorder that may have predisposing factors. Handled tactfully, a discussion of predisposing factors can help parents realize that their child's stuttering was not something they caused. This, in turn, can free them to facilitate the child's development of fluency.

If a parent him- or herself stutters, or used to, he or she may have strong negative feelings about the disorder, including guilt. This may need to be discussed, both in this initial interview and throughout treatment, if the child needs treatment. The way in which the parent handles his or her stuttering is also important because models of this behavior will influence the child. A parent who avoids words or otherwise tries to hide his stuttering may communicate this attitude to the child. This may move a child along to the intermediate level faster than if the parent accepts his disfluency, comments neutrally on it in front of the child, and uses facilitating techniques to handle it.

After obtaining this background information, we then try to learn about the onset and development of the child's stuttering.

5. When was the child's disfluency first noticed?

We have found that, if treatment can begin soon after the child has begun to stutter—within a few weeks or months, rather than a year or more—prognosis for recovery is very good. We therefore take this opportunity to praise the parents for acting promptly in bringing their child in for evaluation, if they have done so soon after they first sensed the child had a problem.

6. Was there anything special going on in the child's life when the disfluency started?

This may give us some leads about pressures to which the child is vulnerable. Knowing about these can help the clinician facilitate changes the parents can make to alleviate the stuttering. Examples of events surrounding the onset of disfluency are: birth of a sibling, moving to a new home, and growth spurts in aspects of language or cognition. Many times, of course, there are no special conditions surrounding onset of stuttering.

7. What was the disfluency like when it was first noticed?

Most stuttering begins with easy repetitions, although some may begin with prolongations, as well. In rare cases, stuttering may begin as complete blockages. This last type of stuttering may have considerable laryngeal tension, which treatment must address.

8. What, if any, changes have there been in the child's speech since the disfluency was first noticed?

Changes we are interested in here include frequency of disfluencies, types of disfluencies, and periods of remission. We are interested in whether the problem is developing or not. Is the frequency increasing? Is there more struggle now? Has the stuttering become chronic, instead of episodic? If the answers to some of these questions are "yes", it indicates that the child is moving toward becoming a beginning stutterer.

We now turn to the disorder in its current form:

9. Does the child appear to be aware of his disfluency?

If there appears to be no awareness, we are more likely to categorize the child as normally disfluent or a borderline stutterer than if he notices or is concerned by his disfluencies. If he is aware that he has difficulty with speaking or shows frustration, he may be a beginning stutterer. Note that this awareness may not be negative, but just a neutral level of awareness at early stages. Indications of this awareness include such things as the child commenting on his stuttering, either when it occurs or at some other time, or the fact that other people have brought it to the child's attention. Awareness may also be suggested if the child stops when he is disfluent and starts again, or if he laughs, cries, or hits himself when he stutters. Even without any of these signs, the child may still be aware of his stuttering.

In some instances, preschool children may have gone beyond neutral awareness and frustration; they may show negative feelings about talking and may have fear of certain words. They may comment that they wished they could speak like someone else, or may show some word avoidances.

10. Does the child sometimes appear to change a word because he expects to be disfluent on it?

Parents are usually able to guess this is happening because they can sense the child's apprehension about saying a word. We may also ask if the child changes words in midstream; that is, does he start a word, get stuck on it, and then change it? Both behaviors are obviously not good signs, and may suggest that the child is moving toward the intermediate stage of stuttering development.

11. Does the child seem to avoid talking in some situations, when he expects to be disfluent?

Again, this is something most parents know because they sense the child's fear of talking. This behavior, like the word avoidance discussed above, may indicate an intermediate level of stuttering.

12. What do the parents believe caused the problem?

In some cases, parents may have ideas, which we believe to be appropriate and accurate, about the possible etiology of their child's stuttering. In other cases, parents may have beliefs, which we think are incorrect, about causal factors and we respond to these with more accurate information. We are particularly sensitive to whether or not the parents blame themselves or each other for their child's stuttering. This is usually a good time to let the parents know that they are not to blame for their child's stuttering. We tell them that some children may have slight differences in their neurological organization for speech and that these may emerge as stuttering during the normal stresses and strains of growing up and learning to talk. The parents didn't cause the stuttering, although the pressures they may have inadvertently created may have precipitated it. But what is more important for them to realize is that they can be a crucial influence in helping their child respond to the stuttering in such a way that it becomes a minor problem, if any.

13. How do the parents feel about the child's disfluency problem?

The kinds of things we are looking for are: Do they feel concern? Guilt? Do they just assume the child will outgrow it? These parental feelings will obviously influence the child. Parent counseling may need to be directed toward these feelings. If the parents feel guilty, counseling to relieve the guilt is important. If the child is normally disfluent, but the parents are overly concerned, counseling may be directed at relieving this concern, so that the child himself does not become excessively concerned and thereby develop stuttering.

14. What, if anything, have the parents done about the problem?

This gives us an opportunity to see how the parents have responded to the child's disfluency. Have they, for example, suggested to the child that he slow down or stop and say the word again? This information will direct us in what we do in parent counseling. If the parents are correcting the child, we may ask them first to observe, then participate in treatment soon after we begin, so that they may develop appropriate ways of responding.

15. Has the child been seen anywhere else for the problem? If so, what were the outcomes?

This can be important in planning our therapy and in counseling the parents. For example, if their family doctor has told them their child will outgrow it, their experience here needs to be dealt with, since they obviously now are less convinced he will outgrow it. If the child has been in other treatment, it is important to know what advice the parents were given. Sometimes, parents have been given what we feel is excellent advice, but were not able to follow it. We need to find out why and to facilitate their changing these responses. We sometimes find that parents have had their child in successful therapy but have moved, and have sought us out for a continuation of the same kind of treatment. In these cases, we will likely contact the previous therapist and will explore with the parents what was done, so that we can continue to work in the same direction as the previous therapy. In some cases, parents may come to us seeking a second opinion, and we are able to reinforce what others have said, if we are in agreement. In other cases, they may have been advised to ignore the child's stuttering, and we might want to tactfully deal with the possibility of going in an entirely different direction.

16. When, and in which situations, does the child exhibit the most disfluency? The least disfluency?

This information will help us identify fluency disruptors and fluency facilitators. We obviously will want to use this information to help the parents facilitate the child's fluency, and we find it effective to point out, whenever possible, all the helpful things that the parents are already doing. Just the awareness that their child's stuttering is responding to environmental cues, and thereby has some logic to it, will help most parents feel more competent to manage it.

Once we feel we understand the child's current stuttering behavior, we ask about his social and emotional development.

17. How does your child get along with his brothers and sisters and other children?

We usually find that children who stutter relate fairly well to others, but we want to find out if the child's stuttering is interfering with his relationships. Sometimes, by asking this question, we learn about pressure and competition from siblings or teasing by a neighborhood bully.

18. What is your child's personality and temperament like?

Some children who stutter are more sensitive and fearful than other children. A child with this temperament may benefit from extra help in developing self-confidence.

We then finish with a very open-ended question, like this:

19. Is there anything else you can think of to tell us that will help us understand your child's stuttering?

Sometimes, it is not possible to direct questions to all areas of concern, and this question provides an opportunity for parents to provide information about which we have not thought of asking.

CLINICIAN-CHILD INTERACTION

One of the most important parts of preschool evaluation is the interaction between the clinician and the child. Here, the clinician can see directly what the child's disfluency is like, how he responds to various cues, and to what extent the child's disfluency is modifiable. We always tape-record this interaction for later analysis, since it is difficult to make notes as we are interacting. If videotape is available, it is preferable to audiotape, since visual cues are sometimes critical in determining a child's developmental/treatment level. If audiotape must be used, the clinician should make every effort to take notes on visual aspects of the child's disfluencies.

We focus our interaction on toys or games suitable to the child's age. The Playskool® farm or airport is a good example. We play alongside the child, letting him direct the action, following his lead, commenting on what he's doing or on what he's playing with. We refrain from questions when we first start, and we talk in an easy, relaxed manner, much like we would advise parents to do. If the child is stuttering similarly to the way the parents have described, we keep the same speech style throughout the interaction. However, if the child is entirely fluent or normally disfluent and the parents have described behaviors we feel are stuttering, we will speed up our speech rate and ask many questions. Occasionally, we interrupt at some point to elicit the disfluent speech, which is perhaps more characteristic. We do this to avoid misdiagnosing a child who is stuttering as a normally fluent speaker. An adult client of ours described an experience that illustrates our concern: When she was 5, she stuttered quite severely, and her parents were understandably concerned. Seeking the best help, her mother took her to a famous midwestern university speech clinic for an evaluation, but for reasons she never understood, she was relatively fluent throughout the entire evaluation. The clinicians observed this temporary fluency, and, despite her mother's protestations that her daughter stuttered at home, labeled her as a normal-speaking child and advised her mother to ignore any disfluency. Her disfluency gradually worsened and she became a severe, chronic stutterer.

We realize that, even by putting pressure on the child, we may not elicit stuttering that the child may have in other settings. Thus, the parent report and the recording made before the evaluation are of vital importance for our full understanding of the child's speech.

Talking About Stuttering.   Prior to the clinician-child interaction, we try to determine if the child is aware of his stuttering. If we think he isn't, we use only our observations in non-directive play to assess his speech. If it is pretty clear, from earlier information or from our own observation, that he is aware, we then try to determine how able the child is to talk about his stuttering. Sometimes, we will ask if he knows why he has come to see us. Most children will answer noncommittally, but some will be very forthcoming and say something like, "Because I don't talk right." This gives us an opening to go further and discuss his stuttering with the child. This is an important opportunity to let the child know he isn't alone—that we have known other children who get stuck on words and we have usually been able to help them. Some clinicians will help a child talk about his stuttering by first telling the child about another child who stutters (Bloodstein, personal communication, 1990). In discussing stuttering with a child, we usually try to use their vocabulary such as "getting stuck" or "having trouble on words." If the child indicates by his answer to the question of why he came to the evaluation that he isn't interested in discussing stuttering, we drop the issue for the moment and return to playing. Then, later, we might insert a few normal-sounding disfluencies in our speech and comment that we sometimes have trouble getting words out. We might play some more and then insert a few more disfluencies and ask the child if he ever has trouble like this. As before, the child's answer will either indicate that he is unwilling to discuss the stuttering or will give the clinician an opening to discuss little by little the child's problem with it. In summary, the goals of these attempts to discuss the child's disfluencies with him are: (a) to see if the child is accepting of himself and his disfluencies enough to discuss them and (b) to indicate to the child that he is not alone with the problem and, moreover, that we may be able to help him.

A Child Who Won't Talk.   At times, we will encounter a preschooler, especially a child who has trouble talking, who is reluctant to be separated from his parents. This may occur after the parent-child interaction has been observed, and we try to take the parents into a separate room to interview them while another clinician interacts with the child. A very shy child may start to cry and cling to his parents. Our suggestion would be not to force the child to separate. It's more important to have the child positively inclined toward the therapy situation rather than having unpleasant memories of his first visit, even if we don't get all the information we want. In this situation, we talk with the parents in one part of the room while the clinician plays with the child in another part. We will talk for a few minutes about general things, such as a typical day in their home or how they handle discipline, letting the child become familiar with the clinician with whom he's interacting. Then we may suggest to the parents that we and they move into an adjacent room but keep the door open. With this arrangement, we can usually talk about sensitive matters without being overheard. An alternative would be to let the child follow, leaving the clinician and toys in the first room and both doors open. The child may then become bored with the room in which his parents are talking, and wander back to the room with the other clinician and the toys. In our experience, it is very rare that a child has more than momentary difficulty separating.

At times, certain children will separate from their parents but won't interact with us during the evaluation. We then avoid asking direct questions. Instead, we take some time to play alongside the child, verbalizing as we do so. After several minutes, we will usually find that the child relaxes and begins to speak spontaneously. After this continues for several more minutes, we begin more direct interactions by asking questions about the toys with which we are playing. Only after the child gets quite comfortable with us do we attempt to discuss his trouble talking, and then only if we're quite sure he is aware of his stuttering. With some children, we do not even attempt to discuss their stuttering with them. We take our cues from the child and go slowly in this area. We can infer many things about the child's feelings from observations rather than direct questions.

A Child Who Is Entirely Fluent.   Some preschool children who stutter may be entirely fluent during the evaluation. In these cases, there are several options. First, the tape recording we asked the parent to send us may have a good enough sample of stuttering to use it for our speech sample. Second, if the child is in a particularly fluent episode, we may reschedule him for evaluation at a later time. If our recommendations to the parents enable them to change the environment enough in the meantime so that the child becomes fluent, the parents may wish to postpone the evaluation until and if the stuttering returns.

Speech Sample

This section describes how to analyze the sample taken of the preschool child's speech. Our procedures usually provide us with more than one speech sample to choose from: a tape recording the parents have sent in, the parent-child interaction, and the clinician-child interaction. We choose the sample that has the greatest amount of stuttering on it for the most detailed analysis, but we also note the extent of stuttering/fluency on the other samples.

Pattern of Disfluencies.   In this analysis, we will get information about whether or not the child is a stutterer and, if so, what developmental/treatment level he belongs in. We analyze six variables, listed below, to begin this determination. Our choice of variables owes much to a number of authors who have written about the differential diagnosis of preschool stuttering (Adams, 1977; Curlee, 1980; Riley & Riley, 1979).

1. Frequency of disfluencies. This is calculated on the entire sample, and is expressed as the number of disfluencies per 100 words (see Chapter 4 for details). Both normal disfluencies and those associated with stuttering are included in this count. Normally disfluent children usually have fewer than 10 disfluencies per 100 words.

2. Types of disfluencies. We identified 8 types of disfluencies in Chapter 4: part-word repetitions, single-syllable word repetitions, multisyllable word repetitions, phrase repetitions, interjections, revisions-incomplete phrases, prolongations, and tense pauses. Children who are normally disfluent are more likely to show revisions and multisyllable whole-word repetitions. Below age three-and-a-half, they will also show interjections. Part-word repetitions, prolongations, and tense pauses are more characteristic of stuttering children.

3. Nature of repetitions and prolongations. There are several dimensions to this variable. First, normally disfluent children are more likely to have only one extra unit to their repetition: li-like this. They may sometimes have two. But, as

the number of repetitions increases, so does the likelihood that the child is a stut-terer. Second, we listen to the tempo of the repetitions. If they are slow and regu-lar, the child is more likely to be appropriately categorized as a normally disfluent speaker. If they are rapid and irregular, it is more likely we will treat the child as a stutterer. Third, we observe the degree of tension in both the repetitions and pro-longations. Both visual and auditory cues help here; tension can be seen in facial expression and heard in increased pitch and more staccato voice quality. Children whom we would label as normally disfluent do not often show tension in their disfluencies.

4. Starting and sustaining airflow and phonation. The child whom we are likely to categorize as a stutterer will show difficulty here. He will have abrupt onsets and offsets of words, especially repeated words. He may also show momen-tary pauses with fixed articulator positions at the onset of words. Moreover, transi-tions between words may be abrupt, jerky, or broken.

5. Physical concomitants. We look for physical gestures that accompany disfluencies, especially those that are timed to the release of the disfluent sound. Examples are head nods, eye blinks, hand or finger movements. Here, we also in-clude extra noises such as the sounds of the child gritting his teeth or clicking his tongue.

6. Word avoidances. Another sign, which we sometimes see in a disfluent preschool child, that suggests that he stutters is word avoidance. This can be bla-tant, as when a child starts a word and then changes it, as in "pu-pu-pu . . . .dog," or it may be more subtle, as in saying "I don't know" when it's clear that he does. We also ask about word avoidances when we interview the child's parents. When the clinician interacts with a child, she may sometimes miss the avoidances in the live interaction. It may take a viewing of the tape of the interaction to pick them up. For example, after a recent evaluation, we were able to see on tape a very subtle avoidance that we had completely missed in the face-to-face interaction. We'd asked the child what he was going to dress as for Halloween. He pursed his lips for a "B," but when he couldn't get the word out, he immediately sang "Nananananah! Batman!"

In our experience, if the child shows any of the characteristics of stutter-ing described above, he should be considered at least a borderline stutterer. The presence of tension, stoppage of airflow or phonation, physical concomitants, or word avoidances will place him on a level above borderline. Details on this place-ment are given in the sections on diagnosis below.

Stuttering Severity Index (SSI). By this time in the proceedings, we should have a fairly good indication as to whether or not the child should be treated as a stutterer. If he is, we will want to obtain a standard sample of the child's speech to analyze with Riley's SSI, shown in Figure 6.3 (see the adult/adolescent evalua-tion section for details on this reference). Riley suggests that any child below third grade should be asked to describe a set of pictures to provide a sample of 150 words for analysis. The child may also be engaged in conversation, and if this sample shows more stuttering than the picture description, it should be used for the analy-sis. We typically use a 5 minute sample, rather than a 150 word sample, because it is easier to ensure that we have a complete sample as we are observing or interacting with the child. Frequency of stuttering, mean duration of the three longest stutters, and physical concomitants are scored, and the total score is computed. The total score permits a labeling ranging from Very Mild to Very Severe.

Speech Rate.   We assess the rate of preschool children's speech using the speech sample obtained for the SSI. Details on the counting and timing procedures were given in the section on assessment of speech rate of adults and adolescents, earlier in this chapter. Speech rates for three age groups of nonstuttering preschoolers have been obtained by Rebekah Pindzola, Melissa Jenkins, and Kari Lokken (1989). Children in their study were asked a series of questions from the Developmental Learning Materials picture cards, and rates were obtained in syllables per minute (SPM) only. Their samples consisted of 6 males and 4 females in each of three age groups. They found, for 3 year olds, 116-163 SPM; for 4 year olds, 117-183 SPM; and for 5 year olds, 109-183 SPM. Differences between age groups were not statistically significant, and no comparisons between males and females were made. Data on words per minute are not available. More research is needed on speech rates of young children before any firm conclusions can be made from assessment of a potentially stuttering preschooler. In the meantime, if the child is stuttering and his speech rate is substantially below the range given for his age, the child's rate of speech may be a problem for listeners, as well as for the child himself.

FEELINGS AND ATTITUDES

We assess the preschooler's feelings about stuttering by asking about them in the parent interview, by observing the parent-child interaction, and by bringing up the topic of stuttering, when appropriate, with the child in our interaction with him. Feelings and attitudes in the preschooler may range from apparent unawareness of difficulty, to mild embarrassment, to extreme hypersensitivity. A child may, for example, look slightly uncomfortable when we ask him why he's here, but he may venture that it's because he has trouble talking. At the other extreme, a child may cry at the prospect of talking to someone about his speech, and he may be deeply embarrassed and uncommunicative even if we gingerly approach the topic of speech or "getting stuck." We are often able to learn a great deal about this by watching the tape of our interaction with the child. With the ability to devote our whole attention to observing and with the possibility of replaying key segments, we find that the taped interaction is a payload of information about the child's feelings. The parent interview is also a valuable source for learning whether the child is simply frustrated at times or whether his feelings are escalating into embarrassment and downright fear.

The assessment of feelings and attitudes of the preschooler leads us to conclude, tentatively, whether the child (*a*) is unaware of his disfluencies; (*b*) is only occasionally aware of them and, even then, is only rarely and transitorily bothered by them; (*c*) is aware of them and frustrated by them; or (*d*) is highly aware of them; is frustrated by them, and afraid of them.

OTHER SPEECH AND LANGUAGE BEHAVIORS

When we evaluate the preschool child's speech for stuttering, we also screen for articulation, language, and voice problems. In addition, we make sure that his hearing has been checked recently and, if not, we arrange to have a hearing screening.

A child's language and/or articulation problems can usually be detected in the parent-child or clinician-child interactions that we sample. When we find apparent delays in these areas, we administer a formal test. The reader may wish to consult Bernthal and Bankson (1988), Hoffman, Schuckers, and Daniloff (1989), or Weiss, Gordon, and Lillywhite (1987) for testing articulatory and phonologic disorders, and Miller (1981) for assessment of language problems. We will discuss the management of concomitant articulation and language disorders in Chapter 10 on the treatment of the beginning stutterer.

Our view of the relationship between language and stuttering, described in Chapter 3, suggests that one of the pressures on a child who stutters may result from language that is significantly advanced over motor development. Thus, in evaluating a child's language and articulation, we explore the possibility that his language is above average for his age. In addition, we observe and question parents about general motor development, as well as about intelligibility of speech.

We believe that, when we find that a child is delayed in motor development relative to language, part of our emphasis in parent counseling should be to reduce some of the external pressures on language development. One indication that motor development might be delayed would be if the child began to use first words well before he began to walk (e.g., started using words at 9 months but did not begin walking until 18 months). Another indication would be if he had a large vocabulary and put together sentences well, but was often unintelligible and had some evident fine or gross motor problems. In these cases, we might work with the parents to reduce the length and complexity of their utterances in their speech to the child. We feel that parents' long, complex utterances may create excess demands, not only because input processing may be strained, but also because the child may sense that he should also speak with the same long and complex utterances. We also explore with parents other ways in which they may be inadvertently putting pressure on their child; for example, through extensive teaching of new vocabulary or by instructions on syntax. Unfortunately, some of the verbal activities that some parents most enjoy with their children, such as puns and other wordplay, as well as teaching them exotic multisyllabic words, may be just the extra pressure that may cause these children to stutter.

We also consider another possibility: rather than the child's language developing "too rapidly," his motor ability may be markedly delayed. A few children, we find, have obvious motor problems that may impair their coordination of respiration, phonation, and articulation with language production. Many of these children are aware that speech for them is difficult; they have already felt frustration and shame—not just about stuttering, but about the way they speak and the way they perform many other fine motor tasks. Therefore, we think it is important to improve their feelings about themselves as talkers as we work on their speech motor skills. These children seem to benefit especially from models of slow speech as well as specific activities that teach the child to speak more slowly.

In addition to exploring the possibility of language and articulation difficulties, we also want to assess the child's voice. A hoarse voice may be especially significant in the preschool stutterer because it may signify that the child is using considerable tension in his laryngeal muscles to cope with stuttering. We look closely at how the child is handling his blocks and listen for signs of excess laryngeal tension, such as pitch rises and hard glottal attacks. Since many of the techniques we will use in the treatment of the young stutterer focus on gentle onset of phonation and a relaxed style of speech, we usually don't treat voice separately from stuttering. However, if the child has other voice problems besides hoarseness or if hoarseness does not diminish with stuttering therapy, the clinician may want to refer the child to an otolaryngologist and follow a treatment approach such as those suggested by Boone (1983) and Wilson (1979).

OTHER FACTORS

In Chapter 3, we described a number of developmental influences on stuttering. In this section, we review them briefly so that they may be recognized if they are important in a particular preschool child's stuttering. Because much of this information usually comes from the parent interview, the reader may wish to consult Chapter 3 for further details about developmental influences before planning or conducting the parent interview.

Physical Development.   We like to ascertain what the child's general physical development was like, both in regard to gross motor skills and to oral motor development. Most children learn to walk at about 1 year, but they do not usually learn to walk and talk at the same time. If the child whom we are evaluating was delayed in walking, while advanced or average in talking, we may further explore the possibility that his stuttering was exacerbated by delayed motor development.

Cognitive Development.   Here we want to rule out retardation, which is associated with increased disfluency. We also would like to know if this child is currently going through a period of intense cognitive growth that, hypothetically, might temporarily take its toll on fluency.

Social-Emotional Development.   As the child grows, various tensions develop between him and his parents and siblings. Between the ages of 2 to 3 and 4 to 5, for example, many children will display a surge of negativism that may be felt throughout the family. When we ask, in the parent interview, about the conditions surrounding the onset or worsening of the child's stuttering, we explore social-emotional factors, as well as many others.

In Chapter 3, we described various life events that may affect a child's stuttering. We now examine the life events surrounding the onset of stuttering to see if upsetting events or difficult ongoing situations can be linked to the child's stuttering. Some events, like the birth of a new sibling, are happy ones, but they can create a disturbance in the psychological "homeostasis" of a family.

Speech and Language Environment.   We have indirectly referred to this factor, but here we are explicit: many children have their hands full trying to compete verbally with fast-talking, articulate adults. Children who stutter may find this particularly hard. We listen to the tape sent in by the parents and watch the parent-child interaction carefully for indications of a complicated verbal environment that may be like rough water to a new swimmer.

Diagnosis

We now turn to the task of pulling together the information we have gathered and making a diagnosis of our young client. We will decide whether the child needs treatment or not, and if he does, into which treatment level he should be placed. These decisions are made on the basis of data from all the sources we have tapped in our evaluation. These are the case history, home tape recording (if available), observation of parent-child interaction (if possible), parent interview, and the clinician-child interaction.

DETERMINING DEVELOPMENTAL/TREATMENT LEVEL

We may categorize the preschool child as normally disfluent, a borderline stutterer, a beginning stutterer, or, in rare cases, an intermediate stutterer. In the following paragraphs, we will present brief reviews of each level, but we recommend reading the relevant sections of Chapter 4 for details.

Normal Disfluency.   All of the characteristics for this level must be met for the child to be considered normally disfluent. This child will have fewer than 10 disfluencies per 100 words, and they will consist of more multisyllable and phrase repetitions, revisions, and interjections. When the disfluencies are repetitions, they will have two or fewer repeated items per instance of disfluency. The repetitions will be slow and regular. All disfluencies will be relatively relaxed, and the child will seem hardly aware of them and will certainly not be upset when he is.

A child may be considered borderline or above if he has any of the characteristics that are described in the following paragraphs. Place him at the level—borderline, beginning or intermediate—that has the child's salient characteristics.

Borderline Stuttering.   The child we place in this category will show more than 10 disfluencies per 100 words. They may be part-word repetitions and single-syllable word repetitions, as well as prolongations. Repetitions may be more than two per instance. Disfluencies will be loose and relaxed.

Beginning Stuttering.   The key features here are the presence of tension and hurry in stuttering. This may take the form of rapid and abrupt repetitions, pitch rises during repetitions and prolongations, difficulty getting airflow or phonation started, and some evidence of facial tension. The beginning stutterer shows signs that he is aware of his stuttering and may be quite frustrated by it. He may use a variety of escape behaviors, such as head nods or eye blinks, to terminate his blocks.

Intermediate Stuttering.   The child we place at this level will have the above characteristics, plus avoidance behaviors. The child will avoid words and situations, and he will feel both fear and shame toward his stuttering.

Although we use information from all sources to determine the child's level, we have found that our own observations of the parent-child and clinician-child interactions provide the most reliable data. Although parents are very helpful in describing the long-term changes in their child's stuttering, they frequently miss the many avoidance behaviors, such as starters, circumlocutions, and postponements, that are critical indicators of the more advanced levels of stuttering. Parents' reports do provide at least as much information about the child's feelings and attitudes as we can gather in observing the interactions in the clinic. Thus, parent reports and our own observations provide complementary and extremely valuable data. A vital adjunct to our direct observations is the videotapes of the parent-child and clinician-child interactions. We have sometimes revised our determination of the child's development/treatment level after viewing videotapes of interactions we have already directly observed.

ASSESSING OTHER FACTORS

In addition to determining how far the child's stuttering has advanced, we assess developmental and environmental factors that may be affecting his fluency. This information is critical for treating the preschool stutterer and for counseling his parents. The reader who is familiar with Chapter 3 will be able to draw from the case history, the parent interview, and the parent-child interaction relevant information with which to formulate hypotheses about developmental and environmental factors.

In a child whom we categorize as normally disfluent, we often find that spurts in physical, cognitive, or linguistic growth may be related to the appearance of disfluencies. We look for these and any other changes in a normally disfluent child's life to help explain to a parent why disfluencies may be occurring or increasing at this time.

In children we call borderline, beginning, or intermediate stutterers, we look for evidence of language growth outstripping motor development or, indeed, for evidence of any developmental asymmetries or delays. These may be important for us to consider as we work out a tentative treatment program. We are also sensitive to aspects of the environment, either normal or unusual, that may be putting enough pressure on the child to bring out stuttering. The most common areas we examine are the communication models of the parents and their standards for the child's speech and language. Do they talk fast and use complex language? Do they correct their child's speech or attempt to teach him more advanced language than he would typically use? We also note any events, such as the birth of a sibling or a pending divorce, that could be creating in the child the kind of anxiety or insecurity that appears to increase stuttering in some children.

The above sections cover most of the sources of information we have about the preschool child. Once we draw together these fragments of data and make some tentative conclusions about the child's speech and how to treat it, we meet with the parents again in a counseling and treatment-planning session. This ends the evaluation.

Closing Interview

We begin by describing the characteristics of the child's stuttering that we have observed in the parent-child and clinician-child observations. We try to stay away from jargon as we briefly describe the child's behaviors. We then review the important information the parents have provided in the case history and interview and give our estimate about how serious the child's problem is. If the stuttering is of serious concern, we say so. If the parents have indicated a feeling of guilt about their child's stuttering, we again reassure them that they aren't to blame for the problem, but that they will be crucial in helping to resolve it, in helping their child to respond to it in a healthy way. At this point, it is important to describe the treatment—environmental changes, indirect treatment, direct treatment. This will differ depending upon the developmental/treatment level of the child's problem.

NORMAL DISFLUENCY

If we believe the child should be considered normally disfluent, we deal with the parents' concern rather than with the child's disfluencies. In some cases, we might give the parents information about normal disfluency, such as this: during the preschool years, many normal children pass through periods of disfluency. Interjections, revisions, pauses, repetitions, and prolongations are commonly heard during this period. These disfluencies are usually fewer than 10 per 100 words spoken. Interjections and revisions are more common than part-word repetitions, and these part-word repetitions typically have only 1 or 2 repetitions per instance of disfluency. Normally disfluent children are generally unaware of their disfluencies and don't develop reactions to them. They gradually outgrow them.

In other cases, we might offer parents the following analogy to help them understand their child's disfluency: learning to speak is like learning many other skills, for example, riding a bike or learning to skate. The learner falls down a lot in the early stages. We try to find situations in the parents' own lives that are analogous and help them realize the value of an accepting environment. Parents who are concerned about their child's normal disfluency are reassured when they find out that it is normal, and they can take it from there. In those rare cases where the parents are still not convinced that their child's normal disfluencies are normal, we teach them to slow their speaking rates, simplify their language, and relieve other pressures that we mutually determine. Then, we set up further appointments to help them make these changes. For all parents of normally disfluent children, we keep the door wide open. This reassures them that help is near at hand, that we realize that it is possible that their child might actually develop stuttering someday, and that we want to help them further if that happens.

BORDERLINE, BEGINNING, OR INTERMEDIATE LEVEL STUTTERING

Our closing interview with these parents is usually the first of many sessions that we will spend together. Consequently, we don't need to accomplish everything in this meeting. Because the treatment of any preschool stutterer is largely focused on the home environment, we often begin our discussion with the things the parents can do at home. The chapter on the beginning stutterer contains more suggestions for parents about ways in which they can change the environment to reduce the pressure on their child. Refer to that section of Chapter 10 to see how you may help parents reduce environmental pressures. We may also discuss general principles and let them decide on specific stresses. We encourage them to first select a small number of potentially critical situations to work on. We find that if they see success at first, they will be highly motivated to continue the changes they have started.

We also give parents reading material to help them better understand stuttering and what they can do to help their child. We have found that two recent publications by the Speech Foundation of America provide a good basis for ongoing discussions. These are: *Stuttering and Your Child: Questions and Answers* (Conture & Fraser, 1989) and the pamphlet *If You Think Your Child is Stuttering* (Guitar & Conture, undated). We also may give parents an excellent publication from the National Easter Seal Society, *Understanding Stuttering: Information for Parents* (Cooper, 1979).

After brainstorming with the parents about changes they can begin to make, we also talk about appropriate treatment. We give a brief overview of the goals of this treatment and describe the important contribution the parents will make to the success of this treatment. We then ask the parents if they have further questions and end by scheduling the next meeting.

Occasionally, we find that, when it is time for the closing interview, we are still undecided about our diagnosis. We may need time to review the videotapes of the interactions with the child. In these cases, we summarize what the possibilities are and give the parents something specific on which to begin work. Then, we reschedule another meeting with them as soon as possible.

ELEMENTARY SCHOOL CHILD

Preassessment

CASE HISTORY FORM

This form is the same as that used for the preschool stutterer (Fig. 6.7). Obviously, many of the questions about speech and language development will be difficult for the parents to recall. We should not be too concerned about these for the elementary school-aged child, but we must remember to probe for those other speech and language delays that may be maintaining factors in an elementary school child's stuttering. An important section of the form for this age child is the one dealing with how the problem has changed since it was first noticed, what has been done about it, and how people have reacted to it. In addition, the section on educational history is valuable in letting us know, ahead of time, whether the child is having problems in school. We will discuss this at greater length below.

Assessment

PARENT INTERVIEW

We begin, as with the preschool parents, by describing the course of the evaluation—essentially getting some history of the child's problem and enlisting the parents' help in identifying things that will enable the child to deal with his problem. We use essentially the same questions used for the preschool child's parents. However, we might also ask the parents of the school-aged child about the child's school experiences. Does he like school? Does his speech seem to bother him in school? Do you think he stutters more at school than he does at home? Has he gotten therapy in his school?

As we ask parents these questions dealing with the child's home environment and school, we listen for answers that help us understand why the child's stuttering has persisted into elementary school. Here are some questions we ask ourselves as we try to integrate the information we are getting: Has this child grown up feeling that talking is hard? Does he feel that he must change what he's doing to make his speech more acceptable to listeners? Have the parents conveyed high expectations to him by saving their approval for evidence of above-average behavior?

We also remember that these parents are probably doing their best with the expectations with which *they* grew up. One of the most important things in the parent interview is to convey acceptance of the parents as they are and point out the many helpful things they have done for their child.

TEACHER INTERVIEW

The more assistance we can get from the child's teachers, the more we can help the child. We must approach the teachers with respect for their heavy responsibilities and their concern for each child, including the one with whom we are working. But we also should anticipate that they may neither understand stuttering nor know what we do to help a child who stutters. As we talk with the teacher, we should try to sense what they might like to know about stuttering and our treatment approach. The following questions serve as a guideline for the types of things we will want to find out:

1. Does the child talk in class? Does he stutter? What is his stuttering like? How does he seem to feel about his stuttering and about himself as a communicator?

Here we are trying to determine how much the child does stutter in class and whether his stuttering might keep him from talking as much as he might otherwise. We also can get a flavor of how the teacher feels about the child and his stuttering.

2. Does his stuttering interfere with his academic progress?

This question is obviously related to the earlier question about how much he talks in class despite his stuttering. But it also will give us some information about how much the child may be avoiding oral performance. We need to ask about disparities between oral and written performance. A big disparity may suggest that the child declines to talk or says "I don't know" when he may know the answer.

3. Do other children tease the child about his stuttering?

Most children who stutter in school get some teasing. We need to find out how extensive it is and how it affects the child.

4. How does the teacher feel about the child's stuttering? How does she or he react to it?

We have probably been able to get this information indirectly, from what she or he may have said before. But, if not, we should ask directly. The teacher is likely to ask how she or he *should* respond to the child's stuttering. This is an important issue, since her response will often influence how the class responds. This and other issues related to the child's speech in the classroom are discussed in Chapter 12.

Classroom Observation

In addition to the information obtained through teacher and parent interviews, some direct observation can help the clinician understand the extent of the child's stuttering and the degree to which it interferes with academic adjustment. In many cases, if the child is to receive services in the schools, the clinician must establish that the child's stuttering is interfering with his learning. What better way to verify this than by first-hand observation of the child in his classroom? Arrange with the teacher to come into the classroom at a time when the child is likely to be participating in class. Observe, unobtrusively if possible, the performance of the class. By observing the class when many students are participating, and not just when the child in question is talking, you do not call as much attention to the child's speech.

Child Interview

After we get the parents' consent to evaluate the child, we ask him to come to the treatment room where we talk with him for a while. In our first encounter, it is important for the child to sense that we are genuinely interested in him as well as in his stuttering. We usually begin by asking him about what he likes to do, with whom he likes to play, and who is in his family. Then we tell him a little about ourselves and how we work with children who sometimes get stuck on words. As he talks, we notice whether he stutters or not and what kind of stutters he has. When the time seems right, we ask him about his speech. The following questions are not asked machine-gun style, one right after another, but over a session or two.

1. Does he think that he has any trouble talking?

We rarely see school-aged stutterers who are unaware of their speech difficulty. However, if the stutterer regards the problem as minor, or is genuinely unaware of any problem, we try not to give it undue emphasis or to create an unfavorable attitude toward it. Thus, when we first talk to the child, we are usually low key, and if he truly doesn't seem to be bothered by his stuttering (although parents and teachers may be), we act in line with his perception and treat it as a relatively minor problem.

2. How would the child describe the problem? When does it happen? What is it like at different times?

The clinician is looking for several things here. One is to find the words that the child uses to describe his stuttering, so that she can use these same words talking with him about his stuttering. She is also finding out if the child is unaware of many of his stuttering behaviors, perhaps because they are too painful for him to face or because he just doesn't like to talk about them. Even more importantly, this question lets the child know the clinician really wants to understand his problem.

3. Does he use any helpers or "tricks" to get words out? Does he avoid certain words?

With this question, the clinician can convey the fact that she understands what people do when they stutter. She can also let the child know that she is nonjudgmental about the "tricks" he uses, by conveying acceptance and interest in his descriptions. She is also exploring to find out which level the child's stuttering has reached, by trying to determine if the child is using escape and avoidance behaviors.

4. Are certain speaking situations more difficult? Does he avoid them?

Again, this question helps the clinician begin to understand what the child is experiencing, and it conveys that understanding.

5. Does anyone ever tease the child about his speech? Who? How does he feel about it? How does he react?

Many children who are teased are not able to talk about it straightaway with a clinician whom they don't know well. This question is just a "feeler," and if the child denies being teased, the clinician should not dwell on it now.

6. How does he feel about his speech?

It is the unusual child who will be able to describe how he feels. To help the child express some feelings about his stuttering, the clinician may want to suggest some possiblities. She may ask "Does it make you mad sometimes?" or "Do you wish you didn't get stuck?" Don't be surprised if the child says it doesn't bother him, because children's feelings are often rejected, perhaps unintentionally, by adults. They may say, for instance, "You don't need to feel that way." or "Why do you let it bother you?" The effective clinician will show the child that whatever he feels is OK, that she is really trying to understand. A real discussion of feelings probably won't begin until the child learns to trust the clinician deeply. But, in this first interview, the clinician may be able to infer what the feelings are and, from that, understand how far the child's stuttering has advanced.

7. How do the child's parents feel about his speech? What do they do when he stutters?

It will help the clinician to determine what sort of learning experiences may have occurred if she can find out what the child has been going through at home. One parent may be less accepting of the child's stuttering than the other. Whatever she can determine will help her when she begins to enlist the parents' participation in treatment.

8. Can you think of anything else important for me to know about you or about the trouble you sometimes have when you talk?

This is a chance for the clinician to let the child know she is really interested in him and that she values his ideas.

Speech Sample

Pattern of Disfluencies. During our interviews with teachers, parents, and the child himself, as well as from the speech samples we describe below, we extract information about when and how the child stutters. The elementary school child is likely to be a beginning or intermediate level stutterer, so we want to know a great deal about the amount of tension in the child's stuttering, the escape behaviors he uses, and the extent to which he avoids words and situations. As with the adult or adolescent stutterer, we use this information not only to decide into which developmental/treatment level to assign the child, but we also use it, when appropriate, to plan the process of unlearning the conditioned responses that once created and now maintain the pattern of stuttering.

Stuttering Severity Instrument.   We need a sample of conversational speech and a sample of reading, from which to calculate a Stuttering Severity Index (SSI). The administration and scoring of the SSI are described in the section on the adolescent and adult above. It should be noted that there is a separate scoring system for children. With the elementary school child, we tape-record him talking for 5 minutes about school and other things. We prefer not to turn on the tape-recorder the moment the child first walks into the room, so we don't use the first few minutes of conversation in the diagnostic interview. Instead, we talk for a few minutes and then ask the child if he would mind if we tape-record as we talk. Then we record a sample which includes, optimally, 5 minutes. If only 3 minutes of the child's speech are available, that is acceptable, but we would not advise using less than that. We also record a sample of the child reading for approximately 3 minutes.

Speech Rate.   In addition to using the samples for calculating the SSI score, we also use them to assess the child's rate. In the section on evaluation of adolescent and adult stutterers, we described how to calculate speech rate, in either words or syllables per minute. The normal rates for school children in Vermont, measured in syllables per minute, are given in Table 6.1. These rates were obtained in children's conversations with a clinician about Christmas, hobbies, school, and home activities. They were calculated by including normal pauses in the conversation speech, but excluding long pauses (longer than 2 seconds) for thought. It is reasonable to expect that children's rates in other states will be similar.

The purpose of assessing rate is to get some idea of how much the child's stuttering is interfering with the rate of speech he might normally be using. As we help the child manage his stuttering, we should expect a steady increase in his speech rate toward normal levels.

FEELINGS AND ATTITUDES

The most reliable measure of the child's feelings and attitudes is your judgment. Obviously, your judgment gets better as you get to know the child better, but you should be able to get a pretty good indication of the child's feelings and attitudes from this first interview. Watch how the child responds when you ask him about his stuttering. Note how much he avoids stuttering. And when he does stutter, note how calm he is, and how good his eye contact is.

After you have gotten to know the child a bit, you may want to administer a paper and pencil assessment of attitude. In Figure 6.8, we present the attitude scale we have occasionally used to assess children's communication attitudes, the A-19 scale (Guitar & Grims, 1977). These are questions which we have found will discriminate between children who stutter and children who do not. Hence, if

Table 6.1   Speech Rates for School Children

Age (yrs)	Range in Syllables per Minute
6	140–175
8	150–180
10	165–215
12	165–220

A-19 Scale for Children Who Stutter

Susan Andre and Barry Guitar
University of Vermont

Establish rapport with the child, and make sure that he/she is physically comfortable before beginning administration. Explain the task to the child and make sure he/she understands what is required. Some simple directions might be used:

> "I am going to ask you some questions. Listen carefully
> and then tell me what you think: Yes or No. There is
> no right or wrong answer. I just want to know what you
> think."

To begin the scale, ask the questions in a natural manner. Do not urge the child to respond before he/she is ready, and repeat the question if the child did not hear it or you feel that he/she did not understand it. Do not re-word the question unless you feel it is absolutely necessary, and then write the question you asked under that item.

Circle the answer that corresponds with the child's response. Be accepting of the child's response because there is no right or wrong answer. If all the child will say is "I don't know", even after prompting, record that response next to the question.

For the younger children (kindergarten and first grade), it might be necessary to give a few simple examples to ensure comprehension of the required task:

a.	Are you a boy?	YES	NO
b.	Do you have black hair?	YES	NO

Similar, obvious questions may be inserted, if necessary, to reassure the examiner that the child is <u>actively</u> cooperating at all times. Adequately praise the child for listening and assure him/her that a good job is being done.

It is important to be familiar with the questions so that they can be read in a natural manner.

The child is given one point for answers that match those given below. The higher a child's score, the more probable it is that he/she has developed negative attitudes toward communication. In our study, the mean score of the K through 4th stutterers (N=28) was 9.07 (S.D. = 2.44), and for the 28 matched controls, it was 8.17 (S.D. = 1.80).

Score one point for each answer that matches these:

1. YES	10. NO
2. YES	11. NO
3. NO	12. NO
4. NO	13. YES
5. NO	14. YES
6. YES	15. YES
7. NO	16. NO
8. YES	17. NO
9. YES	18. YES
	19. YES

Figure 6.8. A-19 Scale of Children's Communication Attitudes. (Printed with permission of Susan Andre.)

A-19 SCALE

Name_____   Date_____

1. Is it best to keep your mouth shut when you
    are in trouble?   YES   NO

2. When the teacher calls on you, do you get
    nervous?   YES   NO

3. Do you ask a lot of questions in class?   YES   NO

4. Do you like to talk on the phone?   YES   NO

5. If you did not know a person, would you
    tell them your name?   YES   NO

6. Is it hard to talk to your teacher?   YES   NO

7. Would you go up to a new boy or girl in your class? YES   NO

8. Is it hard to keep control of your voice when talking? YES   NO

9. Even when you know the right answer, are you afraid
    to say it?   YES   NO

10. Do you like to tell other children what to do?   YES   NO

11. Is it fun to talk to your dad?   YES   NO

12. Do you like to tell stories to your classmates?   YES   NO

13. Do you wish you could say things as clearly as the
    other kids do?   YES   NO

14. Would you rather look at a comic book than
    talk to a friend?   YES   NO

15. Are you upset when someone interrupts you?   YES   NO

16. When you want to say something, do you just say it? YES   NO

17. Is talking to your friends more fun than playing
    by yourself?   YES   NO

18. Are you sometimes unhappy?   YES   NO

19. Are you a little afraid to talk on the phone?   YES   NO

Figure 6.8.—Continued

treatment is effective, you might expect to see a child's attitude about communication change, although this has not been established by research.

In addition to the A-19, the Children's Attitude Test (CAT), shown in Figure 6.9, has been recently developed by Brutten, tested on normal children (Brutten & Dunham, 1990), and shown to differentiate stuttering and normal children (DeNil and Brutten, in press, 1990). Both of these tests are probably ineffective if given too soon, before the child has learned he can trust you.

Name_____

Age: _____
Sex: _____
Grade: _____

Childrens' Attitude Test[1]
Gene J. Brutten, Ph.D.
Southern Illinois University

Read each sentence carefully so you can say if it is true or false _for you_. The sentences are about talking. If _you_ feel that the sentence is right, circle true. If _you_ think the sentence about your talking is not right, circle false. Remember, circle false if _you_ think the sentence is wrong and true if _you_ think it is right.

1.	I don't talk right.	True	False
2.	I don't mind asking the teacher a question in class.	True	False
3.	Sometimes words will stick in my mouth when I talk.	True	False
4.	People worry about the way I talk.	True	False
5.	It is harder for me to give a report in class than it is for most of the other kids.	True	False
6.	My classmates don't think I talk funny.	True	False
7.	I like the way I talk.	True	False
8.	People sometimes finish words for me.	True	False
9.	My parents like the way I talk.	True	False
10.	I find it easy to talk to most everyone.	True	False
11.	I talk well most of the time.	True	False
12.	It is hard for me to talk to people.	True	False
13.	I don't talk like other children.	True	False
14.	I don't worry about the way I talk.	True	False
15.	I don't find it easy to talk.	True	False
16.	My words come out easily.	True	False
17.	It is hard for me to talk to strangers.	True	False
18.	The other kids wish they could talk like me.	True	False

[1]Copyright 1985

Figure 6.9. Children's Attitude Test. (Copyright 1985 Gene Brutten.)

19.	Some kids make fun of the way I talk.	True	False
20.	Talking is easy for me.	True	False
21.	Telling someone my name is hard for me.	True	False
22.	Words are hard for me to say.	True	False
23.	I talk well with most everyone.	True	False
24.	Sometimes I have trouble talking.	True	False
25.	I would rather talk than write.	True	False
26.	I like to talk.	True	False
27.	I am not a good talker.	True	False
28.	I wish I could talk like other children.	True	False
29.	I am afraid the words won't come out when I talk.	True	False
30.	My friends don't talk as well as I do.	True	False
31.	I don't worry about talking on the phone.	True	False
32.	I talk better with a friend.	True	False
33.	People don't seem to like the way I talk.	True	False
34.	I let others talk for me.	True	False
35.	Reading aloud in class is easy for me.	True	False

Score one point for each answer that matches these:

1. True	9. False	17. True	25. False	33. True
2. False	10. False	18. False	26. False	34. True
3. True	11. False	19. True	27. True	35. False
4. True	12. True	20. False	28. True	
5. True	13. True	21. True	29. True	
6. False	14. False	22. True	30. False	
7. False	15. True	23. False	31. False	
8. True	16. False	24. True	32. True	

In a study using this scale on Belgian children (DeNil and Brutten, 1990) mean score of a group of children who stutter (N = 70) was 16.7; mean score of a group of children who do not stutter (N = 271) was 8.71.

Figure 6.9.—Continued

OTHER SPEECH AND LANGUAGE DISORDERS

In our discussion of the preschool child, we described the importance of assessing language, articulation, and voice. The same variables should be assessed in the elementary school child, although, if this child has a language or articulation (and, to a lesser extent, voice) problem, it may have been diagnosed previously and the child may have been in therapy. The clinician should seek out the details of any previous therapy. We have previously suggested articulation assessment procedures which would be appropriate for the elementary school child. Language assessment for this age child is well-described in Lund and Duchan (1988) and Wiig and Semel (1984).

If the child has received articulation or language therapy in the past, the clinician should determine the type of treatment the child received and how he responded. Did he overcome his articulation or language deficit? Did his stuttering first appear or worsen during this previous treatment? If so, the clinician should pay particular attention to indications that the child may think of himself as a poor speaker, and may believe speaking is very difficult. The interviews and questionnaires we have suggested in this section will help you explore this possibility. Moreover, the therapy approach suggested in Chapter 12 is designed to help the child regain confidence in his ability to speak.

OTHER FACTORS

There may be other important factors that will influence the outcome of treatment. We recommend evaluating all factors that may have precipitated and are maintaining the stuttering, so that they may be included in the overall treatment plan.

Physical Development.   Earlier, we voiced our main concern in this area: that motor development may lag behind language development. A child with a speech-motor delay may benefit from fluency shaping therapy designed to help him coordinate respiration, phonation, and articulation, thereby reducing stuttering. He may also benefit from a stuttering modification component, in which he can learn to stutter easily and openly, rather than becoming tense and frustrated, if his fluency breaks down under stress. This child's treatment should also focus on building self-esteem, which may be low in children who are not well coordinated.

Cognitive Development.   As with the preschool child, we need to rule out retardation. Moreover, we examine whether or not the cognitive stresses of school are increasing the general level of demand on this child. This will be discussed further in the section on academic adjustment, below.

Social-Emotional Development.   We are interested in how the child is fitting in with his classmates, how comfortable he feels about talking and relating to others, and to what extent he may feel a need to hide his stuttering. Some children are friendly and outgoing, and they are supported by their classmates, whether they stutter or not. These social skills are a positive factor in their prognosis for recovery from stuttering. Other children have not outgrown their early self-centeredness, and their stuttering compounds their self-concern and keeps them from relating easily to others. Children in the latter category need help learning to relate more easily to their classmates. Evaluation of this component can be done through the teacher, parent, and child interviews. A classroom observation may also help the clinician evaluate this component.

We are also concerned with the extent to which the child's home environment provides support and security. This information comes primarily from the parent and child interviews. The parents can often provide insight into the conditions surrounding the onset of stuttering and the conditions under which it gets better or worse. We sift the evidence, with the parents' help, to determine if there are things that need to be done to improve the child's self-esteem. For some children, we have found school psychologists to be very helpful in building their self-esteem and helping them improve their social adjustment.

Academic Adjustment.   The parent, child, and teacher interviews usually provide information about how well the child is doing in school and how much he likes it. Stuttering may appear for the first time or may worsen when a child is under the additional stress of learning many new things. For example, the process of reading aloud in class when learning to read may put substantial demand on resources for language formulation and speech production. The child must make "second-order mappings of meanings and lexical units from speech"[3] and simultaneously translate the written representation into units appropriate for speech production. Thus, certain academic challenges may be more demanding for the child who stutters, and his stuttering in school should be understood in relation to this. In practical terms, the clinician may want to consider whether the child needs extra help in certain academic areas through discussion with his teachers about which speaking situations in school are most difficult. If the child does have more difficulty in certain academic situations, these should be given extra attention during the planning of generalization of more fluent speech.

Diagnosis

At this point, we pull together the information we have collected from the case history, the parent, teacher, and child interviews, the speech sample, and the classroom observation. We determine what developmental/treatment level the child's stuttering has reached, and this gives us the direction for the specific treatment. We also assess the various developmental and environmental influences still operating on the child and make plans to alleviate those that can be changed and help the child cope with those that can't.

Most elementary school children will be beginning or intermediate stutterers. The major characteristics of these developmental/treatment levels were reviewed in the preceding section on evaluating the preschool child, and they are described in detail in Chapter 4. Important components to include in the treatment for this child may be uncovered as a result of the parent, teacher, and child interviews and from the speech sample. That is, we may learn what developmental or environmental factors may be influences on the child's stuttering. Some of these may be other speech and language disorders, motor problems, or pressures in the child's home. Some can be dealt with in our treatment of the child, but others may require many sessions of parent counseling or referral to other professionals.

Closing Interview

The closing interview is an opportunity to summarize our immediate impressions to parents and to make recommendations about direct treatment. This

---

[3] Gibson, E. (1972). This chapter and others in *Language by Ear and by Eye* (Kavanaugh and Mattingly) make it clear that reading is a resource-intensive process that makes heavy demands on language processing.

also gives us a chance to discuss with the parents the crucial role they may play in reducing environmental pressures. Our comments about the closing interview with parents of preschool children apply here also. We stay away from jargon. We try to let them know the many beneficial things they have done regarding their child's speech, and we say to them that the stuttering was not caused by anything they have done. Although some parents may have created conditions in which a child's predisposition to stutter has been transformed into a serious problem, it does not help if we make an issue of this. We would rather convince them that they are in a key position to help.

After describing clearly and in plain English what we have observed about the child's stuttering, we summarize what we think is appropriate for treatment. This is only in very general terms because parents' main concerns here are not for the details of treatment but about the prospects for their child's future. Therefore, we rely on our experience to describe some possible outcomes. For example, we might say that a combination of many factors will determine the outcome. These include the natural increases in fluency that happen as the child matures, the feeling of self-acceptance the child develops as he finds people accept him whether or not he has a little trouble with his speech, and his learning ways to speak more fluently. When we talk about the child's prognosis, it seems to us appropriate to include some aspect of the parents' role, such as their acceptance of the child's speech or their participation in treatment, as part of the formula for recovery.

After summarizing our impressions and describing some of the ingredients for recovery, we then discuss with the parents the things they can do to promote recovery. Specific suggestions depend upon our findings from our parent, teacher, and child interviews, but the section on parent counseling in Chapter 12 presents ideas for parents' involvement. This discussion is the most important part of the closing interview, and in fact, it may go on for several more meetings. If we treat the child directly, and it is a clinic rather than a school setting, we will meet with the parents on a regular basis as a part of treatment. In these meetings, we will continue helping the parents explore how various changes in the home environment facilitate their child's fluency.

As we have said before, several aspects of evaluation are different when we see a child in a school setting. School clinicians may not always be able to discuss with parents all the details of their findings in person because some parents are unable to come to the school. In these hopefully rare cases much of the continued contact may have to be carried out by telephone. The closing interview follows a staffing team meeting concerning the child, in which teachers, other professionals, and parents discuss the child's speech and develop a treatment plan. The parents' permission to treat the child is then obtained. It is at this time or in a later parent counseling session that the clinician's recommendations for environmental change are discussed. Many times the clinician can continue to meet with the parents throughout the treatment and work with them to facilitate change. It has been our experience that many parents who are tentative at first may become involved in their child's treatment after the clinician has shown her continued interest in the child and an accepting attitude toward the parents. Realistically, however, there will be other parents who are unable for one reason or another to become involved. In these cases, the clinician and others must provide some of the support the parents cannot. We try to give the child enough successful experiences in communication to offset other environmental pressures that cannot be dealt with directly.

SUMMARY

In evaluating a client who may stutter, your task is to decide: (*a*) if his disfluencies warrant treatment; if so, (*b*) what are the important characteristics of his history, current environment, speech behaviors, and reactions, and (*c*) what treatment do these characteristics indicate?

We have provided most of the tools to answer these three questions, but the most critical is your judgment. Whether the person is to be treated as a normally disfluent speaker or as a stutterer depends on interpretation rather than a score. You must weigh what you see and hear about his behaviors to determine if they indicate stuttering, normal disfluency, or even another disorder. Out of the flood of information you gather, you must distill the essential characteristics that lead to a choice of treatment.

To hone your judgment, we urge you to make evaluation a continuing process. The procedures we have suggested for assessment and diagnosis in this chapter will give you a good start, but stuttering is highly variable and an entire individual cannot be glimpsed in an hour or two. Consequently, you will sometimes overlook an important element, and sometimes a vital clue will never appear in the small sample of behavior you see. With good follow-up evaluation of the client, whether you treat him or not, you will be able to change a decision or redirect therapy.

STUDY QUESTIONS

1/ In the section on evaluation of the adult/adolescent, what different pieces of information that you may gather from the interview questions help you to assess the client's motivation?

2/ What various aspects of the client's behavior are assessed by the SSI?

3/ Why is the client's speech rate assessed?

4/ Why is it useful to obtain tape-recordings of a preschool child's stuttering prior to the evaluation, when this is not done for other age levels?

5/ What questions in the interview of the parent of a preschool child assess (a) constitutional, (b) developmental and environmental, and (c) learning factors?

6/ Name 4 of the 7 variables we assess in the speech of a preschooler to determine his developmental/treatment level.

7/ In what various ways do we assess the impact of the school environment on the school-aged child who stutters?

8/ How does the parents' role differ in the diagnosis of preschool versus school children?

9/ What are the benefits of obtaining both a reading and conversation sample with school children and adults?

10/ What are two reasons we suggest continuing evaluation, after the initial assessment, of clients who stutter?

Suggested Readings

Emerick, L. and Haynes, W. (1986). *Diagnosis and evaluation in speech pathology.* (3rd ed.). Englewood Cliffs: Prentice Hall.

The chapters on interviewing and on stuttering are particularly good. Emerick is an intuitive clinician and a down-to-earth writer; these chapters are filled with practical information and they are highly digestible.

Guitar, B. (1981). Stuttering. In J. Darby (Ed.), *Speech evaluation in medicine.* New York: Grune and Stratton.

The sections on differential diagnosis of stuttering versus neurogenic disfluency, psychogenic disfluency, and cluttering will be especially useful to clinicians evaluating adult clients.

Johnson, W., Darley, F., & Spriestersbach, D.C. (1952). *Diagnostic manual in speech correction.* New York: Harper and Brothers.

This manual is admittedly out of date, but its opening sections on the case history, particularly the description of interviewing techniques, are excellent.

Peterson, H. and Marquardt, T. (1990). *Appraisal and diagnosis of speech and language disorders* (2nd ed.). Englewood Cliffs: Prentice Hall.

The chapter on evaluation of fluency is authored by Harold Luper, who is, like Emerick, an experienced clinician and a fine writer. The section of this chapter on differentiating stuttering from normal disfluency is particularly good.

St. Louis, K. (Ed.). (1986). *The atypical stutterer.* New York: Academic Press.

This text contains interesting chapters on fluency disorders that are similar to stuttering, such as cluttering and disfluency associated with retardation. Therapy approaches for these other fluency disorders are also given.

7

THE ADVANCED STUTTERER: STUTTERING MODIFICATION AND FLUENCY SHAPING THERAPIES

In this chapter, we will discuss the treatment of the advanced stutterer. Since most advanced stutterers are adults or high school students, we will be describing therapy procedures for individuals in this age range. After reviewing the characteristics of the disorder at this level, we will discuss stuttering modification and fluency shaping therapies. We will conclude by comparing these two approaches on the clinical issues raised in an earlier chapter.

The advanced stutterer will exhibit any or all of the following core behaviors: part-word or monosyllabic word repetitions that contain excessive tension, vowel prolongations that exhibit tension, and blocks. Secondary behaviors may include escape behaviors, starting behaviors, postponements, word substitutions and circumlocutions, and avoidance of speaking situations. The advanced stutterer will have a well-established self-concept as a stutterer, and he will evidence frustration, embarrassment and fear relative to his stuttering.

STUTTERING MODIFICATION THERAPY

The two key elements in stuttering modification therapy for the advanced stutterer are: (*a*) teaching the stutterer to modify his moments of stuttering, and (*b*) reducing his fear of stuttering and eliminating the avoidance behaviors associated with this fear. To illustrate this approach, we will describe Charles Van Riper's therapy for the advanced stutterer. Van Riper is a leading proponent of stuttering modification therapy and is an excellent representative of this approach. Other contemporary clinicians advocating stuttering modification therapy will also be reviewed, and their therapy will be briefly described.

CHARLES VAN RIPER: FLUENT OR EASY STUTTERING

Clinician's Beliefs

NATURE OF STUTTERING

What position does Charles Van Riper take on the clinical issues we raised in an earlier chapter? With regard to the nature of stuttering, Van Riper (1982) sees stuttering as a disorder of timing. He believes that when a person stutters, there is a disruption in the proper timing and sequencing of the muscle movements involved in producing a word. When this happens, the stutterer exhibits a core behavior, that is, a repetition, prolongation, or block. What accounts for this mistiming of the motor movements involved in speech production? Van Riper suggests this could be due to an organic predisposition, to a faulty feedback system, or to emotional stress. According to Van Riper, secondary behaviors and negative feelings and attitudes are learned.

SPEECH BEHAVIORS TARGETED FOR THERAPY

Since stutterers exhibit these mistimings in their speech, Van Riper believes we should teach them how to cope with these disruptions. His solution is to teach the stutterer how to modify his hard, tense, struggled moments of stuttering into slow, easy, effortless ones. More specifically, the stutterer is to slowly work his way through each sound of the stuttered word. The transition from sound to sound is to be gradual. Van Riper wants "the whole sequence to be slowed down, all sounds and transitions proportionally."[1] Articulatory contacts are to be light,

---

[1] Van Riper notes that some stuttering modification clinicians have the stutterer prolong only the first sound of the word. Van Riper, however, believes it is better for the stutterer not to distort the motoric sequence of the word by using such prolongations.

not tense. Van Riper refers to this new way of stuttering as "fluent stuttering" or "easy stuttering."[2]

FLUENCY GOALS

What are Van Riper's fluency goals for advanced stutterers? Van Riper says that, with therapy, a few advanced stutterers become normal speakers, that is, they exhibit spontaneous fluency all the time. However, in most cases, this does not occur. Thus, ideally, his goal is spontaneous fluency, but realistically, his goal for most advanced stutterers is controlled fluency or acceptable stuttering. These stutterers should be using their new, easy, fluent stuttering to sound relatively fluent or, at least, to exhibit only a minimal level of stuttering.

FEELINGS AND ATTITUDES

Van Riper feels it is very important to consider advanced stutterers' feelings and attitudes toward their stuttering in planning therapy. Because they have been stuttering for many years, he believes that they have developed strong feelings of frustration, fear, and shame focused around their disorder. Van Riper believes it is important to desensitize these stutterers to their stuttering and to other persons' reactions to it. By desensitization, Van Riper implies two things. On the one hand, he means that the intensity of the stutterers' negative feelings need to be reduced. On the other hand, he thinks that the stutterers need to be toughened to the experience of stuttering and to others' reactions to their stuttering. This may be just two ways of saying the same thing; namely, that these stutterers need to become less emotional about their stuttering. If this does not occur, Van Riper feels that advanced stutterers will not be able to successfully modify their stuttering. The reason is that stutterers, like most people, can not perform fine motor acts, like modifying a moment of stuttering, when they are wrought up emotionally.

MAINTENANCE PROCEDURES

Van Riper is very aware of the need to help advanced stutterers maintain the improvements they made during therapy. He puts a great deal of emphasis upon procedures or strategies to help them do this. In fact, one of his four phases of therapy, stabilization, is devoted to this goal. Van Riper has developed a number of clinical procedures that he employs during this phase. For example, he helps the stutterers become their own speech clinicians. Since these stutterers will need to control their stuttering for a long time, possibly forever, they need to know what to do. He teaches them how to keep their speech fears at a minimum and how to keep their stuttering modification skills intact. He also helps the stutterers change their self-concepts with regard to their speech. This will involve the stutterers changing their self-concepts from persons who stutter to persons who speak fluently most of the time but who, occasionally, exhibit mild stuttering.

---

[2] Sources for Van Riper's position on this and the remaining clinical issues were Van Riper, C. (1973). *The treatment of stuttering*. Englewood Cliffs: Prentice-Hall. and Van Riper, C. (1974). Modification of behavior. In *Therapy for stutterers* (pp. 45–73). Memphis: Speech Foundation of America.

Clinical Methods

In terms of clinical methods, Van Riper's therapy would be characterized as a counseling/teaching mode of interaction. It can be implemented in either an individual or group situation. Even though the clinician has definite goals for the therapy session, the session is loosely structured. Many times the clinician and the client go outside the clinical setting into real-life, speaking situations to achieve the goals of the day. The client also has daily therapy assignments that he performs on his own outside of the clinic. These are then discussed with the clinician during a later therapy session. As a general rule, Van Riper has not stressed the collection of data in his discussion of therapy procedures.

Clinical Procedures

Of all Van Riper's contributions to the field of stuttering, he is probably best known for the therapy procedures he has developed for the advanced stutterer. In *The Treatment of Stuttering* (Van Riper, 1973), he provides a very comprehensive discussion of his therapy for the advanced stutterer. In the Speech Foundation of America booklet, *Therapy for Stutterers*, Van Riper (1974) provides a brief, but very good, description of this therapy. In this chapter, we will draw on these two sources for our presentation of his clinical procedures. We plan to describe his therapy in sufficient detail to allow the reader to understand his basic procedures; however, the reader is referred to the above sources for additional information.

Van Riper typically breaks the therapy process down into four phases. The sequence is as follows: (*a*) identification phase, (*b*) desensitization phase, (*c*) modification phase, and (*d*) stabilization phase. Each of these phases will be discussed in turn.

Identification Phase

In the identification phase, the stutterer identifies the core behaviors, secondary behaviors, and feelings and attitudes that characterize his stuttering. If the stutterer is to change, he must become aware of what to change. Clinical activities include oral reading, discussion, modeling of stuttering behaviors by the clinician, self observation in a mirror, and audio and video recordings (Fig. 7.1). During therapy sessions, the clinician is warm, understanding, and accepting of the client's stuttering behaviors and feelings. However, the clinician is also confronting and challenging when she thinks the stutterer is avoiding facing certain aspects of his problem. Yet, even at these times her basic acceptance of the client allows him to become more comfortable with his stuttering. In other words, desensitization is already beginning to occur.

Van Riper recommends that the components of the client's stuttering be identified in a hierarchical order from least to most difficult or stressful for the stutterer. Based upon his experience, he recommends the following hierarchy. First, the clinician helps the stutterer identify easy stutterings in his speech. Most stutterers have some easy or effortless stutterings in their speech. These will become the target or goal behaviors for the stutterer. Next, in order, will come identification of avoidance behaviors, postponement behaviors, starting behaviors, word

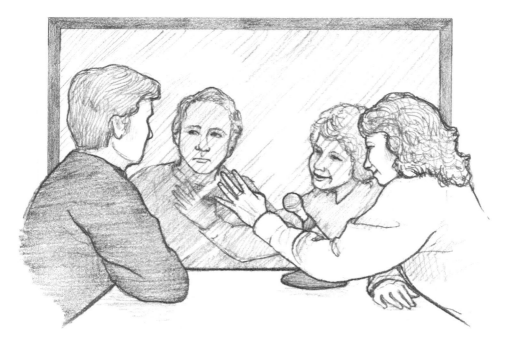

Figure 7.1.   Identification of the core and secondary behaviors.

and sound fears, situation fears, and core behaviors, including escape behaviors. Finally, feelings of frustration, shame, and hostility will be identified and accepted.

These components of the stuttering problem are first identified in the clinic, and then they are identified outside the clinic in the stutterer's own speaking environment. For example, if the goal were to help the stutterer become aware of his use of postponements, the clinician would first help the stutterer become aware of his use of postponements while talking to her in the clinic. Then the stutterer would be given an assignment to gather examples of these behaviors in his everyday speaking situations. At times, it would also be important for the clinician to accompany the client on some outside speaking assignments. This would allow the clinician to verify the validity of the stutterer's self-observation and reporting.

When the stutterer gets to the point where he can identify and knowingly discuss the various aspects of his stuttering, he is ready to move to the desensitization phase.

Desensitization Phase

The goal of the desensitization phase is to reduce the fears and other negative emotions, such as frustration and embarrassment, associated with the stutterer's speech. Van Riper also views it as toughening the stutterer to his stuttering. Specifically, Van Riper believes there are three features of the stuttering problem to which the stutterer needs to be desensitized. These are (*a*) the confrontation with the disorder, (*b*) the core behaviors, and (*c*) the reactions of his listeners. In other words, the stutterer needs to become more comfortable with or tolerant of each of these three aspects of his stuttering problem. The following are examples of typical procedures that could be used to desensitize a stutterer to each of the above three features.

Confrontation with the Disorder.   Most advanced stutterers find it difficult to confront or face up to the fact that they stutter. They tend to deny and run away from their problem. However, by enrolling in a therapy program and by going through the identification phase, which has been previously discussed, the stutterer has gone a long way towards confronting his problem. In other words, much of the desensitization to the confrontation with the disorder has already occurred. However, another strategy the clinician should suggest to the stutterer to help him confront his stuttering is self-disclosure. The clinician encourages the stutterer to be honest and open about his stuttering. She should encourage the stutterer to let people know that he stutters and that he is involved in a stuttering therapy program. When he does this, she should reinforce this behavior with her enthusiastic approval.

Desensitization to Core Behaviors.   The second target for desensitization is the core behaviors, that is, the repetitions, prolongations, and blocks. Van Riper believes that, for many stutterers, these core behaviors are associated with feelings of frustration and fear. Stutterers need to build up their tolerance for them. One technique that Van Riper recommends is called freezing. By freezing, Van Riper means that the stutterer, upon a signal from the clinician, freezes his speech mechanism in the act of what it is doing. The stutterer holds on to the core behavior he was experiencing when the clinician signaled. If he were prolonging a sound, he should continue to do that. If he were repeating a syllable, he should continue repeating it. These activities, like all desensitization activities, should be done in a hierarchical order, that is, from least stressful to most stressful. For example, the first steps might involve the clinician's simulating the client's stuttering and freezing upon the client's signal. At these times, the clinician should remain relaxed as she voluntarily simulates the client's stuttering. Later, when the client begins to freeze in his stutters, the clinician should have him hold his stutters only briefly. While the stutterer is doing this, the clinician should be calm, unhurried, and in no way punishing. Finally, the clinician should have the stutterer hold on to his blocks for longer and longer periods of time. Now, the clinician may introduce some impatience or other mildly aversive behavior into her responses. By experiencing these core behaviors over and over again through such a hierarchy, the stutterer will become less emotional about or more tolerant of his core behaviors.

Desensitization to Listener Reactions.   One procedure that Van Riper might use to desensitize the stutterer to listener reactions is pseudostuttering or voluntary stuttering. The purpose of this is to teach the client that he can experience stuttering without becoming excessively emotional. By stuttering on purpose and by observing his listeners, the stutterer will learn the following things. First, he will learn that most listeners are far more tolerant of stuttering than he thought. Second, he will learn that, even though he may receive an occasional negative reaction from a listener, he can remain relatively calm. Van Riper also recommends the use of hierarchies in doing pseudostuttering. At first, the stutterer uses pseudostuttering that consists of easy repetitions or prolongations. Gradually, the pseudostuttering is changed to approximate his own stuttering. At first, the pseudostuttering is on nonfeared words; later it is on feared words. In the beginning, the pseudostuttering is done in the clinical setting with the support of a sensitive and understanding clinician. The clinician will also engage in and share the pseudostuttering with the client, both inside the clinic and in outside speaking situations. While doing this, it is important that the clinician remain calm and relaxed. Only later will the stutterer have assignments in which he engages in pseudostuttering on his own in outside feared speaking situations. By going through this sequence of activities with the encouragement, sharing, and support of his clinician, the stutterer will gradually become desensitized to his listeners' reactions.

Once the stutterer begins to become less emotional about his stuttering and people's reactions to it, he is ready to move on to the modification phase of therapy.

Modification Phase

During the modification phase, the stutterer learns a new fluent or easy way of stuttering. It is during this phase that the stutterer learns to use Van Riper's well-known techniques of cancellations, pull-outs, and preparatory sets to modify his moments of stuttering (Fig. 7.2). However, before the clinician teaches these techniques, she must help the stutterer reduce or eliminate his use of postponement and avoidance responses to feared words and situations. She must convince the stutterer that, if he is going to learn to stutter more easily, he must learn to tackle his feared words. He can not run away from them. Fortunately, this task has been made easier because the stutterer has already gone through the desensitization phase. Nevertheless, the clinician will probably have to spend some time in helping the stutterer approach feared words, rather than avoid them, before she begins to teach him cancellations, pull-outs, and preparatory sets.

Cancellations. Cancellations are the first step in the sequence of teaching the stutterer a fluent or easy way of stuttering. To begin with, the stutterer needs to have a model of what easy stuttering sounds and feels like. During the identification phase, the clinician may have been able to help the stutterer identify some easy stutterings in his speech. If so, these can be used as models. If the stutterer does not have any easy stutterings in his speech, the clinician will have to model them for him. What Van Riper has in mind is as follows. The word is to be said deliberately and in slow motion. That is, each sound of the word is to be produced slowly. Transitions from sound to sound are to be gradual. Articulatory contacts are to be relaxed or light. Once the stutterer is able to voluntarily produce or model these easy stutterings on single words, he is ready to begin incorporating them into his speech. Cancellations are used for this purpose.

A cancellation goes as follows. After the stutterer stutters on a word, he is to pause for a couple of seconds and then say the word a second time. He is not to say the word fluently this second time; rather, he is to say it using an easy stuttering. The clinician should make sure that the stutterer completes the stuttered word the first time; he should not stop immediately following the moment of stuttering. The clinician should also insist that the stutterer not hurry his pause. It should be a deliberate pause during which the stutterer calms himself, analyzes the way in

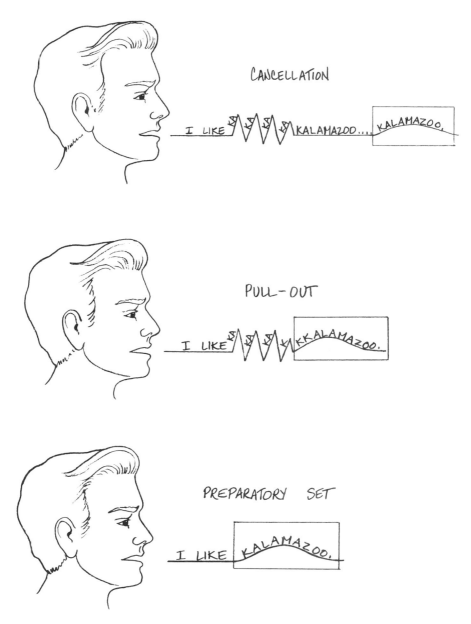

Figure 7.2.   Van Riper's stuttering modification techniques.

which he just stuttered, and prepares to use easy stuttering on the second attempt. Hierarchies are employed in using cancellations. That is, the stutterer will first use cancellations in the clinic with the clinician. Only after he can successfully use them in this context will he begin to use them in daily assignments in outside speaking situations. Once the stutterer has developed skill in cancelling his old stutters, he is ready to move on to pull-outs.

Pull-Outs.   The second step in teaching the stutterer to use easy or fluent stuttering is pull-outs. Now, rather than stuttering the old way on the first attempt at a word, the stutterer is to catch himself while he is still in the act of stuttering and pull or ease himself out of the rest of the word. He is to use the same behaviors that he has already learned. That is, he is to say the rest of the word in slow-motion. Movement from sound to sound should be gradual, and articulatory contacts should be light. Again, pull-outs are first used in the clinical setting and later in outside speaking situations. Once the stutterer has mastered the use of pull-outs, he is ready to move on to preparatory sets.

Preparatory Sets.   Preparatory sets are the third and final step in teaching the stutterer to use fluent stuttering. As the stutterer looks ahead and sees feared words, he now prepares to use the same behaviors he used in cancellations and pull-outs. He works through all parts of the word slowly, and he uses relaxed articulatory contacts. Preparatory sets are also first practiced in the clinical setting and then in outside assignments.

By going through this sequence of cancellations, pull-outs, and preparatory sets, Van Riper has modified the stutterer's old stuttering pattern into a fluent or easy form of stuttering. In operant conditioning terminology, this has been a shaping procedure. The stutterer is now ready for the last or stabilization phase of therapy.

Stabilization Phase

The goal of the stabilization phase is to help the stutterer solidify or stabilize his gains. Van Riper has several subgoals he wants to achieve during this phase. The most important one is to help the stutterer become his own speech clinician. The clinician helps the stutterer take responsibility for developing his own assignments based upon his perceived needs. The clinician will now become more and more of a consultant, and the frequency of contact between the clinician and client will be reduced. In time, the stutterer will develop the ability and confidence to prescribe his own therapy activities.

Another subgoal of the stabilization phase is the automatization of the use of preparatory sets and pull-outs. When the stutterer first began to use these stuttering modification techniques, they required a great deal of concentration. They need to become automatic. Basically, this will involve a great deal of practice using these techniques on feared words and in feared situations, both in the clinic and in everyday speaking situations.

The stutterer also needs to extinguish any residual speech fears. This will involve seeking out any remaining feared situations and employing pseudostuttering, as he did during the desensitization phase, in these situations. Another helpful technique for the stutterer is to purposefully insert brief easy or fluent stutterings on nonfeared words into speech throughout the day.

Finally, Van Riper believes it is important to help the stutterer change his self-concept from being a person who stutters to being a person who speaks fluently most of the time but who occasionally stutters mildly. This self-concept change will go through a series of steps and will involve considerable reality testing. At last, the day will come when the client feels he can manage by himself, and therapy will be terminated.

Other Clinicians

Now we will briefly comment upon the clinical procedures of some other speech-language pathologists who advocate stuttering modification therapy for the advanced stutterer. This list of clinicians is not exhaustive. However, the clinical procedures of these clinicians are representative of the field of stuttering modification therapy, and by being aware of the contributions of these writers, the reader will become more familiar with the stuttering modification literature.

OLIVER BLOODSTEIN

As discussed in a previous chapter, Oliver Bloodstein (1975) views stuttering as an anticipatory struggle reaction. This anticipatory struggle reaction manifests itself as tension and fragmentation in the stutterer's speech. The original tension and fragmentation is caused by continued and/or severe communicative failures and pressures in the young child.

Bloodstein's (1975) treatment goals for the advanced stutterer, or what he calls the "phase 4" stutterer,[3] are (a) the reduction of anxiety about stuttering and (b) the modification of the stuttering behavior. His therapy sessions are loosely structured, and he does not emphasize data collection.

Bloodstein believes it is important to reduce the advanced stutterer's anxiety for two reasons. First, it is often the most handicapping aspect of the problem; and second, if the anxiety is not reduced, the stutterer will not be able to effectively modify his stuttering behavior. Bloodstein does not believe it possible to rid the client of all his anxiety about stuttering; rather, he attempts to reduce the anxiety as much as reasonably possible. Typical procedures for reducing the stutterer's anxiety about stuttering include the following: encouraging the stutterer to discuss his stuttering openly with others, helping the stutterer to evaluate his listeners' reactions realistically, and assisting the client in overcoming his use of avoidance behaviors.

In helping the stutterer learn to modify his moments of stuttering, Bloodstein begins by teaching the stutterer to identify and relax the tension in his speech mechanism. Next, he teaches the stutterer to learn to reduce the fragmentation in his speech. To do this, Bloodstein teaches the stutterer to move through his feared words in a forward-moving and integrated manner. According to Bloodstein, the stutterer needs to learn to keep his speech mechanism moving forward in a deliberate and unhurried manner as he produces a stuttered word.

Bloodstein notes that, as a result of therapy, a few advanced stutterers become fluent speakers; however, most are left with a residue of occasional mild disfluencies or, in other words, acceptable stuttering.

---

[3] Since the terms "advanced stutterer," "beginning stutterer," and "intermediate stutterer" are not used by all clinicians, the authors needed to determine the comparable development/treatment levels of the other clinicians. Whereas the comparisons are not always exact, we believe they are close enough to make our discussions in this and the following chapters valid.

EDWARD CONTURE

Edward Conture (1982, 1990) in his book, *Stuttering*, discusses the remediation of stuttering at different age levels. In terms of clinical methods, his therapy sessions appear to be low structured without a heavy emphasis on data collection. In his chapter on the adult stutterer, he describes his stuttering modification approach for the advanced stutterer. His two goals for therapy are (*a*) identification and (*b*) modification. From his writings, it is apparent that Conture believes it is important to be sensitive to and discuss with the adult stutterer his feelings and attitudes about his stuttering; however, Conture does not have a separate goal for this purpose.

The purpose of identification is to enable the stutterer to accurately and quickly identify when he is stuttering. Conture begins with "off-line" identification. This involves helping the stutterer identify moments of stuttering in the recordings of other stutterers and in the recordings of the stutterer's own speech. Then Conture works on "on-line" identification or helping the stutterer identify his moments of stuttering as he is speaking. Once the stutterer is able to do this accurately and quickly, he is ready for modification.

Modification begins with the more easily recognizable stutters. Conture starts by helping the stutterer become aware of what he is doing when he stutters or, in Conture's words, what he is doing to "interfere with speaking". Conture then helps the stutterer modify this behavior by learning to reduce the duration of these stutters and to move easily into the next sound of the word. Once these skills are acquired in the clinic, they are practiced in the stutterer's own speaking environment. Conture's comments indicate that he believes it will take a lot of time and practice on the part of the advanced stutterer for these modification skills to become automatic. Thus, some may become spontaneously fluent, but many will have to work for a long time to master a controlled fluency or acceptable stuttering.

DAVID PRINS

In a recent chapter on the management of stuttering in adults, David Prins (1984) discusses stuttering as a learned defensive reaction on the part of the stutterer to perceived interruptions in the flow of speech. To help the stutterer manage his stuttering, Prins describes three phases of therapy. They are: (*a*) exploring, understanding, and accepting responsibility for behavior; (*b*) calming the stutterer and stuttering; and (*c*) replacing stuttering with actions that produce fluent speech. Prins' goal for the client is to "speak as fluently as he is able and has the will and motivation to do." Thus, it seems that a client could have spontaneous fluency, controlled fluency, or acceptable stuttering as his goal. Unlike the other stuttering modification clinicians discussed in this section, Prins employs programmed instruction principles in much of his therapy.

The goal of the first phase of therapy is to help the stutterer become aware of what he is doing when he stutters and to help him assume responsibility for it. To help the stutterer do this, the clinician uses video equipment and/or a mirror to provide feedback to the stutterer. The clinician also models the client's stuttering for him. These activities are accompanied by a great deal of discussion of the stuttering behaviors, as well as the feelings and attitudes that accompany them.

In the second phase of therapy, calming the stutterer and stuttering, the goal is to reduce the intensity of the stutterer's overt motor behavior and internal feelings during the act of stuttering. The clinician and the stutterer jointly rate from high to low the intensity of the motor responses during the moments of stuttering. The stutterer also rates the intensity of his feelings during these stutters. The clinician then explains to the stutterer that his goal is to experience all, or nearly all, moments of stuttering with a low intensity rating. To achieve this, the clinician sequences speech activities in a hierarchy from easy to hard, for example, from one word responses to conversation. This feeling of calm during a moment of stuttering is then transferred through a series of hierarchies to everyday speaking situations.

The goal of the final phase is to teach the stutterer to respond to stimuli that previously triggered stuttering with a new response that results in fluency. To do this, the stutterer is taught to identify his moments of stuttering. Then, whenever he anticipates a moment of stuttering, he is to replace the stuttered response with a brief sound prolongation that blends smoothly with the following sound. This response is first practiced in the clinical setting and later transferred to outside speaking situations.

JOSEPH SHEEHAN

Throughout most of his professional career, Joseph Sheehan (1953, 1975, 1984) viewed stuttering as an approach-avoidance conflict. According to Sheehan, the stutterer stutters whenever his tendency to go ahead and talk is equal to his tendency to hold back and avoid talking. Based upon this theory, he sees therapy for the advanced stutterer as having twin goals, namely, increase the stutterer's approach tendencies and decrease his avoidance tendencies. The emphasis, however, is on the reduction of avoidance.

In his discussion of treatment, Sheehan presents five phases of therapy. They are: (*a*) the self-acceptance phase, (*b*) the monitoring phase, (*c*) the initiative phase, (*d*) the modification of pattern phase, and (*e*) the safety margin phase.[4] His therapy sessions are loosely structured or counseling in nature, and he places little emphasis upon data collection.

The goal of the self-acceptance phase is to have the client accept himself as a stutterer. This does not mean that he is to accept for now and evermore his stuttering as it now exists. This will change as therapy proceeds. Typical procedures during this phase involve the stutterer using good eye contact with his listener and discussing his stuttering openly with friends and acquaintances.

During the monitoring phase, the stutterer is to become aware of his stuttering as he is doing it. He is not to modify or control it; just be aware of it.

In the initiative phase, the stutterer is to seek out his feared situations

---

[4] For two excellent chapters on stuttering modification therapy, the reader is referred to the following two references by Sheehan: Sheehan, J. G. (1975). Conflict theory and avoidance-reduction therapy. In J. Eisenson (Ed.) *Stuttering: A second symposium* (pp. 97–198). New York: Harper & Row, and Sheehan J. G., & Sheehan, V. M. (1984). Avoidance-reduction therapy: A response-suppression hypothesis. In W. H. Perkins (Ed.), *Stuttering disorders* (pp. 147–151). New York: Thieme-Stratton.

and to enter them. He is to seek out his feared words and go ahead and stutter openly on them.

During the modification of pattern phase, the stutterer is to learn to stutter openly and easily. Stuttering openly and easily, according to Sheehan, requires the stutterer to let his listener see and hear that he is having trouble in saying a word. Sheehan recommends the stutterer use a "slide" or a prolongation of the first sound of the word. There should be a smooth release into the next sound of the word. The stutterer is to use the slide on feared words as an alternative method of stuttering.

The goal of the safety margin phase is the development by the stutterer of a tolerance for disfluency. He is to get to a point where he is comfortable in exhibiting more disfluency than he would naturally have. When the stutterer is comfortable putting more stuttering into his speech than he would typically have, he develops a sense of security. This is his "margin of safety." Sheehan recommends that the stutterer voluntarily stutter by using the slide on nonfeared words throughout his speaking day. The more he does this, the more solid his fluency will become. By doing this, Sheehan believes that some advanced stutterers will become spontaneously fluent; most, however, will have acceptable stuttering.

Summary of Stuttering Modification Therapy

At the beginning of this section on stuttering modification therapy for the advanced stutterer, we stated that this form of therapy was characterized by two key elements: (*a*) teaching the stutterer to modify his moments of stuttering, and (*b*) reducing his fear of stuttering and eliminating the avoidance behaviors associated with this fear. Based upon our description of Van Riper's clinical procedures and upon our comments about Bloodstein's, Conture's, Prins', and Sheehan's clinical procedures, it should be apparent to the reader that all of these clinicians' treatments share these two key components. These clinicians' specific clinical procedures may vary, but they all share the above two clinical beliefs.

FLUENCY SHAPING THERAPY

The essence of fluency shaping therapy is that some form of fluency is first established in the clinical setting. While still in the clinic, this fluency is reinforced and gradually modified to approximate normal sounding conversational speech. This new fluency is then generalized to the person's everyday speaking environment. Also, as a general rule, fluency shaping clinicians do not put a great deal of emphasis upon reducing the stutterer's fear and avoidance of words and speaking situations.

We have chosen the fluency shaping approach of William Perkins to illustrate this therapy. Perkins has been involved in developing fluency shaping programs for many years and is an excellent representative of this approach to therapy. We will also briefly describe the clinical procedures of several other fluency shaping clinicians to give the reader a broader understanding of fluency shaping therapy.

William Perkins: Replacement of Stuttering with Normal Speech

CLINICIAN'S BELIEFS

Nature of Stuttering

William Perkins has been a prolific writer on the topic of stuttering for many years. What are his beliefs with regard to the clinical issues we raised in the last chapter? To begin with, Perkins (1986) views stuttering as discoordination of phonation with articulation and respiration. In other words, stutterers have difficulty coordinating or timing the process of phonation with the processes of articulation and respiration during speech. He implies that this discoordination has a constitutional or organic basis, but he cautions that this has not been substantiated. Why is this belief about the nature of stuttering important clinically? Perkins gives us his answer. He suggests that, if stutterers are constitutionally limited in their ability to be fluent, then they would have to rely on compensatory skills to sound fluent.

Speech Behaviors Targeted for Therapy

What are these compensatory skills that Perkins believes stutterers need to use? They include seven fluency skills in all. First of all, there is reduced rate. Second, there are five breathstream management skills. They are: phrasing, phrase initiation, soft contact, breathy voice, and blending. Finally, prosody or rhythm skills are also important.[5] All of these skills will be described when we discuss Perkins' clinical procedures. Perkins believes that, when stutterers use these fluency skills, they will facilitate the coordinations between phonation, articulation and respiration. Fluent speech will be the by-product.

Fluency Goals

What is Perkins' fluency goal for the advanced stutterer? Perkins' (1981) first choice is spontaneous fluency, but he admits this is unrealistic in most cases. Therefore, his goal for this stutterer is not to have controlled fluency all the time; rather, it is to have the ability to use controlled fluency whenever he expects to stutter and would rather not. In other words, his goal is to help the stutterer maintain his fluency skills so that he can use controlled fluency in any difficult speaking situation he chooses.

Feelings and Attitudes

Even though Perkins (1979) believes that attitude change is important in maintaining improvement, he does not focus on this aspect of therapy the way that stuttering modification clinicians do. He does not attempt to desensitize the stutterer to his problem. Rather, Perkins attempts to give the stutterer a sufficient num-

---

[5] Perkins describes these fluency skills in Perkins, W. H. (1973b). Replacement of stuttering with normal speech: II. Clinical procedures. *Journal of Speech and Hearing Disorders, 38,* 295–303, and Perkins, W. H. (1984). Techniques for establishing fluency. In W. H. Perkins (Ed.) *Stuttering disorders* (pp. 173–181). New York: Thieme-Stratton.

ber of experiences in successfully using his fluency skills to prove to the stutterer that he can use controlled fluency in any situation he wants, no matter how scared he is. Perkins relies upon these positive experiences to reduce the stutterer's negative feelings and attitudes about his speech. Perkins notes that, if this strategy is to be successful, the stutterer should not engage in any avoidance behaviors.

Maintenance Procedures

To help his clients maintain their fluency skills, Perkins (1984) prepares them to recover from relapse. For example, in the later stages of therapy, he will have the stutterers discontinue their use of fluency skills until they regress and begin to stutter again. He will then have them practice their fluency skills until they regain their ability to use controlled fluency. He wants them to know that, if they do regress after discontinuation of therapy, they have the ability to recover.

Clinical Methods

Finally, what clinical methods does Perkins employ? In his original fluency shaping program (Curlee & Perkins, 1969), he relied heavily upon operant conditioning and programmed instruction principles; however, in his most recent modification of his fluency shaping therapy (Perkins, 1984), he relies much less on these methods. Perkins, however, has continued to systematically obtain data relative to his clients' frequency of stuttering, rate of speaking, and attitudes about their speech. Now, let us look at how he implements these beliefs in his clinical procedures.

CLINICAL PROCEDURES

Perkins' original fluency shaping therapy program was published with Richard Curlee in 1969, over twenty years ago (Curlee & Perkins, 1969). Several years later, Perkins (1973a, 1973b) described the rationale and clinical procedures for his "replacement of stuttering with normal speech" program. In a recent chapter, Perkins (1984) discussed some modifications to his replacement of stuttering with normal speech program. In essence, the recent modifications appear rather similar to those procedures originally presented. We will describe, for the most part, his 1973 procedures. Where there appear to be important changes, we will note these. We will describe the procedures in enough detail to provide a basic understanding of the program, but the clinician who is interested in using this approach will want to read Perkins' original publications.

In this program, normal-sounding speech is first shaped in the clinical setting, and then it is generalized to everyday life. We will first describe the sequence of goals involved in the shaping of normal-sounding speech in the clinical setting, and then we will discuss the generalization of normal-sounding speech or controlled fluency to everyday speaking situations.

Shaping of Normal Speech

The sequence of goals involved in the shaping of normal speech in the clinical setting is as follows: (a) establish fluent speech, (b) establish normal breath flow, (c) establish normal prosody, (d) shift responsibility for taking all subsequent steps to the stutterer, (*e*) establish slow-normal speech in conversation, (*f*) incorporate psychotherapeutic discussion, (*g*) establish normal speech rate, (*h*) establish normal speech without DAF, and (*i*) establish a clear voice. The delayed auditory feedback machine (DAF) is used to facilitate movement through these goals.

During the first six sessions, or so, the clinician moves the client through the first three goals. The client develops normal-sounding speech in slow-motion (250-msec DAF). He also learns proper breathstream management skills and the use of normal prosody. Once this is achieved, the progression through the remaining goals is determined by the stutterer. He is instructed to move from step to step only when he is comfortable and confident in his use of slow-normal speech. Perkins charts the client's progress during this shaping phase of therapy on a form that he developed for this purpose. Each of the nine goals will now be discussed in some detail.

Establish fluent speech.   The rate skill is the first fluency skill to be taught (Fig. 7.3). The DAF machine, which is set at 250-msec delay, is used to facilitate this goal. The clinician demonstrates to the client that he can overcome the disrupting effects of the DAF machine if he speaks by sufficiently prolonging each syllable. She will also point out to him that when he speaks in this slow-motion manner, approximately 30 words a minute, his stuttering disappears. Reading is usually used at this step because it allows the stutterer to focus on the motor skills of speech production. When the client is able to read without stuttering in this slow-motion pattern, he is ready for the second goal.

Establish normal breath flow.   Five fluency skills are taught in meeting this goal. They are taught in the original program, and Perkins seems to give them even more emphasis in his recent chapter. These fluency skills are as follows: phrasing, phrase initiation, soft contact, breathy voice, and blending. In developing the phrasing skill, the clinician instructs the stutterer to limit his phrase length to 3-8 syllables. This insures sufficient respiratory capacity so that the stutterer does not become tense trying to squeeze extra air out. In teaching the phrase initiation skill, the clinician instructs the client to initiate the first syllable of each phrase

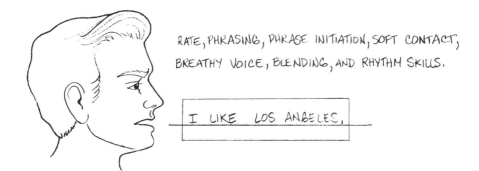

Figure 7.3. Perkins' fluency skills.

with an easy vocal onset. The soft contact skill involves soft or easy articulatory contacts, and the breathy voice skill involves breathy or soft voice. Finally, in presenting the blending skill, the clinician instructs the stutterer to maintain continuous airflow from the beginning of a phrase to the end. All the syllables in a phrase are to flow together smoothly and effortlessly. When the client has mastered these skills, he is ready for the next goal.

Establish normal prosody.   The last fluency skill to be taught is the prosody or rhythm skill. One of the results of speaking in a slow-motion manner is monotonous-sounding speech. This type of speech will not be generalized to everyday speaking situations. Thus, the clinician needs to help the stutterer use normal inflections and syllable durations proportional to normal stress patterns even at this slow rate. When this has been done, the stutterer is ready to move on.

Shift responsibility for taking all subsequent steps to the stutterer.   To foster their self-management and self-confidence, stutterers are given the responsibility for taking all subsequent steps. The criteria they use are subjective, but they appear to be based upon the stutterer's confidence, comfort, and ability to use the fluency skills described above.

Establish slow-normal speech in conversation.   With the DAF machine still set at 250-msec delay, conversation is introduced. The clinician cautions the stutterer that he should not use any avoidance behaviors to maintain his fluency. When the stutterer is able to engage in conversation at this slow-motion rate, he is ready for the next step.

Incorporate psychotherapeutic discussion.   This goal is in the original program, but Perkins does not discuss it in his recent chapter. Basically, his strategy in the original program is for the clinician to respond positively to any statements the client makes that are deemed beneficial to therapeutic progress. In addition to client statements that indicate successful experiences with fluency skills, this includes client statements that reflect growing insights into his stuttering problem and that indicate increased talking on his part. The purpose behind these procedures is to facilitate attitude changes on the part of the stutterer.

Establish normal speech rate.   In achieving this goal, the DAF is gradually phased out. The first step involves reducing the delay to 200 msec. This will allow the stutterer to increase his rate to 45 to 60 words per minute. When the stutterer feels he is ready, the delay is reduced to 150 msec. At this point, the stutterer is allowed to increase his phrases to normal length. Some stutterers will achieve normal rates, 90 to 120 words per minute, at this 150-msec delay. If this is true for her client, the clinician will begin to gradually reduce the volume of the DAF. If normal rates are not achieved for her client at 150-msec delay, the clinician will continue to reduce the DAF in 50-msec decrements until a normal rate is achieved. Then the volume of the DAF will be gradually reduced. At this point, it is important to stabilize a "home base" rate to which the stutterer can return when he encounters problems. This rate should be fast enough to sound normal, but it should be slow enough to allow the stutterer to successfully use his fluency skills.

Establish normal speech without DAF.   At this point, the DAF machine is turned off. Then one earphone is removed at a time, and finally, the headset is removed.

Establish a clear voice.   If the client's voice sounds satisfactory, and if he is using the fluency skills acquired above, then the shaping of normal-sounding speech is concluded. However, if he is using an excessively soft or breathy voice, then voice therapy procedures will be required.

In his 1984 chapter, Perkins suggests that it is impossible for any stutterer to use all seven of the fluency skills at the same time at normal rates. Therefore, he now helps each stutterer to discover which skills are most effective for himself. These are the ones that he will use from here on.

Generalization of Normal Speech

In his original program, Perkins discusses 3 goals or strategies to facilitate the generalization of normal sounding speech. These are: (*a*) to prepare the stutterer to recover normal speech when it is disrupted or when disruption is anticipated, (*b*) to extend stimulus control of normal speech to daily life, and (*c*) to facilitate living pattern changes to foster permanence of normal speech. These goals are not pursued sequentially. In fact, goal 1 can only be achieved while working on goal 2. Goal 3 should be pursued whenever it seems appropriate.

In his recent chapter, Perkins discusses another strategy, which he believes has promise, to help the client maintain his improvement. This is preparation for recovery from relapse. All four of these strategies will now be presented.

Prepare the stutterer to recover normal speech when it is disrupted or when disruption is anticipated.   As the stutterer works his way up the hierarchies involved in meeting goal 2 below, he is to evaluate his speech in terms of fluency, rate, breath flow, prosody, and self-confidence. Perkins has developed a rating form for this purpose. The client is to do this during each therapy session. Tape-recordings should be used so that he and his clinician can consensually validate their judgments. If the stutterer falls below certain criteria in terms of these five dimensions, he is to return to appropriate shaping procedures. It is important to train the stutterer to apply his fluency skills to regain normal-sounding speech whenever it is disrupted or when disruption is anticipated.

Extend stimulus control of normal speech to daily life.   This is done through the use of a series of hierarchies. A hierarchy is a series of speaking situations sequenced from easy to difficult. These speaking situations are changed very gradually so that the stutterer is able to maintain his feeling that speaking is easy. For example, the first hierarchy involves changing the site and social complexity of speaking situations within the clinic and in the presence of the clinician. This is done by changing rooms, by increasing audience size, and so on. Another hierarchy would involve "real" speaking situations that the stutterer typically encounters in everyday life. Again, these would be ranked from easy to difficult. The stutterer would work his way through this later hierarchy by himself. By the use of these and other hierarchies, the stutterer generalizes his new speech pattern to his daily life.

Facilitate living pattern changes to foster permanence of normal speech. This involves exploring with the stutterer social and vocational activities that he would enjoy if he didn't stutter and encouraging him to participate in these and other activities that require speaking.

Preparation for recovery from relapse.   Perkins now prepares the stutterer for the certain eventuality of relapse. Perkins will encourage the stutterer to reverse the use of his fluency skills, that is, to do just the opposite of what he is supposed to do to have normal-sounding speech. For example, Perkins will have the stutterer increase his rate. When he has relapsed, Perkins will have him use the fluency skills he learned in the treatment program to regain his use of normal-sounding speech or controlled fluency. By going through this procedure repeatedly, the stutterer develops confidence in his ability to recover from a relapse. As the stutterer feels he is able to function more independently, the frequency of sessions is reduced. Finally, therapy is terminated.

Other Clinicians

As we did in the stuttering modification section of this chapter, we will now briefly comment upon the therapies for the advanced stutterer of some other representative fluency shaping clinicians. This will increase the reader's familiarity with the fluency shaping literature.

EINER BOBERG

For a number of years, Einer Boberg (1984) has conducted intensive three-week therapy programs during the summers at the University of Alberta in Canada. The program is divided into seven phases: (*a*) baseline, (*b*) identification, (*c*) early modification, (*d*) prolongation, (*e*) rate increase and cancellation, (*f*) self-monitoring and transfer training, and (*g*) transfer. Throughout his therapy program, Boberg puts a great deal of emphasis upon the objective measurement of speech behaviors and the use of criterion levels for movement from one phase to the next. He uses electronic counters and timers to aid in this process.

The purpose of the baseline phase is to establish a baseline from which to measure subsequent changes as the client moves through the program.

During the identification phase, the stutterer learns how to accurately identify his moments of stuttering. He does this from audio tapes, video tapes, and while he is actually speaking.

In the early modification phase, the stutterer is introduced to the following fluency skills: prolongation, easy onset of phrases, soft contact on consonants, short phrases, and continuous airflow throughout the phrases. These skills are first practiced in vowels, then consonant-vowel combinations, then one- and two-syllable words, and finally, in short phrases.

During the prolongation phase, the stutterer is to speak in a prolonged manner at approximately 60 syllables per minute. While doing this, he must incorporate the fluency skills he learned in the previous phase. This slow speech must be struggle free.

In the rate increase and cancellation phase, the stutterer systematically increases his speaking rate in 4 steps from approximately 90 syllables per minute to approximately 190 syllables per minute. The criterion for moving from one rate to the next is less than 1% disfluency. Cancellation, a procedure wherein the stutterer smoothly repeats any syllable on which he struggles, is also introduced.

The goal of the self-monitoring and transfer training phase is for the stutterer to learn to talk at normal rates with less than 1% disfluency and without any feedback from the clinician or the electronic counters.

The purpose of the last phase, the transfer phase, is to transfer the normal-sounding speech or controlled fluency from the clinic to a variety of nonclinical situations. A series of standard and personal assignments are used for this purpose.

BRUCE RYAN

Bruce Ryan (1974) has been involved in programmed therapy for stuttering for many years. His programs are based very heavily upon operant conditioning and programmed instruction principles. Ryan organizes his treatment programs into the following three phases: (*a*) establishment, (*b*) transfer, and (*c*) maintenance. During therapy, Ryan continuously collects data on the client's speech performance, that is, his stuttered words per minute (SW/M) and his words spoken per minute (WS/M). These data are used to determine if the client meets the criterion, usually 0 SW/M for a given period of time, to move on to the next step of the program.

The goal of the establishment phase is to establish fluency with the clinician in the clinical setting. Ryan has a number of establishment programs; however, he usually employs his delayed auditory feedback (DAF) program with adults. In this program, the DAF machine is used to help the stutterer speak in a slow, prolonged, fluent manner. The delay times on the DAF machine are systematically changed to allow the stutterer to gradually increase his speaking rate by reducing his prolongation of speech sounds until he approaches a normal rate. In this program, Ryan sequentially moves the stutterer through a series of steps, or delay times on the DAF machine, in each of the following three modes: reading, monologue, and conversation. He begins with a slow, prolonged, fluent oral reading and gradually shapes it into a fluent conversational speech, or controlled fluency, in the clinical setting.

The goal of the transfer phase is to transfer the client's fluency from the clinical setting to a wide variety of other settings and other people. To do this, Ryan uses a number of hierarchies, or sequences of speaking situations arranged from easy to difficult, in which the client talks and meets the fluency criterion of 0 SW/M. The client obviously needs to be exhibiting spontaneous or controlled fluency, not acceptable stuttering, to meet this criterion.

The goal of Ryan's last phase, the maintenance phase, is for the client to maintain his fluency in all situations for approximately 2 years. This involves the client returning to the clinician for a series of maintenance checks.

GEORGE SHAMES AND CHERI FLORANCE

George Shames and Cheri Florance (1980) are authors of a fluency shaping program for adults that has as its goal "stutter-free speech." Their program is fairly structured, but a little less so than that of some other fluency shaping clinicians. They obtain a substantial amount of data on their stutterers before, during, and after treatment. Shames and Florance divide their therapy into the following five phases: (*a*) volitional control, (*b*) self reinforcement, (*c*) transfer, (*d*) training in unmonitored speech, and (*e*) follow-up.

The goal of the first phase is for the stutterer to gain volitional control over his speech. The two skills that Shames and Florance believe are the most important for the stutterer to acquire, if he is going to volitionally control his speech, are control of rate and continuous phonation. Shames and Florance use the delayed auditory feedback (DAF) machine to help the stutterer learn these skills. They begin with the DAF machine set at its maximum delay and instruct the stutterer in the use of rate control and continuous phonation to produce a slow, prolonged, stutter-free speech. Shames and Florance then gradually increase the stutterer's speaking rate by systematically reducing the delay times on the DAF machine. By the end of this phase, the stutterer is producing stutter-free speech at a near normal rate. In other words, he is using a controlled fluency.

In the self reinforcement phase, the stutterer learns to monitor, evaluate, and reinforce himself for using stutter-free speech in the clinical setting. The reinforcement is gradually shifted from the clinician to the client. The reinforcement that Shames and Florance use in this program is the opportunity for the stutterer to use brief units of unmonitored speech. This is a very interesting clinical procedure, which is based on the Premack Principle (Premack, 1959). This principle states that a frequently occurring behavior can serve as a reinforcer for a less frequently occurring behavior. In other words, after the stutterer uses monitored, stutter-free speech for a period, being able to use unmonitored speech is reinforcing.

The third phase involves the systematic transfer of monitored, stutter-free speech or controlled fluency into the client's environment. At first, this involves only a few situations each day, but by the end of this phase of therapy, it will involve the stutterer using monitored, stutter-free speech for the entire day. Shames and Florance do not use hierarchies, as many clinicians do, to transfer the monitored, stutter-free speech; rather, they use a contract plan. This involves the client preparing a daily contract that specifies the situations in which he will be using monitored, stutter-free speech and then reinforcing himself with some unmonitored speech.

In the fourth phase, the stutterer gradually replaces his monitored, stutter-free speech with unmonitored speech. Shames and Florance indicate that, by this time in treatment, the stutterer's monitored, stutter-free speech and his unmonitored speech are both generally fluent. In other words, the stutterer is now exhibiting both controlled fluency and spontaneous fluency. The important difference, however, is that the stutterer finds the unmonitored speech to be much more reinforcing.

Following the completion of the training in the unmonitored speech phase, the client is placed in a five year follow-up program.

RONALD WEBSTER

Ronald Webster's (1974, 1979, 1980) Precision Fluency Shaping Program at Hollins College has received a great deal of national attention in recent years. Many stutterers from across the country have gone there to participate in his three week intensive treatment program.

Webster believes that the core behaviors of stuttering reflect distorted activities on the part of the muscles involved in voicing and articulation and that these distorted activities probably have a physiological basis. He further believes that the secondary behaviors and feelings and attitudes are most likely learned.

The goal of Webster's Precision Fluency Shaping Program is to teach the stutterer to use fluency-generating target behaviors that, when used correctly, will result in fluency. The two most important target behaviors appear to be slightly increased syllable duration and gentle voice onset. The program begins by teaching the stutterer to prolong or stretch out syllables. A stopwatch is used to measure the duration of the syllables. The stutterer is then taught to coordinate diaphragmatic breathing with these prolonged syllables. Following this, gentle voice onsets are taught. A specially designed voice onset computer, the Voice Monitor, is used to evaluate this target behavior. Once the above target behaviors are established in syllables, they are practiced in one-syllable words; two-syllable words; three-syllable words; short, self-generated sentences; and finally, spontaneous conversation. As the length of the linguistic unit is systematically increased, the duration of the syllables is gradually reduced. By the time the stutterer is practicing his target behaviors in conversation, his speech rate is up to a slow-normal rate; he is using a controlled fluency.

Now, the stutterer is ready to transfer this controlled fluency to outside situations. This involves the following interactions with merchants: single-message telephone calls, single-message personal contacts, double-message telephone calls, double-message personal contacts, and multiple messages both by telephone and personal contact.

Webster's entire program is a very structured or programmed instruction approach to therapy. Every client goes through the same set of explicitly defined procedures. During the 3-week program, the typical stutterer practices his fluency-generating target behaviors approximately 100 hours. Progress from one step of the program to the next depends upon the stutterer meeting certain criterion levels, and a record of correct and incorrect responses is kept for each step.

Summary of Fluency Shaping Therapy

When we began this section on fluency shaping therapy for the advanced stutterer, we stated that the essence of this approach to therapy is the establishment of some form of fluency initially in the clinical setting. It is then reinforced and gradually modified to approximate normal-sounding speech. Following this establishment of fluency in the clinical setting, the fluency is generalized to the client's everyday speaking environment. We also said that, as a general rule, fluency shaping clinicians do not emphasize the reduction of the stutterer's fear and avoidance of words and situations. Based upon our discussion of Perkins' clinical procedures and upon our brief descriptions of Boberg's, Ryan's, Shames and Florance's, and Webster's programs, it should be clear to the reader that all of these clinicians share the above clinical beliefs.

COMPARISON OF THE TWO APPROACHES

Now that we have completed our discussions of stuttering modification and fluency shaping therapies for the advanced stutterer, it would be appropriate to

Table 7.1   Similarities and Differences between Stuttering Modification and Fluency Shaping Therapies for the Advanced Stutterer

Clinical Issue	Therapy Approach	
	Stuttering Modification Therapy	Fluency Shaping Therapy
Speech behaviors targeted for therapy.	Moments of stuttering.	Fluency skills.
Fluency goals.	Spontaneous fluency, controlled fluency, or acceptable stuttering.	Spontaneous fluency or controlled fluency.
Feelings and attitudes.	Considerable attention given to changing feelings and attitudes.	Little attention given to changing feelings and attitudes.
Maintenance procedures.	Emphasis upon maintaining stuttering modification skills and changes in feelings and attitudes.	Emphasis upon maintaining fluency shaping skills.
Clinical procedures.	Therapy characterized by loosely structured interaction.	Therapy characterized by tightly structured interaction or programmed instruction.
	Little emphasis upon collection of objective data.	Considerable emphasis upon collection of objective data.

compare these two approaches on the five clinical issues on which they often differ. As will be recalled, these five issues are as follows: (*a*) speech behaviors targeted for therapy, (*b*) fluency goals, (*c*) attention given to feelings and attitudes, (*d*) maintenance procedures, and (*e*) clinical methods. See Table 7.1 for an overview of the similarities and differences between these two therapy approaches for the advanced stutterer.

With regard to the first issue, speech behaviors targeted for therapy, stuttering modification clinicians teach the stutterer to modify the moments of stuttering to reduce their severity; fluency shaping clinicians, on the other hand, teach the stutterer to use certain fluency enhancing skills to increase the fluency.

Stuttering modification clinicians have spontaneous fluency as their fluency goal for a few advanced stutterers, but for most advanced stutterers, these clinicians have controlled fluency or acceptable stuttering as their goal. Like stuttering modification clinicians, fluency shaping clinicians have spontaneous fluency as their goal for a few advanced stutterers. For the rest, however, their goal is controlled fluency.

Stuttering modification and fluency shaping clinicians differ significantly with regard to targeting feelings and attitudes in therapy. Stuttering modification clinicians give considerable time and energy to reducing the advanced stutterer's negative feelings and attitudes toward his speech. They also stress the elimination of avoidance behaviors. Fluency shaping clinicians give relatively little attention to changing these feelings, attitudes, and avoidance behaviors.

To help the advanced stutterer maintain his improvement following the termination of therapy, stuttering modification clinicians emphasize maintaining the reduction of negative feelings and attitudes and maintaining the elimination of avoidance behaviors. They also emphasize maintaining proficiency in the use of stuttering modification skills. Fluency shaping clinicians emphasize maintaining proficiency in the use of fluency shaping or fluency enhancing skills.

On the last issue, clinical methods, these two therapy approaches usually, but not always, differ. Stuttering modification therapy is usually characterized by loosely structured interaction between the clinician and the client. It is a counseling/teaching type of interaction. Fluency shaping therapy, on the other hand, is often characterized by tightly structured interaction between the clinician and the client. It often occurs in a programmed instruction format. These two approaches often differ, as well, with regard to data collection. Stuttering modification clinicians usually put little emphasis upon the collection of objective data, while fluency shaping clinicians usually put considerable emphasis upon this aspect of therapy.

Even though stuttering modification and fluency shaping therapies differ to some degree on all of the above issues with regard to the treatment of the advanced stutterer, we believe the two most clinically significant differences have to do with the speech behaviors targeted for therapy and the attention given to feelings and attitudes. Thus, when we discuss the integration of these two approaches in the next chapter, we will concentrate much of our effort upon the integration of these two aspects of therapy.

STUDY QUESTIONS

1/ What are the two key elements in stuttering modification therapy for the advanced stutterer?

2/ What are the goals for the following phases of Van Riper's therapy for the advanced stutterer: (a) identification phase, (b) desensitization phase, (c) modification phase, and (d) stabilization phase?

3/ Briefly describe Van Riper's clinical procedures for the advanced stutterer during the identification phase.

4/ Describe one clinical procedure Van Riper uses to desensitize the advanced stutterer to each of the following features of the disorder: (a) confrontation with the disorder, (b) core behaviors, and (c) listener reactions.

5/ Describe the following procedures Van Riper uses to modify the advanced stutterer's moments of stuttering: (a) cancellations, (b) pull-outs, and (c) preparatory sets.

6/ Briefly describe Van Riper's clinical procedures for the advanced stutterer during the stabilization phase.

7/ Describe the key elements of fluency shaping therapy for the advanced stutterer.

8/   Summarize the goals for the following phases of Perkins' therapy for the advanced stutterer: (a) shaping of normal speech and (b) generalization of normal speech.

9/   Describe the following 7 fluency skills as used by Perkins: (a) reduced rate, (b) phrasing, (c) phrase initiation, (d) soft contact, (e) breathy voice, (f) blending, and (g) normal prosody.

10/   Compare stuttering modification and fluency shaping therapies for the advanced stutterer on the following five clinical issues: (a) speech behaviors targeted for therapy, (b) fluency goals, (c) attention given to feelings and attitudes, (d) maintenance procedures, and (e) clinical methods.

Suggested Readings

Perkins, W. H. (1973). Replacement of stuttering with normal speech: I. Rationale. *Journal of Speech and Hearing Disorders, 38,* 283–294.

This is an excellent article in which Perkins discusses a rationale for teaching the advanced stutterer fluency enhancing skills.

Perkins, W. H. (1973). Replacement of stuttering with normal speech: II. Clinical procedures. *Journal of Speech and Hearing Disorders, 38,* 295–303.

In this article, which is a companion article to the above suggested reading, Perkins describes his clinical procedures for teaching fluency enhancing skills.

Sheehan, J. G. (1975). Conflict theory and avoidance-reduction therapy. In J. Eisenson (Ed.), *Stuttering: A second symposium* (pp. 97–198). New York: Harper & Row.

This chapter is a thorough presentation of Sheehan's stuttering modification approach for the advanced stutterer. A great deal of emphasis is placed upon avoidance-reduction techniques.

Van Riper, C. (1973). Our therapeutic approach. In C. Van Riper, *The treatment of stuttering* (pp. 201–370). Englewood Cliffs: Prentice-Hall

In the last half of this book Van Riper presents a very comprehensive presentation of his therapy for the advanced stutterer. For any serious student of stuttering modification therapy, these chapters are "must" reading.

Van Riper, C. (1974). Modification of behavior. In *Therapy for stutterers* (pp. 45–73). Memphis: Speech Foundation of America.

This is a brief, but very good, description of Van Riper's therapy for the advanced stutterer.

8

THE ADVANCED STUTTERER: INTEGRATION OF APPROACHES

Like many other clinicians, we adopt and integrate ideas and clinical procedures from both stuttering modification therapy and fluency shaping therapy. This is true relative to all of the clinical issues on which these two approaches often differ. However, as we indicated in the last chapter, we think it is particularly helpful, with the advanced stutterer, to integrate work on both the modification of moments of stuttering and the teaching of fluency enhancing skills. We also believe it is important to reduce negative feelings and attitudes and eliminate avoidances. We will describe our clinical procedures for integrating stuttering modification and fluency shaping therapies in sufficient detail to allow the clinician to implement them with her clients. We will also discuss the clinical procedures of some other clinicians who integrate stuttering modification and fluency shaping therapies with the advanced stutterer.

Before we begin to discuss our approach, however, it may be helpful to review the characteristics of the advanced stutterer. This client will be either an adult or a high school student. In terms of core behaviors, he will exhibit any of the following: part-word repetitions that contain excessive tension, vowel prolongations that have excessive tension, and blocks. In terms of secondary behaviors, he may exhibit escape behaviors, starting behaviors, postponements, word avoidances, and situation avoidances. The advanced stutterer will evidence frustration, embarrassment, and fear relative to his stuttering. Finally, he will have a definite self-concept of himself as a stutterer.

OUR APPROACH

Clinician's Beliefs

Although our beliefs about the nature of stuttering were stated in Section I of this book, and our views on the other clinical issues were briefly stated in Chapter 5, we have not focused in one place our beliefs regarding the advanced stutterer. Therefore, it seems appropriate that, before we discuss our clinical procedures for the advanced stutterer, we clearly state our clinical beliefs.

NATURE OF STUTTERING

As we stated in Section I, we believe that predisposing physiological factors interact with environmental influences to produce and/or exacerbate the original core behaviors. The child responds to these early core behaviors, or disfluencies, with a tension response in an effort to inhibit them. As the child matures and attempts to cope with these core behaviors, he acquires a variety of escape and starting behaviors. We believe that these are reinforced through operant conditioning. During this same period, a variety of negative feelings, such as frustration, shame, and fear, begin to become associated with the stuttering. These negative feelings generalize through classical conditioning to more and more words and situations. Finally, the child begins to avoid these feared words and situations. These avoidances, we believe, are reinforced through avoidance conditioning. If these underlying processes continue to develop until the individual has reached adolescence or young adulthood, the client will have become an advanced stutterer.

Since the tension response, the secondary behaviors, and the feelings and attitudes are learned, we believe they can be unlearned or modified. Operant and classical conditioning principles are employed in doing this. However, inasmuch as predisposing physiological factors may be contributing to the core behaviors, we believe it is also important to help the advanced stutterer learn to cope with these disruptions in his speech. This is important if he is going to maintain the improvement in his fluency.

SPEECH BEHAVIORS TARGETED FOR THERAPY

Which speech behaviors should be targeted in therapy? We believe that most advanced stutterers have developed a substantial tension response and that associated with this tension response is a considerable overlay of learned secondary behaviors. To cope with these learned behaviors and to speak more fluently, we believe it is beneficial for the advanced stutterer to learn to modify the given mo-

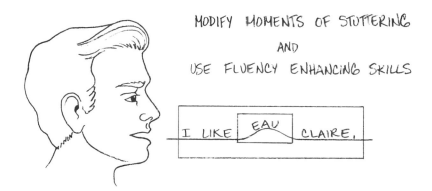

Figure 8.1. Integration of stuttering modification and fluency shaping therapies.

ments of stuttering, as well as to learn to use certain fluency enhancing skills. We believe these two skills can complement one another. After all, the slow movements and light articulatory contacts involved in Van Riper's pull-outs or preparatory sets are identical to the slow, prolonged sounds and soft articulatory contacts involved in Perkins' fluency skills. The only difference is that the former involves modifying the stuttered word, and the latter involves modifying the overall speech pattern. To state this another way, the stuttering modification clinician teaches the stutterer to modify words on which there is actual or anticipated stuttering, and the fluency shaping clinician teaches the stutterer to modify the whole sentence in an effort to keep any stuttering from arising. Why not teach the stutterer to do both (Fig. 8.1)?[1]

Whether the clinician is teaching the stutterer to modify given moments of stuttering or teaching him to use fluency enhancing skills, operant conditioning principles, especially reinforcement principles, will be helpful in achieving either of these goals. Examples of the application of operant conditioning principles will be presented in our discussion of clinical procedures.

Finally, since we believe that the core behaviors may have a physiological basis, we believe that both stuttering modification skills and fluency enhancing skills will help the advanced stutterer cope more effectively with these physiological disruptions in his speech. By using these skills, he will be able to maintain his fluency more effectively.

Fluency Goals

What are our fluency goals for the advanced stutterer? We believe the ultimate goal for the advanced stutterer is spontaneous fluency in all situations or, in other words, normal speech. In our opinion, though, most advanced stutterers

---

[1] As we (Guitar and Peters, 1980) have previously observed, stuttering modification and fluency shaping therapies often produce speech patterns that sound similar. As clients receiving either therapy become more fluent, "they pass through a stage of controlled fluency in which words are spoken with a prolonged, gradual onset. The pull-outs and preparatory sets of stuttering modification therapy may be indistinguishable from the gentle onsets or slow, prolonged patterns of some fluency shaping therapies."

do not reach this level of fluency. The stutterer will probably have periods of spontaneous fluency lasting from a few hours to a month or more, but usually some stuttering will return, especially in stressful situations. At these times, we would like the stutterer to have the following three options available to him.

First, when the stutterer feels it is important to sound fluent, we would like him to be able to successfully apply either stuttering modification skills or fluency shaping skills or both to achieve controlled fluency.

Second, when he feels it is important to sound fluent but is unable to achieve controlled fluency, we would like him to, at least, be able to apply and feel comfortable with either stuttering modification skills or fluency shaping skills or both to achieve acceptable stuttering.

And third, when he feels it is not important to sound fluent and he does not want to put the effort into doing so, we would like him to be comfortable with acceptable stuttering. These fluency goals seem realistic to us. Further, it is important to note that, in the final analysis, it will be the stutterer who chooses which of the above options he will use in a particular situation.

FEELINGS AND ATTITUDES

We believe that the advanced stutterer's avoidance behaviors and negative feelings and attitudes need to receive considerable attention in therapy (Fig. 8.2). He needs to eliminate his use of avoidances. This is because the stutterer will never reduce his fear of certain words and certain speaking situations as long as he continues to run away from them. Furthermore, it is very important that these fears be reduced. If the stutterer is going to successfully use either stuttering modification or fluency shaping techniques to improve his fluency, these speech fears need to be diminished. If the stutterer is too fearful, the result will be excessive muscular tension. Under these conditions, his motor control will break down, and he will not be able to alter his speech production.

We also believe that these avoidances and speech fears need to be substantially reduced if the stutterer is going to maintain his improvement over the long run. If these avoidances and fears are not significantly diminished, we believe

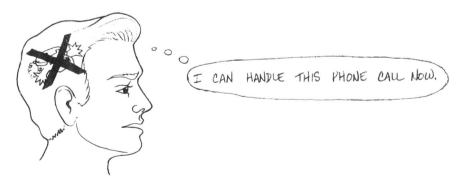

Figure 8.2. It is important to target feelings and attitudes.

they will become the seeds for relapse, which is so prevalent among advanced stutterers.

It is important for the clinician to understand classical conditioning principles when attempting to eliminate the client's avoidance behaviors and reduce his negative feelings and attitudes. How do these changes occur? They occur when the clinician employs counterconditioning and/or deconditioning procedures. Counterconditioning takes place when conditioned stimuli, that is, words and situations that elicit fear, are experienced over and over again in the presence of positive feelings. For example, when the stutterer confronts and explores his stuttering in the presence of an accepting and understanding clinician, counterconditioning occurs. Deconditioning, on the other hand, takes place when words and situations that elicit relatively low levels of fear are experienced over and over until the fear becomes dissipated or extinguished. This is why we use hierarchies of least to most fearful stimuli in helping the stutterer reduce his negative emotions. By beginning with the client's least fearful words or situations and gradually working our way up his hierarchies, his fears are systematically reduced. Examples of these procedures will be presented in the discussion of our clinical procedures.

MAINTENANCE PROCEDURES

What procedures do we use to help the stutterer maintain the gains he made in therapy? We believe it is very important for the stutterer to become his own speech clinician. This involves a number of things.

We need to help the stutterer keep his speech fears and avoidances at a very low level.

We need to help him thoroughly master stuttering modification and fluency shaping techniques so that he can effectively modify both his moments of stuttering and enhance his fluency.

It is even more important that we help him learn to evaluate his own performance with regard to these goals and to give himself assignments to maintain these goals. This will involve gradually shifting more and more of the responsibility of therapy to him as he improves. We also believe that it is important for the stutterer to have a realistic understanding of what he might expect in terms of long-term fluency. In other words, we want him to understand the concepts of spontaneous fluency, controlled fluency, and acceptable stuttering. We want him to set his own fluency goals. It is also important that he come to realize the relationship between the conscientiousness with which he applies what he has learned in therapy and the attainment of his fluency goals.

CLINICAL METHODS

Our clinical procedures for the advanced stutterer are implemented primarily in a counseling/teaching type of interaction. The only exception to this is teaching the stutterer fluency shaping or fluency enhancing behaviors. At this time, we often use a loose application of programming principles. We accompany our clients on many outside speaking assignments, and we also give our clients a great many outside speaking assignments to do on their own. We have applied our clinical procedures in both individual and group therapy.

In terms of data collection, we measure our client's frequency of stuttering and rate of speech before treatment begins and at the termination of treatment. At times, we measure our client's speech during each therapy session. This is especially true when we are teaching the client a new skill, such as fluency shaping or fluency enhancing behaviors. We also attempt to assess our client's speech in his daily speaking environment and to evaluate his feelings and attitudes about his speech. The particular measures that we use were described in chapter 6 in our discussion of assessment.

Clinical Procedures

We have been integrating or combining components of stuttering modification therapy and fluency shaping therapy in a number of ways in our clinical work over the past several years.[2] In the following pages, we will describe what we are currently doing.

Based upon our present beliefs, we think it is important that treatment for the advanced stutterer contain the following components or phases: (*a*) understanding stuttering, (*b*) reducing negative feelings and attitudes and eliminating avoidances, (*c*) using fluency enhancing skills and modifying the moments of stuttering, and (*d*) maintaining improvement. We usually sequence the components as they are listed above. However, at times we have found it beneficial with some stutterers to have phase 3, using fluency enhancing behaviors and modifying the moments of stuttering, precede phase 2, reducing negative feelings and attitudes and eliminating avoidances. This has been especially true with some advanced stutterers who resist confronting their speech fears. This resistance is usually manifested by the stutterer either being tokenly involved in therapy or discontinuing therapy.

We typically provide the client with a set of handouts that describes the procedures used in each of the above phases (Peters, 1987). These handouts are written for the stutterer. In the following pages, we will be reproducing these handouts.

UNDERSTANDING STUTTERING

The goal of this first phase is to help the stutterer understand some basic information about his stuttering. Besides identifying his core behaviors, secondary behaviors, and feelings and attitudes about his stuttering, he will also become familiar with our beliefs about the nature of stuttering. If he is to change his stuttering, we believe he needs to understand what he can change about his stuttering. Also, by becoming familiar with his stuttering, he will lose some of the discomfort associated with it. In other words, some of his fears will become deconditioned. The reader will see the obvious similarities between what we do in this phase and what Van Riper does in his identification phase.

---

[2] The reader is referred to Guitar, B., & Peters, T. J. (1980). The high school and adult stutterer. In B. Guitar & T. J. Peters, *Stuttering: An integration of contemporary therapies* (pp. 31–47). Memphis: Speech Foundation of America for an earlier version of an integrated or combined approach to treatment for the advanced or adult stutterer.

When the clinician first meets the stutterer, she should be warm and friendly. Her behavior should also indicate that she is comfortable with stuttering. Finally, she should be well prepared. That is, she should be thoroughly familiar with the overall goals of therapy and the procedures that will be used to achieve these goals. This will give her an air of competence and will foster the client's developing confidence in her clinical ability. This is important. We all want to believe that the person we are going to for help knows what she or he is doing. The stutterer is no different.

During the first session, it is usually beneficial to familiarize the client with the overall plan of therapy, that is, to briefly explain to him the purpose and nature of the 4 phases enumerated above. The clinician should also answer any questions the stutterer may have regarding any of the above phases or about therapy in general.

Then, it would be appropriate to begin working on the first phase. One strategy that seems to work well is to have the stutterer read the "Understanding Your Stuttering" handout, which appears below. He could read this to himself. If he is like most stutterers, he will have questions, or he will comment upon some of his own behaviors that are described in the handout. The clinician should carefully answer his questions and enthusiastically reinforce any insights he shares about his own stuttering. She should be careful to be understanding and accepting of his comments and feelings.

UNDERSTANDING YOUR STUTTERING

We want to better understand your stuttering, and we want you to do the same. You may not know what you do or how you feel when you stutter. Because it's unpleasant, you have probably attempted to hide it from yourself as well as others. Let's begin to explore your stuttering by discussing the following components of the problem. Once you explore and better understand your stuttering, it will lose its mystery, and you will be less uncomfortable with it.

CORE BEHAVIORS: These are the repetitions, prolongations, and/or blocks (getting completely blocked on a word) that you have. These are the core or heart of the problem. These were the first stuttering behaviors you had as a child.

Why do you have these core behaviors? An increasing amount of research suggests that persons who stutter may have "timing" problems related to the control of the speech mechanism. For fluent speech to occur, muscle movements involved in breathing, in voice production (voice box), and in articulation (tongue, lips, jaw) must all be well coordinated. There is evidence to suggest that persons who stutter experience a lack of coordination between these muscle groups during speech. Further, the research implies that these physical "timing" problems are so slight that they show up as stuttering only when feelings and emotions are strong enough to cause a breakdown in the coordination of the speech mechanism. We know that our ability to perform any physical skill can be affected by our emotions at the time. When our feelings and emotions are strong, they usually interfere with our performance. This is especially true with regard to the fine coordinations of the speech mechanism in the person who stutters. In therapy, we will teach you techniques to more effectively cope with these core behaviors.

SECONDARY BEHAVIORS: Secondary behaviors are tricks or crutches that you use to avoid your stuttering or to help you get a word out. They are behaviors you have learned over the years to help you cope with the core behaviors. They can be unlearned. There are different types of secondary behaviors. Which of the following do you use?

Avoidance Behaviors: Avoidance behaviors include: substituting words, rephrasing sentences, not entering feared speaking situations, pretending not to know the answer, etc. There are many ingenious ways stutterers avoid talking when they expect to stutter.

Postponement Behaviors: These are tricks stutterers use to postpone saying a word until they can say it fluently. Examples include: pausing, repeating a word like "well" over and over, etc.

Starting Behaviors: Starters are tricks you may use to help you begin a feared word. Common starters include: beginning a sentence with unnecessary words like "you know" or "um," body movements like tapping your foot or moving your head at the same time you start the word, etc.

Escape Behaviors: These are things the stutterer does to get out of a word once he is stuttering. It could be a nod of the head, jerk of the jaw, etc., to help him out of the word.

Disguise Behaviors: These are tricks stutterers use to hide their stuttering. Some common disguise behaviors include: covering your mouth with your hand when you stutter, turning your head when you stutter, etc.

FEELINGS AND ATTITUDES: When you began to stutter as a child, you were probably unaware of your stuttering. However, because you have been stuttering for many years, you may have had many frustrating and embarrassing speaking situations. Consequently, if you're like most stutterers, you have probably developed or learned some negative feelings and attitudes about your speech. You may feel embarrassed, guilty, fearful, or even angry. Fear is the most common. Stutterers typically fear certain speaking situations and certain sounds or words. What feelings and attitudes do you have regarding your stuttering? As part of your therapy, we will help you reduce these unpleasant feelings and attitudes.

With the help of your clinician, explore and describe the various components of your stuttering problem. Before you can change something, you need to understand what you are changing.

After the clinician has answered any questions the stutterer may have had about the handout and after the stutterer has shared any insights he may have had, it is a good idea for the clinician to go through the handout section by section with the stutterer to begin cataloging all the various aspects of the stutterer's problem. This may take several sessions. It is important that the stutterer become familiar with the components of his stuttering. If he is going to change, he needs to know what to change. This will involve the clinician's questioning the stutterer about his stuttering. It will involve explanations by the clinician. It will include the clinician's modeling the client's stuttering behaviors, doing mirror-work, and making audio and video recordings. It will also include outside assignments in which the stutterer identifies various components of his stuttering problem in his everyday speaking environment. During these sessions, the clinician must attempt to be understanding and accepting of the stutterer's behaviors and feelings. She needs to show interest in what he is doing and saying. At times, however, if she thinks he is avoiding facing some aspect of his problem, she may need to confront him on it. Nevertheless, throughout this process she must convey to the stutterer a basic interest in and acceptance of him and his stuttering. This is important if counterconditioning of his speech fears is going to occur. Although much of the work of this phase of therapy will be done in a few sessions, the stutterer will continue to learn new things about his stuttering and himself throughout the remainder of treatment.

REDUCING NEGATIVE FEELINGS AND ATTITUDES AND ELIMINATING AVOIDANCES

The goal of this second phase of therapy is to help the stutterer reduce his fear and other negative emotions associated with his stuttering. Another goal is to help him change his attitudes about his speech. We want him to become more open and accepting of his disfluency. Finally, we want him to eliminate his use of all speech avoidance behaviors. We have found the following four techniques particularly helpful in meeting these sub-goals: (*a*) discussing stuttering openly, (*b*) using feared words and entering feared situations, (*c*) freezing or holding on to moments of stuttering, and (*d*) using voluntary stuttering. The reader will see the strong influence of Van Riper and Sheehan in these procedures.

Discussing stuttering openly.   We usually begin this second phase by encouraging the stutterer to discuss his stuttering openly with others. We have found the following handout for the stutterer helpful in introducing this activity.

DISCUSSING STUTTERING OPENLY

One way to become more comfortable with your stuttering is to discuss stuttering openly with your family, friends, and acquaintances. When you get to the point of being open about your stuttering, you will lose much of your fear of it. You will be more relaxed. In most cases, your listeners know you stutter, you know you stutter, but nobody ever says anything about it. It's like the ostrich sticking his head in the sand. If the ostrich can't see the danger, he pretends it's not there. He would be much better off if he got his head out of the sand and dealt directly with his problem. This is true for stuttering, too. You would feel much more comfortable about your stuttering if you could talk about it openly. Your listener would also be more comfortable if you were open and at ease with your stuttering. Your listener often takes his cue from you regarding how to respond. If you look uncomfortable, he will probably be uncomfortable. On the other hand, if you are open and comfortable with your stuttering, you will put your listener at ease.

How can you be more open about your stuttering? It is important to tell family and friends that you are in speech therapy. Explain to them what you are doing in therapy and why you are doing it.

It is important for you to discuss with your family and friends how you feel about your stuttering. Do they know you are afraid to talk in some situations? Do they know you get embarrassed when you stutter?

Do any of your family or friends respond to your stuttering in ways that make you uncomfortable? Do they say words for you? Do they look away when you stutter? It is important for them to know how you would like them to respond.

It would also help you and your listeners—family, friends, and acquaintances—to feel more relaxed about your stuttering if you could briefly comment on your stuttering from time to time. If you had a particularly hard block, you could make a brief comment about it. This would let your listener know that you can cope with the problem, and that they don't have to feel uneasy for you. Along this same line, many stutterers find it helps to start a speech or presentation to a group by announcing at the very beginning that they stutter. This breaks the ice and puts everyone more at ease.

The above examples are only some of the ways that you can be more open with your stuttering. With the help of your clinician, you can come up with many more. The more you are able to do this, the more comfortable you and your listeners will become. You will feel much less fear and tension, and you will speak with less stuttering.

A few advanced stutterers will find these assignments easy to do; however, most advanced stutterers will find them somewhat difficult. They will need the help of a supportive clinician. Here are some of the things the clinician can do to help the stutterer implement these assignments. She can help the stutterer generate a list of speaking situations in which he will talk openly about his stuttering. She can explore with him what he will say in these situations. For example, he can casually comment upon his stuttering to some strangers, he can take a survey of people's reactions to stuttering, he can inform his friends that he is enrolled in speech therapy, or he can talk to his parents or spouse about his feelings about stuttering. Before the stutterer does any of the above assignments on his own, it is usually helpful if the clinician accompanies him on some outside assignments where first she, and then he, carry out the assignments. For example, they could jointly take a survey of people's reactions to stuttering. The clinician and the stutterer can also role-play situations in the clinic before the stutterer does them on his own in real life. Finally, it is very important to arrange all of these tasks or assignments in a hierarchical order from least to most stressful as perceived by the stutterer. This will increase the probability that the stutterer's fear will be kept at a minimum. In other words, as the stutterer successfully completes the easier tasks on the hierarchy, the apprehension or fear associated with these tasks will be reduced. This desensitization, or reduction of negative emotion associated with these less stressful tasks, will generalize to the more stressful tasks. Consequently, when he gets to these more stressful tasks, they will no longer be as difficult. As the stutterer does the assignments on his hierarchy, he should discuss the outcomes with his clinician. She should give him a great deal of praise for confronting his fears and discussing his stuttering openly. At other times, she may need to encourage or even push him to move on to the next step. However, she should be sensitive to the intensity of his feelings so that she does not expect too much from him too soon.

The stutterer will probably never be completely finished with this activity. That is, discussing his stuttering openly will be an important strategy for him to use throughout therapy. It will also be a beneficial strategy for him to use long after therapy is ended to help him maintain his improved fluency. Thus, the clinician does not stay on this activity until the stutterer completes his hierarchy before moving on to the next technique. Rather, she gets the stutterer started on his hierarchy, and then she moves on to the next technique. The stutterer will continue to work on discussing his stuttering openly in his outside assignments in conjunction with his work on other techniques or procedures.

Using feared words and entering feared situations.   Again, we introduce this procedure by having the stutterer read the accompanying handout. This handout appears below.

USING FEARED WORDS AND ENTERING FEARED SITUATIONS

An important goal for you to achieve in overcoming your stuttering is to eliminate your use of avoidance behaviors. You must eliminate your avoidance of feared sounds and words and your avoidance of feared situations. You will make much more progress if you keep seeking out feared words and feared situations instead of running away from them. An "approach set" is incompatible with an "avoidance set." You must replace your avoidance set with an approach set.

Avoidance of feared sounds and words must be eliminated. You should stop using substitutions of easier words for words on which you expect to stutter. You should discontinue rephrasing sentences to get around feared words. You should no longer pretend to not know an answer when you do know the answer. Instead of using these tricks, you should have an approach set to say exactly what you want to say. Once you are aware of some fear on a word, you should commit yourself to saying that word. In time, you will find your old fears decreasing, and, with this decrease in word fears, you will find your word and sound avoidances decreasing and your fluency increasing.

From this day on, you should try not to avoid talking while in the clinic. If you want to talk about a topic or ask a question, do it. You should not avoid or postpone saying feared words in therapy. If you think you are going to stutter on a word, go ahead and stutter. In the long run, this is much better than avoiding or postponing. You will learn that you can tolerate your stuttering, and you will be more comfortable with it. You will also be more fluent.

Avoidance of feared situations must also be eliminated. You must begin to talk in all those situations you have avoided in the past. You must begin to introduce yourself to strangers. You must begin to use the telephone, and you must begin to speak in groups. Once you are aware of any fear of a speaking situation, this should be a red flag to you that indicates that you should approach and enter that speaking situation. Your willingness to speak in these situations will make things much easier for you in the long run. You will find your situation fears decreasing; consequently, you will find your wanting to avoid these speaking situations also decreasing. A by-product will be increased fluency.

Besides not avoiding here in the clinic, you should begin today to eliminate the use of word and situation avoidances in the real world. You will need to develop an approach set in your own speaking environment. Your clinician will help you do this. You and your clinician will set up a series of outside speaking assignments—from least fearful to most fearful—to help you overcome your use of avoidances. Now and then, the old speech fears will be too strong; you will avoid, but come back the next day and try again. In time, you will find the old fears decreasing. Your tolerance for stuttering will increase. You will be more comfortable with yourself as a speaker, and you will be speaking more fluently. You will need to keep working on this approach attitude for a long time. It is important that you eliminate your avoidances—and keep them eliminated.

After the stutterer has read the handout, the clinician should answer any questions he may have. Then she should instruct him to try not to use any postponements or word avoidances in therapy from then on. If he does, she should again remind him. When she sees him deliberately using a word that he appeared to want to avoid, she should strongly reinforce him for this approach behavior. The clinician can also set up activities where the stutterer purposively uses his feared words, which have been previously identified. This can involve the stutterer's reading word lists or text loaded with his feared words or involve his making up sentences loaded with these words. The clinician should warmly praise him each time he does not postpone or avoid a feared word. She should remain calm when he stutters. She should also be sensitive to his feelings and let him know that she understands the frustration or anxiety he is probably experiencing. This will help him become more comfortable with these words and will reduce his tendency to want to avoid them.

To help the stutterer eliminate his use of avoidances outside the clinic, the clinician needs to help him set up a hierarchy of word and situation avoidances that he uses in his daily life. Like all hierarchies, it should be sequenced from least to most difficult for the client. By using this strategy, the stutterer's fears will be kept to a minimum. A typical step or assignment in the hierarchy would be the stutterer's deliberate use of certain feared words on purpose throughout the day. How often should the stutterer use these feared words? He should use them over and over until he no longer is prone to avoid them. Another step in the hierarchy involves the stutterer's entering the feared situations that he usually avoids in his daily life. Again, he should enter these situations often enough so that he loses his motivation to avoid them. Many of the above assignments can be done as the stutterer goes through his daily routine. That is, they will not take extra time on the part of the stutterer. He just needs to answer the telephone whenever it rings with his feared word "hello" or to introduce himself to a different person in his class each day. Other assignments may have to be created, and the stutterer will need to go out of his way to perform them. For example, the stutterer may have to go shopping for an item with a name that contains one of his feared sounds or to prefabricate telephone calls to local businesses. To help the stutterer get started on his outside hierarchy, it is helpful for the clinician to join him in some of the assignments. Thereafter, the stutterer can do the assignments by himself, but he is to discuss his progress with his clinician during their regular therapy sessions. She should make sure he keeps on track in completing his hierarchy, and she should provide him with the necessary support, and possibly gentle nudging, to help him do so.

Like discussing stuttering openly, eliminating avoidances is a strategy that the stutterer will use throughout therapy and beyond. So, once the stutterer is beginning to do this in his outside assignments, it is time to move on to the next procedure.

Freezing or holding on to moments of stuttering. The next technique we will discuss is referred to as freezing or holding on to a moment of stuttering. See the handout below.

FREEZING OR HOLDING ON TO THE MOMENT OF STUTTERING

The experience of being caught in a core behavior can be very unpleasant. Experiencing a repetition, a prolongation, or a block can be very frustrating and scary. When the mouth doesn't do what you want it to do, it can be very traumatic. However, you need to increase your tolerance for these core behaviors. You need to learn that you can experience these core behaviors without becoming panicky. Instead of avoiding or hurrying out of one of these core behaviors, you need to learn that you can experience them and still remain relatively calm.

How do you learn to remain relatively calm while experiencing a moment of stuttering? We use a technique called "freezing" or "holding on." By freezing we mean that when you are stuttering, and we signal, you are to hold on to that moment of stuttering until we again signal you to come out of it. If you are repeating a syllable, you are to continue repeating it; if you are prolonging a sound, you are to continue prolonging it; and if you are having a block, you are to maintain that phonatory arrest or articulatory posture. By experiencing these core behaviors over and over again while remaining relatively calm, you will find your tolerance for them increasing. You will no longer become fearful at the thought of getting stuck on a word. You will find the core behaviors becoming more relaxed.

You will begin by holding on to a core behavior for only a brief period of time, possibly a second or two. When you get caught in a stutter, your clinician will signal you to hold on to that stutter. You are to hold on to that core behavior and keep it going until she signals you to complete the word. While holding on to the repetition, prolongation, or block, you are to try to be as calm as possible. Just experience the stutter and be as composed and relaxed as you possibly can be. As your tolerance increases, your clinician will gradually increase the length of time you are to hold on to your stutters. Eventually, you will hold on to your stutters until the tension and struggle have dissipated. This will involve your signaling yourself—and your clinician—when you begin a stutter and when you will come out of a stutter. She will also have you watch yourself in a mirror and listen to yourself on a tape recorder as you are holding on to your stutters. Again, just experience your stuttering and try to be as calm as possible.

By experiencing these moments of stuttering over and over again in this manner, you will gradually lose your fear of them. You will find yourself feeling more comfortable when you are talking, and you will be talking more fluently.

After the clinician has made sure that the stutterer understands the concept and procedures involved in freezing, she explores with the stutterer the sequence of activities they will follow. Freezing, like the other procedures in this phase of therapy, is most effectively implemented in a hierarchical order. Will the stutterer be able to stop in the middle of a block and hold on to it when the clinician signals, or will this be too stressful? Possibly, the clinician will first have to put some stutterings into her speech and have the stutterer signal her to freeze. How long will the stutterer be able to hold on to a core behavior in the beginning? Will it be more unpleasant for the stutterer to watch himself in a mirror as he holds on to a block, or will it be more difficult to listen to himself on a tape recorder? Once these questions are explored and a hierarchy tentatively established, the clinician begins on the first or easiest task.

Suppose it was decided to begin by having the stutterer hold his stutters for 1 to 2 seconds. This activity would go something like this. Whenever the stutterer has a moment of stuttering during a conversation, the clinician signals him, by raising her finger or tapping on the table, to freeze or to hold on to whatever he is doing at that time. She has him hold his repetitions, prolongations, or blocks for only a second or two. Then she signals him to continue. If his tension and struggle have dissipated before the clinician's signal, the stutterer is to voluntarily keep his stuttering going until she signals. During these periods, the clinician remains calm and shows interest in what the stutterer is doing. She encourages the stutterer to remain calm, too. If the stutterer appears to be frustrated, fearful, or angry, she verbalizes these feelings for him, and she accepts these feelings. If the stutterer looks away when he is holding his stutters, she encourages him to maintain eye contact with her. She also strongly reinforces him for his successes in hanging on to his stutters. When the stutterer is successful with this step, the clinician moves on to more stressful steps.

These more stressful steps include gradually increasing the duration with which the stutterer holds on to his core behaviors. They also include having the stutterer assume the responsibility for signaling when he begins and when he will end a stutter. He should signal the end when the tension and struggle have dissipated. These steps also include having the stutterer listen to himself on a recorder and watch himself in a mirror as he holds on to moments of stuttering. Throughout all of these steps, the clinician continues to be understanding, accepting, and reinforcing of the stutterer's feelings and behaviors. By spending a number of sessions in the clinic doing activities such as these, the stutterer will gradually lose much of the strong negative emotion associated with his moments of stuttering; that is, he will gradually become counterconditioned to his stutters. When this has occurred, it is time to move on.

Using voluntary stuttering.   Voluntary stuttering can be a very potent procedure in the desensitization process. Every clinician should be familiar with it. Our handout explaining voluntary stuttering to the advanced stutterer appears below.

USING VOLUNTARY STUTTERING

One of the most important goals for you to achieve in overcoming your stuttering is to reduce the negative feelings, such as fear and embarrassment, associated with it. The more embarrassed you are by your stuttering and the more fearful you are of talking, the more you try to hide the stuttering. The more you try to hide your stuttering, the more tense you become and the more you tend to stutter. This process needs to be reversed.

One way to reduce these feelings is to stutter voluntarily. If you are afraid of something and constantly run away from it, you will always remain afraid of it. The way to overcome being afraid of something is to gradually confront it and discover that it's not that scary. By confronting your fear, you will learn that you are tougher than you think you are. This is true for stuttering, too. By stuttering on purpose, first in easy situations and later in more difficult situations, you will learn that you can stutter without becoming overly emotional about it.

You will begin using voluntary stuttering in the clinic. You and your clinician will begin by putting easy repetitions and prolongations in your speech. You will do this on nonfeared words. Don't be alarmed if you begin to stutter on some words on which you use voluntary stuttering. This is a common experience when beginning voluntary stuttering. Just keep on stuttering voluntarily until you can finish the word comfortably and without struggling. We will continue to practice this until you are able to remain calm while voluntarily stuttering here in the clinic.

The next step will involve you and your clinician's going out into the real world to do voluntary stuttering together. Again, you will use easy repetitions or prolongations with strangers on nonfeared words. While doing these activities, you will find out that most people are accepting of stuttering. Most people will simply wait for you to say what you want to say. Very few listeners have any reactions. While testing reality in this way, you will learn that you are able to tolerate stuttering and any listener's reactions to it without becoming overly emotional about it.

You will also need to do the above type of activities by yourself in your own speaking world. You will need to do a great many of these voluntary stuttering activities in your own environment to reduce your old fears. Old feelings die slowly! However, if you conscientiously do voluntary stuttering sufficiently often over a long period of time, you will find your old fears decreasing. You will no longer be hiding your stuttering. You will be less tense. You will be talking more comfortably and more fluently. When you are ready to do voluntary stuttering on your own in your everyday speaking situations, we will help you prepare assignments for yourself.

Upon being introduced to voluntary stuttering by their clinician, many stutterers believe their clinician must be crazy. After all, they came to therapy to rid themselves of stuttering, not to do more of it. At this point, the clinician needs to carefully explain to the stutterer the rationale behind the use of voluntary stuttering. We have often found the following analogy to be helpful in this regard. Suppose a person wanted to overcome being afraid of snakes. They would not overcome being afraid of snakes by constantly running away from them. Rather, the person would have to begin seeking out contact with snakes. The best way to do this would be as follows. First, the person would need the guidance of another person who was an expert on snakes and who was not afraid. Second, the person should gradually come into contact with snakes through a series of small steps. For example, the first step might involve only looking at a harmless, little grass snake in a tank. The next step might involve briefly touching the little snake. Next, the person might pick up the grass snake and hold it for a short period. Finally, this process would be repeated over and over again with larger and more fearsome snakes until the person had totally overcome his fear of snakes. This is true with stuttering, too. With the clinician's guidance and with the use of voluntary stuttering and hierarchies, the stutterer will begin to approach stuttering on purpose and learn that he has nothing to fear.

After explaining the rationale behind voluntary stuttering, the clinician begins teaching the stutterer how to do voluntary stuttering. The clinician models brief, easy repetitions or prolongations. She is calm and relaxed when she does this. She encourages the stutterer to attempt some voluntary stuttering. If he does, she enthusiastically reinforces his efforts. If he finds it too difficult, she can suggest that they do them together. That is, the stutterer can imitate her while she is doing some voluntary stuttering. With this sort of modeling and support, most stutterers will be able to do some voluntary stuttering within the session. The clinician continues to give the stutterer lots of praise for his courage in doing this frightening thing. She points out to him that what seemed so fearful before, no longer seems so.

After the stutterer becomes comfortable with voluntary stuttering with the clinician in the clinic, it is time to move out into the world. With input from the stutterer, the clinician establishes a hierarchy of situations in which the stutterer will use voluntary stuttering. The beginning steps involve the clinician. That is, she goes out into situations with the stutterer and puts voluntary stuttering into her speech. These situations might include asking directions from strangers or asking information from store clerks. She remains calm as she does this. Then she accompanies the stutterer as he does some voluntary stuttering in similar situations. She continues to give him a lot of support and reinforcement during these activities. She also points out to the stutterer that the large majority of listeners do not respond negatively to his stuttering. If he does receive some occasional adverse responses, she accepts his feelings of embarrassment or anger. She also notes that, even though this happened, he was strong enough to handle it. He did not wither and blow away. The stutterer and the clinician continue doing these activities until the stutterer feels comfortable with them. Then the stutterer works his way up through the rest of the situations in his hierarchy on his own. He continues putting voluntary stuttering into his speech in a given situation until his fear subsides. Then he goes on to the next situation. The clinician continues to check with the stutterer regarding his progress during therapy sessions. She commends him when he is successful and supports, encourages, and counsels him when he runs into problems. Voluntary stuttering is a procedure that the stutterer will continue to employ throughout active treatment and maintenance. It is not an activity that will soon be discontinued.

By introducing and implementing the above four techniques or procedures, the clinician has the stutterer on the way toward reducing his negative feelings and attitudes toward his stuttering and eliminating his use of avoidance behaviors. It is an intensive counterconditioning/deconditioning process, which will take continued effort.

Using Fluency Enhancing Behaviors and Modifying the Moments of Stuttering

The goal of this phase of therapy is to help the stutterer learn to use both stuttering modification skills and fluency shaping skills. As we have previously stated, we believe that these two skills can complement one another. We will now describe the two procedures that we use during this phase. They are: (*a*) using fluency enhancing behaviors, and (*b*) modifying the moments of stuttering.

With regard to the sequencing of these procedures, we have done it both ways. That is, we have first taught stuttering modification skills and then taught fluency shaping skills; and vice versa. The results seem to be equally effective. In the following pages, we will describe the latter sequence.

Using fluency enhancing behaviors.   Fluency shaping clinicians, particularly Perkins, have strongly influenced our thinking with regard to this procedure. This will be apparent in the following handout.

USING FLUENCY ENHANCING BEHAVIORS

We know that stutterers can increase their fluency by modifying their speech patterns in certain ways. For example, one of the most common modifications that stutterers use is to slow down their rate of speech. Many stutterers have discovered on their own that if they speak more slowly, they will speak more fluently. Other techniques that stutterers have found helpful are to begin speaking with a gentle onset of voice after each breath and to use soft articulatory contacts. We call these modifications or changes in the manner of speaking "fluency enhancing behaviors" (FEBS). Now let's talk about these FEBS in more detail.

The first FEB we will discuss is "slower rate." There are at least two ways to use a slower rate. One way is to put more and longer pauses in your speech. The other way is to prolong or stretch out the sounds in your words. We prefer this latter approach. More specifically, by slower rate we mean speech characterized by a reduction in rate involving a relaxed prolongation of all sounds. We are not expecting you to speak abnormally slowly, but we are suggesting that you speak at a slow-normal rate when you want to increase your fluency.

The second FEB is the use of "gentle onsets." By gentle onsets we mean that after each breath you begin producing your voice slowly and with as little tension in your larynx (voice box) as possible.

The third FEB is "soft contacts." By this, we mean that the movements of the articulators (tongue, lips, jaw) should be slow, prolonged, and relaxed. These articulatory movements should not be fast and tense. By using these FEBS, you will have a feeling of fluency as you are speaking.

We're sure by now you're wondering how you are going to learn to use these FEBS. Your clinician has a machine called a delayed auditory feedback (DAF) machine that will help you. The DAF machine delays your hearing your own speech by a fraction of a second. Usually, this delay has a disrupting effect upon a person's speech. Normal speakers will often begin to exhibit stuttering-like behaviors. However, if you slow down and prolong your speech sufficiently until your speech coming from the DAF machine through the headset and your on-line speaking are at the same rate, it will not disrupt your fluency. In fact, you will be able to speak with a great deal of fluency, but in a slow, prolonged, relaxed manner. Besides slowing your rate by prolonging all the speech sounds, the DAF machine will help you use gentle onsets and soft contacts. We will begin with the DAF machine set at the maximum delay. This will help you speak at a very slow rate and use gentle onsets and soft contacts, too. As you develop skill in using these FEBS, we will gradually reduce the delay time of the DAF until you get to the point where you are able to speak fluently at a slow-normal rate off the DAF machine using your FEBS.

You and your clinician will spend time over the next several weeks learning how to use FEBS. Your clinician will show you how to do this. Once you have mastered the use of your FEBS on the DAF machine, you will practice them off the machine with your clinician here in the clinic and in outside situations. Next, you will begin to use these FEBS on your own in your everyday speaking situations. Eventually, these FEBS will be tools you will use for years to come to increase your fluency in certain speaking situations.

One word of advice in using these FEBS. You should not use them to hide the fact that you are a stutterer. You should be open and honest about your problem. Let your listener hear and see you speaking slower and using gentle onsets and soft contacts. Be open about the fact that you are using these techniques to improve your fluency in a given speaking situation.

At this point, the clinician will introduce the stutterer to the DAF machine. Since most clients will be curious about how the DAF affects them, it is a good idea to let the stutterer read aloud on the DAF machine. The clinician has the machine set at 250-msec delay, the maximum delay. Most likely, the DAF will have a disrupting effect upon the stutterer's speech. The clinician now explains to the stutterer that, if he slows his rate way down by prolonging each sound, he will be able to read fluently. She notes that, if he slows down and prolongs each sound sufficiently, the DAF will not disrupt his speech. Rather, it will do just the opposite; it will facilitate fluency. The clinician models what this speech pattern will sound like. Besides each sound being prolonged, the words will be run together; that is, there will not be breaks between words. The only breaks will occur when the clinician naturally needs to take a breath. The rate will be approximately 30 to 40 words per minute. The clinician then has the stutterer try reading aloud in this slow, prolonged, fluent pattern. She reinforces him if he is doing it right, and gives him corrective feedback if he is off target. She may have to do more modeling for him. With the DAF set at 250-msec delay, most stutterers are able to use this slow, prolonged pattern, or slower rate FEB, within the first session. Finally, the clinician will explain and model gentle onsets and soft contacts. She explains that both of these FEBS involve using slow, prolonged, relaxed movements in either voice initiation (gentle onsets) or articulation of consonant sounds (soft contacts). She points out to the stutterer that he is often already using these FEBS in his speech when he is using the slow, prolonged speech pattern. She encourages the stutterer to be aware of and to also use these FEBS while he is reading aloud. Once the stutterer has acquired some rudimentary skill in using FEBS while reading aloud with the DAF set at 250-msec delay, the clinician explains to him the sequence of tasks outlined in the program in Table 8.1.

The goal of this program is to help the stutterer establish or acquire the ability to use FEBS without the aid of the DAF machine while engaged in a conversation with the clinician. We have found the use of such a structured program very useful for this purpose. The clinician tells the stutterer that he is to read aloud any material that is of interest to him. While doing this, he is to practice using the FEBS, that is, slower rate, gentle onsets, and soft contacts. She gives him feedback regarding how well he is doing. If he does well, she positively reinforces him. If he is not using the FEBS, she reminds him to do so. If he seems uncertain as to how they should sound, she explains them again and provides him with the correct models. The clinician tells the stutterer that, if he is using the FEBS correctly, he will be almost totally fluent. At this point, she informs him that he must obtain 30 minutes of fluency with no more than one stuttered word per minute (SW/M) at the maximum delay of 250 msec before he can move on to the next delay time. The clinician uses a stopwatch to measure the stutterer's oral reading time, and she records the number of words on which he stutters. When he completes this first 30 minutes, the delay is decreased to 200 msec. This allows the stutterer to slightly increase his oral reading rate. He will progress through all the succeedingly lower delay times in this manner until he reaches zero delay. With each change in the delay, the stutterer slightly increases his oral reading rate. By the time he gets to zero delay, or possibly sooner, his rate should have reached 100-120 words per minute, a slow-normal rate.

Table 8.1 DAF Establishment Program

Antecedent Event	Response	Consequent Event	Criterion
Oral Reading:			
DAF: 250 msec	30 minutes of fluency using FEBS.	Intermittent social reinforcement.	1 SW/M or less.
DAF: 200 msec	"	"	"
DAF: 150 msec	"	"	"
DAF: 100 msec	"	"	"
DAF: 50 msec	"	"	"
DAF: 0 msec	"	"	"
Conversation: Repeat the above sequence.			

The stutterer now repeats the same sequence of tasks as above, but this time he and the clinician engage in conversations on a wide variety of topics. During these conversations, it is helpful if the clinician uses the same slower rates, and gentle onsets and soft contacts, the stutterer is using at that point in the program. This facilitates the client's ability to use FEBS. The clinician continues to reinforce the stutterer for his use of FEBS, and she reminds him when he forgets. Besides meeting the criterion of 1 SW/M or less, it is very important that the stutterer develop the ability to use the FEBS while engaging in conversation. These are the skills he will be using from now on in therapy and well beyond.

After the stutterer completes the above establishment program, the clinician moves on to the following 2 activities. She devotes about equal amounts of therapy time to each one. In other words, they are done in parallel fashion. First, she begins to transfer the stutterer's ability to use these FEBS to other locations and other people in the clinic. This is the first hierarchy that is employed in transferring the stutterer's use of FEBS to his everyday speaking environment. Second, she introduces the stutterer to the next procedure, "stuttering easily." Before discussing stuttering easily, however let us say more about this first hierarchy.

We have found the use of hierarchies to be very effective in helping the stutterer transfer his use of FEBS to his everyday speaking situations. We typically use four hierarchies: (a) inside the clinic with the clinician hierarchy, (b) outside the clinic with the clinician hierarchy, (c) everyday speaking situation hierarchy, and (d) telephone hierarchy. We will only discuss the first hierarchy at this time. After presenting the stuttering easily procedures, we will return to the remaining hierarchies.

The inside the clinic with the clinician hierarchy involves varying the physical location and social complexity of the therapy session in the clinic. This involves conducting therapy in other locations in the clinic. It also involves bringing other people into the therapy session. The size of the audience can be increased. People from the stutterer's world, such as family and friends, can be brought into therapy. The stutterer and the clinician rank these situations from easiest to most difficult as perceived by the stutterer. Then the stutterer, with the clinician present, goes through these situations in this sequence. He is to use his FEBS and meet the fluency criterion of 1 SW/M or less in each situation for a set period of time before he goes on to the next, more difficult situation. The clinician continues to reinforce the stutterer's successful use of FEBS. It is important that his confidence in using FEBS continues to increase during these activities. As previously mentioned, the clinician spends about half the therapy time on moving the stutterer through this hierarchy. The other half of the time she spends on teaching the stutterer to stutter easily. Let us now go on to stuttering easily.

Stuttering easily.   Stuttering modification clinicians, particularly Van Riper, have strongly influenced us on this procedure. However, the work of the fluency shaping clinicians has also affected our approach to this procedure. As we previously pointed out, the strategies or physiological movements involved in modifying a moment of stuttering are very similar to those involved in using fluency enhancing behaviors to modify the overall speech pattern. We attempt to make this clear to the stutterer in the following handout.

STUTTERING EASILY

What do we mean by stuttering easily? We mean several things. First, we mean saying the word without using any of your secondary behaviors, such as postponement, starting, or escape behaviors. Don't use these tricks to help you get started or to help you get out of a word.

Second, we mean you should stutter and/or say the word in a slow and relaxed manner. This is done by slowly prolonging each syllable of the word. Stutter or say the word in slow-motion. Don't be in a hurry to complete it. In other words, you should use your slower rate FEB on the word. Instead of slowing down your whole speech pattern, you are to just slow down the word on which you stutter or expect to stutter.

Third, by stuttering easily, we also mean using your other two FEBS, gentle onsets and soft contacts, to say a troublesome word. The word should begin slowly and in as relaxed a manner as possible. Phonation (voice) should be initiated slowly and with as little tension in your larynx (voice box) as possible, that is, use a gentle onset. Movement of the articulators (tongue, lips, jaw) should also be slow, prolonged, and relaxed. In other words, use soft contacts on consonant sounds.

How does one learn to do this? The first step involves the use of "cancellations." By cancellations, we mean the following. After completing a stuttered word, you are to pause for a couple of seconds. Then you are to say the word again, but this time you are to say the word in a slow, prolonged, relaxed manner. You should use a gentle onset or soft contact at the beginning of the word. Each syllable of the word should be prolonged. Soft contacts should be used on consonant sounds. In other words, you are to say the word again, but this time you are to say it as if you were stuttering easily on it. Don't say it fluently, even if you could. Don't use any of your old tricks. You will practice these cancellations here in the clinic.

The next step in learning to stutter easily involves the use of "pull-outs." This involves catching yourself in a stutter and then pulling yourself out of it. Rather than struggle and hurry out of the word, you should say the rest of the word in a slow, prolonged, relaxed manner. Each remaining syllable should be slowly prolonged (slower rate). Consonant sounds should be produced with a soft contact. These pull-outs will be practiced first in the clinic and then in outside situations around the clinic. You will also use these in your everyday speaking situations.

The last step in learning to stutter easily involves the use of "preparatory sets" (prep sets). When you anticipate stuttering on a word, you should prepare to use either a gentle onset or soft contact at the beginning of the word, and then each syllable of the word should be slowly prolonged. These prep sets will also be practiced in the clinic and in outside speaking situations. You may need to use these throughout the rest of your life when you expect to stutter on a word.

Once you have learned to use prep sets and pull-outs, you will have another strategy or technique to use if you don't want to use FEBS to modify your overall speech pattern. You can just go ahead and talk spontaneously. If you expect to stutter on a word, you can use a prep set to stutter easily on it. If you unexpectedly get caught in a stutter, you can use a pull-out to come out of it easily.

One word of advice in using these techniques. You should not use them to hide your stuttering. You should be honest and open about the fact that you stutter. In other words, you should let your listener know that you are having some difficulty in getting a word out. You should not use these techniques to hide your stuttering; rather, you should use them only to modify your stuttering in the direction of an easier, more relaxed form of stuttering.

After the stutterer reads this handout, the clinician makes sure that he understands that he will now be applying his FEBS only to words on which he either stutters or anticipates stuttering. The clinician then explains and models cancellations. She simulates the client's stuttering on a word, and then she cancels it by slowly prolonging each sound within the word, by using a gentle onset of phonation at the beginning of the word and by applying soft articulatory contacts on the consonant sounds in the word during this second attempt. She points out to the stutterer that he should be sure to complete the stuttered word the first time he says it. He is not to stop part way through the word. She should also point out to the stutterer that the pause between the first and second attempt on the word should be an unhurried pause. During this pause, he is to calm himself and plan how he will apply his FEBS on the second attempt. She then has the stutterer try to use some cancellations as they engage in conversation. At first, it may be difficult for the stutterer to catch himself and cancel his stutters. However, with reminders to cancel, feedback regarding his performance, and ample reinforcement from the clinician, the stutterer will soon be able to use some good cancellations while conversing with the clinician. The clinician then explains to the stutterer that his goal is to use good cancellations on 90% of his stuttered words while they are engaged in conversation for a therapy session or two. The clinician needs to count the number of stuttered words and the number of successful cancellations the stutterer has during these sessions. After the stutterer has demonstrated this level of competency in using cancellations, it is time to introduce pull-outs.

The clinician explains to the stutterer that now he is to catch himself while he is still in the moment of stuttering. Then he is to slowly prolong the rest of the sounds in the word. He is to use soft contacts on the remaining consonants in the word. The clinician also models pull-outs. After the stutterer experiments with the use of pull-outs, the clinician again informs the stutterer that he is to use pull-outs on at least 90% of his stuttered words during conversation for a session or so. She positively reinforces his use of good pull-outs and gives him corrective feedback when he is having difficulty using them.

The final step in learning to stutter easily is preparatory sets. In other words, the stutterer is to use his FEBS on words on which he anticipates stuttering. Many stutterers have learned to do this on their own on some words by this time. They approach a feared word by initiating it with a gentle onset or a soft contact. They slowly work their way through the word by prolonging each sound. They use soft contacts on the consonant sounds in the word. If the stutterer is already doing this, the clinician points out to him that he is using prep sets, and she strongly reinforces him for it. If the stutterer has not yet acquired this skill on his own, the clinician explains and models prep sets for him. As with pull-outs, the stutterer needs practice using prep sets in the therapy room before he begins to transfer them to the outside speaking world. To provide this practice, the stutterer is to use either a good prep set or a good pull-out on 90% of his stuttered words during conversation with the clinician for a therapy session or two. The clinician reinforces the stutterer for the use of either of these two behaviors and gives him appropriate corrective feedback as needed. The reason we accept either a prep set or a pull-out in this activity is that stutterers do not always anticipate all of their moments of stuttering. Consequently, it is unrealistic to expect a stutterer to use preparatory sets on all of his stutters.

The stutterer is now ready to begin transferring his stuttering easily skills to his own speaking environment. To do this, we employ the same 4 hierarchies that we use in transferring FEBS. As will be recalled, these are: (*a*) inside the clinic with the clinician hierarchy, (*b*) outside the clinic with the clinician hierarchy, (*c*) everyday speaking situation hierarchy, and (*d*) telephone hierarchy. By now the stutterer has probably almost completed the inside the clinic with the clinician hierarchy using his FEBS. When he does, he completes the same hierarchy again, but this time he uses the stuttering easily skills. In other words, the stutterer goes through the same speaking situations with the clinician in the clinic as he did before, but this time, instead of using FEBS, he uses a prep set or a pull-out to modify any moments of stuttering he may have. His criterion for success in each situation is using a good prep set or pull-out on 90% of his stutters. The clinician continues to reinforce his stuttering easily during this hierarchy.

Once the stutterer has completed this first hierarchy using both FEBS and stuttering easily skills, it is time to move on to the next hierarchy, that is, the outside the clinic with the clinician hierarchy. It involves situations in which it is possible for the clinician to accompany the stutterer. The clinician and the stutterer jointly select and sequence items for this hierarchy. Examples of situations include asking directions from strangers and obtaining information from store clerks (Fig. 8.3). The stutterer will move through this hierarchy using both FEBS and prep sets or pull-outs. First he will use one, and then he will use the other. The stutterer could initially complete the entire hierarchy using one set of skills, and then repeat the hierarchy using the other set of skills. On the other hand, he could alternate using FEBS and stuttering easily on each step of the hierarchy. It is important, however, that the stutterer begins to generalize both of these sets of skills from inside the clinic to outside the clinic. Whichever set of skills is being worked on in a given situation, the criterion for success is the fact that both the stutterer and the clinician agree that the stutterer used the skills as well as he used them in the clinic. By this, we mean that his use of FEBS or prep sets or pull-outs felt and sounded as good as when he used them in the clinic. This is a subjective evaluation, but realistically, it is the type of evaluation the stutterer will use on his own in the future. It is also important that the stutterer be successful in using each set of skills in each situation a number of times so that he gains confidence in his ability to use them. After gaining skill and confidence in using FEBS and prep sets or pull-outs in outside situations with his clinician present, it is time for the stutterer to move on to the next, more difficult hierarchy.

The everyday speaking situation hierarchy involves situations from the stutterer's own environment, and thereby requires his completing it on his own. Usually the stutterer ranks, from least to most difficult, 2-3 dozen speaking situations that he encounters in a typical week. The stutterer may first go through this hierarchy using his FEBS, and then go through it again using prep sets or pull-outs, or he may do it vice versa. He may also choose to use both sets of skills on one step or situation of the hierarchy before going on to the next situation. Most importantly the stutterer must begin to generalize his use of both of these sets of skills to his everyday speaking situations. As a general rule, before moving on to a more difficult step or situation on the hierarchy, the stutterer should feel that he has

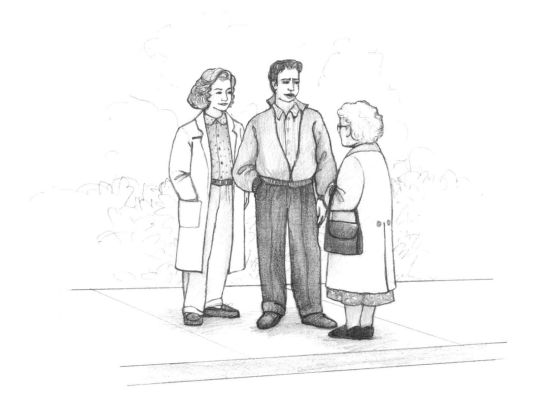

Figure 8.3. Transferring stuttering modification and fluency shaping skills.

successfully used his FEBS or stuttering easily skills a number of times in the immediately preceding or easier situation. This is important in developing his skill and confidence in using these techniques. During their regular therapy sessions, the clinician monitors the stutterer's progress through this hierarchy. She praises him when he has successes, encourages him when he has failures, and gives him suggestions when he has problems. In time, the stutterer will be reporting to the clinician that his speech is becoming much better in his everyday encounters.

We have also found that most advanced stutterers need a separate hierarchy involving the telephone. The same strategies or principles involved in implementing the above hierarchies are applied here as well. In other words, telephone calls, with and without the clinician present, are arranged in a hierarchical order. The stutterer practices both his FEBS and his stuttering easily skills during these calls until the success criterion is met. The clinician continues to support and reinforce the stutterer during these activities. Soon, the stutterer may be reporting successes in his use of the telephone.

By now, the stutterer will be speaking much better in most situations. He is not yet out of the woods, but he is on his way. We now move on to the last phase of therapy, increasing and maintaining improvement.

Maintaining Improvement

The goal of this last phase of therapy is to help the stutterer generalize his improvement, that is, his reduced negative feelings, attitudes, and avoidances and his increased fluency, to all remaining speaking situations. It is also to help the stutterer maintain his improvement following termination of therapy. We introduce the following 2 procedures during this phase: (*a*) becoming your own clinician and (*b*) establishing long-term fluency goals.

Becoming your own clinician. If the advanced stutterer is going to generalize his improvement to all speaking situations, and if he is going to maintain his improvement, we believe that he must assume responsibility for his own therapy. We attempt to make this clear to the stutterer in the following handout.

BECOMING YOUR OWN CLINICIAN

Now that we have covered all the therapy techniques you will need to meet your therapy goals, it is time for you to become your own speech clinician. This is important for two reasons. First, we have helped you reduce much of your negative feelings and attitudes about your stuttering, and we have helped you reduce a lot of your avoidance behaviors. We have also helped you improve your fluency in many situations by using FEBS and prep sets or pull-outs. Yet, there are probably still some situations that give you trouble. You have now come to the point in therapy where you need to go to work on these remaining difficult situations. You will have to apply on your own the techniques you have learned in therapy. You are the only one who can apply these techniques in these difficult, everyday speaking situations. This is true for all the techniques you have learned, that is, discussing stuttering openly, using feared words and entering feared situations, using voluntary stuttering, using fluency enhancing behaviors, and using prep sets and pull-outs. You need to assume the responsibility for applying these techniques throughout your daily life and, thereby, completing your therapy.

Second, it is even more important for you to become your own speech clinician if you are to maintain your improvement in the long run. The reason for this is that adult stutterers very often relapse or slip back after they leave therapy. This does not have to happen, but it is not surprising that it does. You have been stuttering for a long time. You have had a lot of practice at it. In fact, you are an expert! You have used avoidance behaviors for a long time. Your negative feelings and attitudes about your speech are well learned. Finally, you may always have some core behaviors, and you will just have to successfully cope with them. In other words, you will need to keep applying—on your own—long after you leave therapy—the techniques you have learned in therapy. Therefore, you need to become your own speech clinician.

What is involved in becoming your own speech clinician? You will need to learn to give yourself assignments to overcome any remaining difficult speaking situations. If you are still avoiding speaking in a certain situation, you will need to design assignments that will eliminate this avoidance. If you are still fearful while talking in some situation, you will need to give yourself assignments to reduce this fear. If you are still doing a lot of stuttering in a given situation, you will need to come up with assignments to improve your fluency in this situation. In the beginning of therapy, your clinician helped you create these assignments, but as you improved, your clinician has turned more of the responsibility over to you. She will continue to do this. With additional practice, you will be able to determine your therapy needs and to make up assignments to meet these needs. When you can do this, you will have become your own speech clinician.

We have found the following approach effective in meeting this goal. Every day you need to do some meaningful work on your therapy. Every day you need to work at reducing any remaining speech fears and eliminating any remaining avoidances. For example, if you are still fearful while talking in a certain situation, you could give yourself a daily quota of voluntary stuttering in that situation. Every day you also need to work on improving your fluency. If you are still doing a lot of stuttering in a given situation, you could set a daily quota of talking time in that situation during which you use prep sets and pull-outs. These are only examples, but the important thing is that everyday you ask yourself which situations are still giving you problems and then give yourself assignments designed to overcome these problems. Let's get started in helping you become your own speech clinician.

By this time, the stutterer is probably getting close to completing his everyday speaking situation hierarchy. The clinician points out to him, however, that completing this hierarchy is not enough. The stutterer needs to become aware of any other situations that are still giving him trouble. The clinician asks the stutterer the following questions. Is he avoiding talking in any situations? Is he still unduly afraid while talking in some situations? Is he unable to successfully use FEBS and prep sets or pull-outs in some situations? If the answer to any of these questions is "yes," then the stutterer needs to target these situations in his assignments.

If the stutterer is still avoiding some situations, the clinician reminds him of the importance of using feared words and entering feared situations. She has the stutterer reread this handout. She then helps him prepare assignments to overcome these avoidances. The clinician does not assume any more responsibility than necessary in helping the stutterer prepare these assignments. She asks helpful questions. She wants him to be able to figure out, on his own, what he needs to do. As time goes on, she will gradually have the stutterer assume more and more responsibility for making up his own assignments.

If the stutterer is still unduly apprehensive while talking in some situations, the clinician reminds him of the importance of discussing stuttering openly and using voluntary stuttering as techniques to reduce these negative feelings. She has him reread these handouts. She helps him create assignments in which he uses these techniques to become more comfortable in these situations. Here again, she does not assume any more responsibility for these assignments than necessary. She wants him to eventually become his own speech clinician.

If the stutterer is having difficulties using FEBS and prep sets or pull-outs in some situations, the clinician explores with him the nature of his difficulties. She attempts to help him determine what types of assignments he needs to have to be successful. Maybe he just needs more practice in some less difficult situations before he can reasonably expect to be successful in these more difficult situations. Possibly he needs to further reduce his speech fears, and resulting muscular tension, in these difficult situations so that his motor control does not break down as readily. We have also found that some stutterers prefer to use fluency enhancing behaviors, while some other stutterers prefer to use preparatory sets and pull-outs. There is no reason why all stutterers need to use both. If the stutterer wants to use only one of these sets of skills, the clinician accepts this. During all of these discussions, the clinician keeps in mind that her goal is to help the stutterer become independent of her. She becomes less directing and gradually turns the total responsibility for the assignments over to him.

Throughout this phase of therapy, the stutterer is working daily on his outside assignments. During the therapy sessions, he discusses his progress with the clinician. During this same period, she is becoming more and more of a consultant. The time is soon coming when the stutterer will feel that he can go out and fly on his own.

Establishing long-term fluency goals.   Before therapy comes to an end, we believe it is very important for the stutterer to be made aware of what he can expect in terms of fluency following termination from therapy. By understanding what are realistic goals for himself, we believe he can substantially decrease the possibility of his becoming disappointed and frustrated with his speech. These feelings lead to relapse. To begin this topic, we share the following handout with the stutterer.

ESTABLISHING LONG-TERM FLUENCY GOALS

You are at the point in therapy where you need to consider your long-term fluency goals. Before you do this, however, we need to define some terms we will be using. These are "spontaneous fluency," "controlled fluency," and "acceptable stuttering."

By spontaneous fluency, we mean speech that contains no more than an occasional number of disfluencies and does not contain tension or struggle. This fluency is not maintained by paying attention to or controlling your speech. In other words, you don't use FEBS or prep sets and pull-outs to be fluent. You just talk and pay attention to your ideas. It is the fluency of the normal speaker.

Controlled fluency is similar to spontaneous fluency except that you must attend to or control your speech to maintain relatively normal-sounding fluency. You must use FEBS and/or prep sets and pull-outs to sound relatively fluent. You sound fluent only because you are working on your speech at the time.

Finally, acceptable stuttering refers to speech that contains noticeable, but mild, stuttering. Furthermore, you feel comfortable with this stuttering. You are not doing any avoiding. You may or may not need to use FEBS and/or prep sets and pull-outs to have this acceptable stuttering. In other words, sometimes you will have this acceptable stuttering without having to work on or control your speech. At other times, despite your use of FEBS and/or prep sets and pull-outs, you will still have some mild stuttering.

Now, let's consider long-term fluency goals. A few adult stutterers become spontaneously fluent in all speaking situations on a consistent basis; they become normal speakers. In our experience, though, most adult stutterers do not reach this goal. Typically, these remaining stutterers have situations, like talking to a friend, in which they are spontaneously fluent. However, in other situations, like speaking in a group, their stuttering tends to return and give them trouble. In these troublesome situations, we think it is important for these stutterers—and possibly you—to have the following options.

First, if it is important to you to sound fluent in one of these situations, we want you to be able to use either FEBS and/or prep sets and pull-outs to achieve controlled fluency. We know this is possible in most situations; we also know there will be some situations in which you will not be totally successful. In these situations, we want you to feel comfortable with acceptable stuttering.

Second, if it is not important to you to sound fluent in a situation, and you do not want to put the effort into using FEBS and/or prep sets and pull-outs, we would like you to feel comfortable with acceptable stuttering.

These options or goals are both realistic and acceptable. In other words, you don't have to sound perfectly fluent all the time. You don't have to work on your speech constantly. In fact, attempting to sound fluent all the time by using FEBS and/or prep sets and pull-outs can become burdensome. Where are you now with regard to these fluency goals? Are you satisfied with your present fluency? Where would you like to be in the future with regard to these goals? You should discuss these questions with your clinician and begin to make plans based upon your answers.

The clinician makes sure that the stutterer understands the concepts of spontaneous fluency, controlled fluency, and acceptable stuttering. When the clinician is convinced that the stutterer understands what she means by these terms, she explores with him the types of fluency he now has in his various, everyday speaking situations. If he is unsure, he gives himself assignments to find out the answers. She then explores with him whether or not he is satisfied with the types of fluency he has in these daily speaking situations. If the stutterer is satisfied with his fluency in all situations, then he has met his goals, and the end of therapy is getting near. If he is not satisfied, then he needs to continue to work along the lines discussed in the previous section, becoming your own clinician, until his goals are met.

We have observed a couple of problems that frequently occur relative to stutterers' fluency expectations or goals. First, many stutterers at this point in therapy are experiencing a great deal of spontaneous fluency. They expect, and want, this spontaneous fluency to last forever without any effort on their part. It will not. It can last, but it will require continued work on the part of the client. He will need to continue to give himself assignments to keep his negative feelings and attitudes at a minimum and his avoidance behaviors eliminated. He will also need to continue to work on his FEBS and/or prep sets and pull-outs so that he has confidence in his ability to use them when he chooses. Spontaneous fluency will be a by-product of these efforts. The clinician must help the stutterer understand this. If the stutterer doesn't understand this, he will be disappointed, and possibly panicked, when he begins to lose some of his spontaneous fluency. This often leads to relapse.

The second problem frequently involves the more severe advanced stutterer. This stutterer often does not obtain a great deal of spontaneous fluency. If he is going to talk better, he needs to constantly use FEBS or prep sets and pull-outs. Even then, he often only achieves acceptable stuttering. This gets to be discouraging. It is too much of a burden to constantly monitor and modify his speech. In time, he becomes tired of the task, and he gives up doing anything at all. Relapse soon follows. The clinician needs to help this stutterer accept and become comfortable with his acceptable stuttering. She also needs to help him realize the substantial amount of effort he will need to expend to stay at this level of fluency.

Once the stutterer gets to the point where he feels he is meeting his fluency goals, and he has become his own clinician, the frequency of therapy contacts is systematically reduced. We typically fade our contacts to once a week for a month or two, then to once a month for several months, and finally, to once a semester for two years. This gradual transition provides the stutterer with some continued support. If he is doing well, he is reinforced. If he is having a few problems, we can help him find the solutions. If he has totally relapsed, he can be reenrolled in therapy. Finally, the day comes to say "goodby." We commend him for all his efforts, and we let him know that, if he ever needs us again, he should feel free to contact us. If we have done our job well, we will not be hearing from him.

OTHER CLINICIANS

We will now discuss the clinical procedures of two other clinicians that integrate stuttering modification and fluency shaping therapies for the advanced stutterer. These two clinicians do not integrate the two approaches in the exact manner as we do, but the reader will see from this discussion that this integration of the two approaches can occur in a number of ways.

Hugo Gregory

For the last 20 years, Hugo Gregory (1968, 1979, 1986a) has been integrating stuttering modification and fluency shaping therapies. In his most recent discussion of his therapy for the advanced stutterer, he describes four general areas of therapeutic activity. They are: (*a*) changing the attitudes of the stutterer, (*b*) diminishing excessive bodily tension, (*c*) analyzing and modifying speech, and (*d*) building new psychomotor speech patterns and improving speech skills. Gregory states that, although the four areas are interrelated, changing attitudes and diminishing excessive bodily tension usually precede modifying speech and building new psychomotor speech patterns.

Gregory believes that it is important for the advanced stutterer to change his attitudes about his problem. Thus, Gregory provides the stutterer with an accepting and understanding relationship in which the stutterer feels free to explore and clarify his feelings and attitudes about his problem. These discussions likewise help to reduce the stutterer's negative feelings about his speech. During this period, Gregory also provides the client with information about stuttering. Toward the end of therapy, as the client's speech improves, Gregory helps the client integrate his new fluency into his life patterns.

Gregory thinks that diminishing excessive bodily tension is beneficial for many stutterers. To help the stutterer do this, Gregory employs Jacobson's (1938) progressive relaxation techniques. Briefly, this involves having the stutterer systematically tense and relax his muscles in one part of his body at a time. By going through this process over and over again, the stutterer learns to identify the feelings associated with relaxation and to voluntarily relax his muscles. Gregory reports that many stutterers, as they enter a feared speaking situation, are able to consciously reduce bodily tension and to carry this over to the muscles involved in speaking.

Gregory's third area of therapeutic activity is analyzing and modifying speech. At this time, Gregory helps the stutterer analyze what he does when he stutters. Audio and video recordings are used for this purpose. Besides having the stutterer become aware of what he does when he stutters, Gregory also helps the stutterer become aware of other aspects of his speech pattern, such as rate, phrasing, and prosody. Following this analysis, Gregory teaches the stutterer to modify his stuttering by relaxing the tension, by slowing the repetitions, and by using other similar techniques. Van Riper's cancellations, pull-outs, and preparatory sets may sometimes be used. Gregory also teaches the stutterer to use an "easier, more relaxed approach with smooth movements" (ERA-SM) in the initiation of speech. These relaxed, smooth movements are first practiced in words, then in phrases, and finally, in phrases in connected speech. Since ERA-SM are used on nonstuttered words, they are much more akin to Perkins' fluency skills than to Van Riper's stuttering modification techniques.

The last area that Gregory works on in therapy with the advanced stutterer is building new psychomotor speech patterns. His goal is to make the person who stutters a good speaker. The emphasis is upon strengthening normal fluency. Some of the aspects of speech production that are targeted are rate control, loudness, phrasing, and prosody.

In the introduction to this section on the integration of stuttering modification and fluency shaping therapies, we said that we believe it is important to reduce the advanced stutterer's negative feelings and attitudes and eliminate his use of avoidances. We further stated that it is helpful to integrate work on modifying both the stutterer's moments of stuttering and enhancing his fluency skills. It should be clear by now that Gregory shares many of these beliefs.

C. Woodruff Starkweather

C. Woodruff Starkweather (1980) views stuttering as being due to multiple conditioning processes, namely operant, classical, avoidance, and vicarious conditioning. Consequently, he takes a multiprocess behavioral approach to its treatment. Specifically, he recommends that treatment for the advanced stutterer have the following 5 goals: (a) reversing conditioning processes currently maintaining the disorder, (b) reducing or eliminating avoidance behavior, (c) modifying stuttering to reduce abnormality, (d) rate reduction and/or monitoring, and (e) rate reduction and monitoring in situations.

To achieve the first goal, it is necessary to determine which conditioning processes are currently maintaining the disorder. Starkweather suggests this becomes apparent from the evaluation. The two following examples depicting how conditioning processes can maintain the disorder and how the conditioning can be reversed should clarify what Starkweather has in mind in meeting this goal. In one situation, parents may be unintentionally reinforcing an adolescent's stuttering by giving him more attention when he stutters. In this case, the parents will need to be advised to discontinue this behavior. In another situation, the spouse of a stutterer may be responding negatively toward his stuttering and, consequently, increasing his tendency to use avoidance behaviors. If this is so, then the spouse should be counseled to change her responses so that she reflects more acceptance of the disorder.

Starkweather suggests that there are 3 principles that should guide clinicians in their efforts to reduce or eliminate the stutterer's use of avoidance behaviors. The first principle involves reducing the fear on which the avoidance behavior is based. Starkweather believes this fear is the fear of stuttering itself and/or the fear of listener reactions. To reduce this fear, he recommends many of the identification and desensitization procedures advocated by Van Riper. Among the desensitization procedures, Starkweather believes that pseudostuttering is the most effective. The second principle that should guide the clinician in reducing avoidance behaviors involves motivating the stutterer to approach his fear. The stutterer is encouraged to enter his feared situations and to stutter openly in them. The third principle for eliminating the stutterer's avoidance behaviors is response prevention. The purpose here is to have the stutterer not use his avoidance behaviors and to force him to experience his stuttering. Starkweather suggests this can be achieved by the use of both pseudostuttering and freezing. At the beginning of this section on the integration of approaches, we stated that we believe it is important to reduce the stutterer's negative feelings and attitudes and eliminate his use of avoidances. It is obvious that Starkweather believes this, too.

Starkweather's procedures for modifying stuttering are very similar to Van Riper's. First, the stutterer is taught to vary his stuttering. He is to stutter with more tension, as well as with less tension. When he has learned how to do this, he is introduced to cancellations. In other words, he is to say a stuttered word over, but the second time he is to stutter on it with less tension and struggle. Starkweather believes that, as the stutterer gets better at using cancellations, he will be able to move his modification forward in time to catch himself while he is still in a stutter. This is a Van Riper pull-out. Based upon his experience, Starkweather suggests that some, but not all, stutterers will then be able to move this modification forward in time even more and will be able to ease into anticipated stutters or use a Van Riper preparatory set.

Starkweather's fourth goal is to teach the client a form of controlled fluency to use in those situations where he feels it is important for him to sound fluent. Based upon his experience, Starkweather does not believe it is necessary to use a structured fluency shaping program like Perkins' to do this. Rather, he believes that, with modeling and instructions, the clinician can help the client achieve a carefully monitored, slower rate of speech in the clinical setting.

Starkweather's last goal is rate reduction and monitoring in all situations. To facilitate the client's ability to use this monitored slower rate, or controlled fluency, in all speaking situations, Starkweather recommends the use of hierarchies. Once the client has developed the ability to both modify his stutters and use a monitored, slower rate of speech in everyday speaking situations, he is ready to go out on his own.

From Starkweather's last 3 goals, it is apparent that he believes, like we do, that it is beneficial to teach the advanced stutterer to both modify his moments of stuttering and to use certain fluency enhancing skills.

SUMMARY OF INTEGRATION OF APPROACHES

When we began this chapter on the integration of stuttering modification and fluency shaping therapies for the advanced stutterer, we stated that we thought it was important to reduce the stutterer's negative feelings and attitudes and eliminate his avoidance behaviors. We also indicated that we thought it was beneficial to integrate work on both modifying the stutterer's individual moments of stuttering and enhancing his fluency skills. From the presentation of our clinical procedures and from the comments on Gregory's and Starkweather's clinical procedures, the reader should recognize that we all share the above clinical beliefs. Further, the reader should see that there are a number of ways these two major approaches to the treatment of the advanced stutterer can be integrated.

STUDY QUESTIONS

1/ In integrating stuttering modification and fluency shaping therapies for the advanced stutterer, what position do Peters and Guitar take with regard to the speech behaviors targeted for therapy and the attention given to feelings and attitudes?

2/ List the 4 phases of Peters and Guitar's therapy for the advanced stutterer. What is the goal for each of these phases?

3/ Briefly describe the methods involved in Peters and Guitar's understanding stuttering phase.

4/ List and briefly describe the procedures used in Peters and Guitar's reducing negative feelings and attitudes and eliminating avoidances phase.

5/ How do Peters and Guitar integrate stuttering modification and fluency shaping therapies with regard to the speech behaviors targeted in therapy?

6/ List and briefly describe the procedures in Peters and Guitar's maintaining fluency phase.

Suggested Readings

Starkweather, C. W. (1980). A multiprocess behavioral approach to stuttering therapy. *Seminars in Speech, Language and Hearing, 1,* 327–337.

This is an excellent article in which the author applies various learning paradigms to the treatment of the advanced stutterer.

9

THE BEGINNING STUTTERER: STUTTERING MODIFICATION AND FLUENCY SHAPING THERAPIES

In the previous chapter on the treatment of the advanced stutterer, we described how stuttering modification clinicians teach the stutterer to modify his moments of stuttering in order to reduce the severity of the stuttering. This contrasts with fluency shaping clinicians who teach the stutterer to use certain fluency enhancing skills to increase fluency. We also noted that, besides differing with regard to the speech behaviors targeted for therapy, these two therapy approaches generally differ with regard to fluency goals, attention given to feelings and attitudes, maintenance procedures, and clinical methods. In this chapter, it will become apparent that, in the treatment of the beginning stutterer, the differences between these two therapy approaches become less, and their similarities become greater.

However, before presenting the therapies of these two approaches, we will briefly review the characteristics of the beginning stutterer. Children at this treatment level are usually between 2 to 8 years of age. Thus, they are either preschool or early elementary school children.

In terms of the core behaviors, the beginning stutterer may exhibit part-word or monosyllabic word repetitions produced rapidly and with irregular rhythm. He may have vowel prolongations. Some of these core behaviors may have excessive tension present. The beginning stutterer may also exhibit blocks. Secondary behaviors probably include escape behaviors and possibly some starting behaviors. This child may have a self-concept as someone who has trouble talking; however, he has little, or only occasional, concern about this. He may also be experiencing frustration because of his stuttering. Now let us present stuttering modification therapy for the beginning stutterer.

STUTTERING MODIFICATION THERAPY

To illustrate stuttering modification therapy for the beginning stutterer, we will describe Charles Van Riper's therapy in detail. We will also comment briefly upon the clinical procedures of several other stuttering modification clinicians.

Charles Van Riper: Creation of Basal Fluency Levels and Desensitization to Fluency Disrupters

CLINICIAN'S BELIEFS

Nature of Stuttering

As previously noted, Charles Van Riper (1982) views stuttering as a disorder of timing. He believes that, when the child stutters, there is a disruption in the proper timing and sequencing of the muscle movements involved in producing a word. When this happens, the child exhibits a core behavior, that is, a repetition or prolongation. What accounts for this mistiming of the motor movements involved in speech production? Van Riper suggests this could be due to an organic predisposition, to a faulty feedback system, or to communicative and emotional stress. Van Riper further suggests that the child's motor speech system is less mature and less stable than that of the adult's; therefore, it is more subject to disruption by stress, especially communicative stress. By communicative stress, Van Riper is referring to such fluency disrupters as losing listener attention, being consistently interrupted, speaking under time pressures, or attempting to reproduce speech and language models that are too difficult. The focus of Van Riper's therapy for the beginning stutterer is on facilitating the child's acquisition of normal fluency and on increasing the child's tolerance for communicative stress. To achieve these goals, Van Riper will work directly with the child, as well as counsel the child's parents. Finally, Van Riper believes the secondary behaviors, such as escape and starting behaviors, are learned.

Speech Behaviors Targeted for Therapy

At this treatment level, Van Riper does not teach the child to modify his moments of stuttering. Rather, his goal is to create a "basal level of fluency" in the clinical setting.[1] Van Riper accomplishes this by manipulating the clinical conditions to cause the child to become fluent. By providing a simple fluency model, by engaging in certain fluency facilitating activities, and by reinforcing fluency, Van Riper establishes a basal level of fluency in the clinic. Then, by gradually introducing fluency disrupters while the child is experiencing this basal fluency, Van Riper little by little increases the child's tolerance for these communicative stresses. As a result of this process, the child's fluency has often been observed to improve at home and at school.

Fluency Goals

What are Van Riper's fluency goals for a beginning stutterer? Quite simply, he believes the prognosis is excellent for this child to gain or regain normal or spontaneous fluency in all speaking situations.

Feelings and Attitudes

As will be recalled, we stated that a child at this treatment level is probably aware that, at times, he has some problems in talking. However, he has little or only occasional concern about this. We also suggested that this child may occasionally be experiencing some frustration because of his stuttering. Van Riper generally agrees with this description. Furthermore, he believes that, if a child is exhibiting signs of concern or frustration about his speech, this should be responded to in therapy. Van Riper's way of doing this is to engage the child in play activities in which the goal is to make talking fun again. He wants to remove any unpleasant association that speech may have acquired for the child. More will be said about this when we discuss Van Riper's "making speech pleasant" procedure later in this chapter.

We also believe that, in some cases, Van Riper's "desensitizing the child to fluency disrupters" procedure involves responding to the child's feelings and attitudes about his speech. For example, when Van Riper desensitizes the child to speaking under emotionally disruptive conditions, we believe Van Riper is, to some degree, dealing with the child's feelings.

Maintenance Procedures

Van Riper does not discuss maintenance procedures for the beginning stutterer. This fact, coupled with his belief that the prognosis for this child to achieve normal or spontaneous fluency is excellent, leads us to conclude that Van

---

[1] The reference for Van Riper's point of view on this and the remaining clinical issues is Van Riper, C (1973). *The treatment of stuttering*. Englewood Cliffs: Prentice-Hall.

Riper does not believe maintenance procedures are necessary with the beginning stutterer.

Clinical Methods

In terms of the structure of therapy, Van Riper's interaction with the beginning stutterer is characterized by play activity. Even though Van Riper has definite goals for a therapy session, the session is loosely structured. This will become apparent when we discuss his procedures in the next section. Van Riper does not address the collection of data in his discussion of therapy procedures.

CLINICAL PROCEDURES: DIRECT TREATMENT OF THE CHILD

The reference for the material in this section is the chapter on therapy for the beginning stutterer in Van Riper's (1973) *The Treatment of Stuttering*. We plan to describe his therapy in sufficient detail to allow the reader to understand his basic procedures; however, the reader is referred to the above chapter for additional information.

As mentioned earlier, Van Riper's therapy for the beginning stutterer involves a two-pronged attack on the problem: (*a*) direct treatment of the child and (*b*) parent counseling. We will first discuss his direct treatment of the child.

In working with the beginning stutterer, Van Riper stresses the importance of establishing a relationship with the child in which the child feels accepted and supported. The young stutterer must feel secure in this relationship. In his interactions with the child, Van Riper does not call attention to the child's stuttering. As Van Riper is developing this relationship, he is working on the following goals: (*a*) making speech pleasant, (*b*) creating suitable fluency models, (*c*) integrating and facilitating fluency, (*d*) reinforcing fluency, (*e*) desensitizing the child to fluency disrupters, (*f*) counterconditioning integrative responses to fluency disrupters, and (*g*) preventing stuttering from becoming a stimulus for struggle and avoidance.

Before discussing the clinical procedures used to achieve the above goals, we should point out that Van Riper encourages the parents to observe and then participate in the therapy sessions. By doing this, he is providing modeling and guidance for them on ways they can help their child at home.

Making Speech Pleasant

Not every beginning stutterer will need help in this area. Only if the child is exhibiting some signs of frustration or concern about his speech will Van Riper plan activities aimed at reducing these negative feelings. How does Van Riper do this? One of his favorite activities with a shy child, for example, is to have 2 boxes of toys, one for the child and one for himself. They sit on the floor and begin to take the toys out of their respective boxes. At this point, they engage in "solo play." Both are involved with only their own toys and play activities. At first, Van Riper is silent and puts no demands upon the child to speak. After a while, Van Riper begins to vocalize as he plays. For example, he may make animal noises or car noises as he plays with his toys. Soon, he may begin to use one-word commentaries upon what he is doing as he plays, but he is still careful not to put demands upon the child to talk. If things continue to go well, Van Riper moves into "tangential play," where his toys occasionally bump into the child's or Van Riper and the child intermittently interact. Van Riper may now begin to use short phrases and sentences as he comments upon the activities. Gradually, their play becomes more and more "co-operative play," and, little by little, the child begins to verbalize (Fig. 9.1). This may take a number of sessions, but in time, the child is talking more and more. Once this stage is reached, Van Riper begins to engage the child in a variety of children's games and activities where the goal is having a good time and a by-product is having fun talking. He has the parents observe and possibly participate in these activities, with the intention of having them carry out similar ones at home.

Creating Suitable Fluency Models

As previously noted, Van Riper believes that, when a child attempts to use speech and language patterns that are too difficult for him to produce, he becomes disfluent. Thus, while he is interacting with the child in play activities, Van Riper provides the child with simple speech and language models. In the early sessions, he uses single words. Later, he uses simple phrases, and still later, he uses short, simple sentences as he talks with the child. Van Riper uses a normal speech rate; however, he does put a lot of pauses and silent periods into his speech. He believes it is very important for the child's acquisition of normal fluency for him to be bombarded by unhurried, simple speech and language patterns. Van Riper also expects that the parents will follow this model, which they have heard him use, when they talk with their child at home.

Integrating and Facilitating Fluency

As discussed previously, Van Riper believes that the beginning stutterer's motor speech system is prone to breakdown or disfluency. Consequently, Van

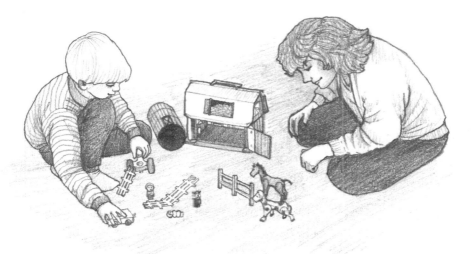

Figure 9.1. Making speech fun.

Riper believes it is important to provide this young stutterer with activities that will integrate and stabilize his motor speech fluency. To do this, Van Riper uses rhythm or timing techniques. It is well known that various rhythm or timing techniques, such as tapping a finger on the table for each syllable spoken, speaking in unison with another person, or echoing or repeating what someone else says, facilitates fluency for the stutterer. Van Riper does not teach these techniques as methods the beginning stutterer uses to become fluent; rather he embeds these procedures in games to provide the young stutterer with fluent speaking experiences. Van Riper tells the child to talk this way only when they are playing their speech games together. A typical game may be playing "Indian." Both Van Riper and the child clap their hands against their mouths as they speak. At first, each movement is accompanied by a syllable, later a word, and eventually a short phrase or sentence. Other activities may involve the use of puppets, who need to echo or repeat everything that is said to them, and again, Van Riper begins by having the child repeat words, then phrases, and finally short sentences. By these and similar games, Van Riper provides the beginning stutterer with experiences that facilitate fluency.

Reinforcing Fluency

Van Riper's goal here is to reinforce the child's fluency without making the child aware of why he is being reinforced. How does Van Riper do this? One way is to show interest and enthusiasm in the child's fluent communication and only ordinary acceptance of the child's stuttered speech. Another way Van Riper achieves this goal is to play games like "Say the Magic Word." During this game, the child is to tell what he sees out the window or in a picture book. When he says the magic word, a bell is rung and the child wins a reward, like a peanut. Van Riper does not have a particular magic word in mind. Rather, he reinforces the child only after the child has been especially fluent, and Van Riper then chooses one of the fluent words as the magic word. In these ways, Van Riper reinforces the child for fluency without the child being made aware of why he is being reinforced.

Desensitizing the Child to Fluency Disrupters

By this time, Van Riper has developed a warm, friendly relationship with the child, and the child feels comfortable talking with him. Van Riper has also learned how to create a basal level of fluency—a few minutes of fluent, continuous speech on the part of the child—by providing simple fluency models, by engaging in rhythm or timing activities, and by reinforcing fluency. Van Riper is now ready to begin desensitizing the child to the fluency disrupters or conditions that have been identified by the parents and himself as being particularly important in disrupting this child's fluency. We will discuss the common fluency disrupters identified by parents of young stutterers later when we discuss Van Riper's parent counseling, but for now, let us assume Van Riper wants to desensitize the child to being interrupted. How does he do this?

Van Riper first interacts with the child until he achieves a basal level of fluency. Then he gradually begins to interrupt the child. In the beginning, he does this only occasionally. If the child's fluency does not break down, Van Riper begins to interrupt him a bit more frequently. Van Riper continues to do this until just before the child begins to stutter. How does Van Riper know where this point is? It varies with the child, but usually the child's speech becomes less spontaneous and freeflowing. It may become somewhat halting and jerky. Once this point is reached, Van Riper discontinues interrupting the child and returns to the basal fluency level. After letting the child experience this basal fluency for a few minutes, Van Riper repeats the above cycle once more. In other words, he again gradually and systematically interrupts the child until just before he begins to stutter, and then again, Van Riper returns the child to the basal fluency level for a few minutes. In the beginning of this desensitization process, Van Riper goes through only two such cycles during a therapy session. Later as the child becomes able to handle more and more interruptions, he will be able to tolerate several such cycles during a session. By using similar strategies or procedures, Van Riper desensitizes the beginning stutterer to the major fluency disrupters that he and the parents are able to identify. Van Riper suggests that these desensitization procedures also increase the child's tolerance for fluency disrupters in his home and school environments, and thereby increase his fluency in these situations.

Counterconditioning Integrative Responses to Fluency Disrupters

Now we are going to discuss Van Riper's procedures for counterconditioning integrative responses by the child to fluency disrupters. In other words, Van Riper's goal is to have the child establish new competing integrative responses to situations that disrupt his fluency. Suppose a young stutterer responds to direct questions with increased stuttering, like most beginning stutterers do. How would Van Riper countercondition an integrative response to this fluency disrupter?

One way is to play "Can't catch me." In this game Van Riper has a jar of peanuts and tells the child that one of them will get a peanut when the other one asks a question. However, the person who gets a peanut has to put it back in the jar if he begins to answer the question before he eats his peanut. Van Riper sees to it that he loses a lot of his own peanuts because he answers too soon and that the child is asked a lot of questions and wins a lot of peanuts. Thus, at least two things are happening here. First, the child begins to associate a pleasant experience with answering questions. Second, the child is responding to the questions slowly; he is not giving in to time pressures. Both of these things facilitate fluency. Through games such as this, Van Riper counterconditions more adaptive and integrative responses to the child's usual fluency disrupters.

Preventing Stuttering from Becoming a Stimulus for Struggle and Avoidance

Van Riper believes it is very important to keep the child from reacting to his moments of stuttering with frustration and concern. Van Riper thinks that, once a child begins to do this, the next step is for the child to respond to these moments of stuttering with struggle and avoidance behaviors. If this can be prevented, Van Riper believes the chances are very good that the stuttering will tend to disappear. Much of the work done in meeting this goal is done by the parents, and we will return to this topic when we describe Van Riper's parent counseling in the next section. For now, we will discuss what Van Riper does with the child directly.

Since the beginning stutterer's stuttering may vary in severity from time to time, Van Riper likes to see the child more frequently during the periods of increased stuttering. At these times, Van Riper wants to create for the child as many basal level of fluency experiences as possible. Procedures used to create a basal level of fluency were discussed earlier. Van Riper feels it is important for the child to have these fluent experiences during the periods of increased stuttering in his life.

Another technique Van Riper uses to reduce the stimulus value of the child's moments of stuttering is "restimulation." By restimulation, Van Riper means the following. After a moment of stuttering to which the child responds with apparent frustration or concern—and after the child completes his utterance—Van Riper casually reflects or paraphrases what the child says. By calmly restimulating the child with the stuttered word said normally, Van Riper hopes the memory of the unpleasant experience is soon forgotten. This completes the list of goals and procedures that Van Riper employs in his direct, or face to face, treatment of the child.

CLINICAL PROCEDURES: PARENT COUNSELING

The second component of Van Riper's treatment for the beginning stutterer is parent counseling. Van Riper believes it is very important to provide the child with an environment that is conducive to fluency, and this involves working with the significant persons in the child's life. In all his interactions with the parents, Van Riper endeavors to develop a supportive and helping relationship. He encourages the parents to join him in solving this problem.

In the early sessions, Van Riper attempts to do a number of things. He obtains information about the child and the family. He provides the parents with some basic information about the nature of stuttering, and he informs them about the overall plan of treatment. He advises the parents that neither they, nor anyone else, is to correct or call negative attention to their child's speech. Van Riper also gives the parents absolution for any past mistakes they may have made in their handling of the child's stuttering. He is more concerned with the present and the future. Finally, he encourages the parents to observe and participate in the child's therapy sessions. This is important because Van Riper wants the parents to implement at home some of the same procedures he uses in direct therapy with the child. It is especially desirable to have the parents provide the child with unhurried, simple speech and language models when they interact with him throughout the day.

The main thrust of Van Riper's parent counseling is to help the parents decrease those conditions that disrupt the child's fluency and to increase those that facilitate his fluency. If the parents are to decrease the conditions that disrupt the child's fluency, they first need to identify those conditions. To help them do this, Van Riper discusses with the parents the fluency disrupters most frequently identified by other parents of young stutterers. These include the following: losing listener attention, being interrupted, competing for the conversational floor, speaking under time pressures, using display or show-off speech, attempting to use speech and language patterns that are too difficult, answering questions, speaking under emotionally disruptive conditions, and, last but not least, speaking when excited. The parents are then asked to observe their child in his daily activities to determine which conditions are associated with increased stuttering. When these fluency disrupting conditions have been identified, Van Riper explores with the parents ways to eliminate or decrease their occurrence. In a similar manner, Van Riper helps the parents identify and increase those situations that appear to facilitate the child's fluency.

Finally, Van Riper suggests to the parents ways they can help prevent the child from becoming more aware of his stuttering and, thereby, help prevent his moments of stuttering from becoming stimuli for struggle and avoidance reactions. One way is for the parents to arrange things so that there is little need for the child to talk on days when he is having a lot of stuttering, and vice versa, creating many opportunities for the child to talk on days when he is being more fluent. In addition, Van Riper gives the parents ideas for handling those times when the child is having frequent or severe moments of stuttering. He recommends to the parents that they attempt to distract the child from his speech at these difficult times. If this is not possible, he recommends that they reassure the child. He also recommends that they use the restimulation technique, which they have seen him use in therapy.

It may appear as if Van Riper's treatment of the beginning stutterer is long and complex; however, Van Riper indicates that neither is the case. He suggests that he has often been successful with only brief periods of therapy or by working on only a few of his goals. In conclusion, Van Riper reports that, by using these procedures, he has been very successful with the beginning stutterer.

Other Clinicians

Let us now take a brief look at the treatment procedures for beginning stutterers of some other clinicians who have been associated with the stuttering modification approach in recent years. By being aware of these authors' contributions, the reader will have a broader appreciation of stuttering modification therapy for the beginning stutterer.

OLIVER BLOODSTEIN

Oliver Bloodstein (1975) discusses his therapy for the beginning stutterer, or what he calls the "phase 2" stutterer, in a chapter in which he also discusses his viewpoint of stuttering as an anticipatory struggle reaction. In line with this anticipatory struggle theory, which we described earlier in this book, Bloodstein's primary objective with the beginning stutterer is to combat the child's concept of himself as a defective speaker. As will be recalled, the essence of Bloodstein's anticipatory struggle theory is that stuttering is caused by the child's development of the belief that he is a defective speaker or communicator. This attitude grows out of a background in which the child is subjected to continued and/or severe communicative failures and pressures. Bloodstein wants to reverse this belief on the part of the child. Consequently, his therapy goals for the beginning stutterer are (*a*) general speech improvement designed to establish a self-image as an effective speaker, (*b*) general personal development, (*c*) subtle and appropriate use of suggestion, and (*d*) parent counseling.

The first goal is designed to improve the child's self confidence as a communicator. All areas of communication with the exception of fluency are targeted. For example, a treatment program may involve improving the child's voice and diction or improving his conversational skills.

Bloodstein's second goal, general personal development, is aimed at increasing the child's sense of personal worth by helping him develop new interests and abilities, minimizing his old liabilities, and enhancing his image with his friends and classmates.

With regard to the third goal, Bloodstein conjectures that almost any form of suggestion to the child that he is doing well in therapy will be effective in improving his confidence in his speaking ability and will, thereby, improve his fluency.

The goals of Bloodstein's parent counseling for the beginning stutterer are to remove environmental pressures and reinforce the child's anticipation of fluency. In removing environmental pressures, Bloodstein insists that the parents remove all speech pressures upon the child. He also suggests, when necessary, that the parents be less restrictive in their child-rearing practices. In reinforcing the child's anticipation of fluency, Bloodstein recommends that the parents provide more situations for their child where he is fluent and eliminate those situations where he is disfluent.

Like Van Riper, Bloodstein believes the prognosis for the beginning stutterer is excellent. Also like Van Riper, his therapy is characterized by a low level of structure and little emphasis upon data collection.

EDWARD CONTURE

In his book, *Stuttering*, Edward Conture (1982) presents his therapy for the beginning stutterer under the heading of "children who clearly stutter and parents who are (un)concerned." From his description, his therapy appears to be a form of stuttering modification. His clinical methods are loosely structured, certainly not programmed instruction.

Conture begins by making an analogy between the speech mechanism and a garden hose. Conture equates the larynx or voice box with the faucet at the house, the throat and tongue with the hose, and the lips with the nozzle at the end of the hose. He and the child then practice stopping the water or air at various points. Next, Conture introduces the notion of "air stoppers" in the child's speech. Once the child understands that he is stopping the air at various points in his speech mechanism when he stutters, Conture explains to the child that the tightness or pressure he feels when he stutters is similar to the pressure in the garden hose when he "squeezes" the hose to stop the water. Conture then explains to the child that he can change these feelings of tightness by doing things differently with his speech mechanism.

At this point, Conture introduces another analogy. He explains to the child that speech requires movement from one sound to the next much like the frog jumping from one lily pad to the next as he crosses the stream. If the frog jumps up and down on a lily pad (repetition) or stays too long on one pad (prolongation), he will get wet and not get across the stream. Similarly, if the child wishes to say a word, he needs to keep moving from sound to sound; he can not stop too long on one sound. Conture then helps the child learn to do this by using "smooth, easy movements" as he says his words.

Conture believes it is very important for the parents to be kept informed regarding their child's therapy; they need to understand what is happening. Conture also believes it is important to provide the parents with information about stuttering and to relieve their guilt about the child's speech problem.

CARL DELL

Carl Dell (1979) was trained by Van Riper to become a stuttering specialist in the public schools. After receiving this training, Dell worked as a stuttering specialist for several years in the schools around Grand Rapids, Michigan. Based upon this training with Van Riper and upon his experiences in the schools, he wrote a booklet, *Treating the School Age Stutterer: A Guide for Clinicians.* Dell describes his therapy procedures for the beginning stutterer, or what he refers to as the "mild stutterer," in a chapter in that booklet. Dell discusses his therapy under the following headings or goals: (*a*) gradual but direct confrontation, (*b*) making stuttering more voluntary, (*c*) exploring the emotional nature of the child, (*d*) exploring struggle and tension, and (*e*) reducing the severity of repetitions and prolongations. Dell implements these goals in a low structured, play interaction with the child. He places little emphasis upon data collection.

In describing the first goal, gradual but direct confrontation, Dell discusses how he inserts pseudostuttering into his own speech and makes comments about it. This helps Dell open the door to talk to the child in an objective and relaxed manner about the child's stuttering. Dell also encourages the child to engage in some pseudostuttering with him at this point.

Once the child has done some pseudostuttering, Dell helps him learn that he can make stuttering more voluntary. Dell does this by having the child try different types of pseudostuttering. By doing this, the child learns that stuttering is not completely involuntary; rather, he has some control over it.

In meeting the third goal, exploring the emotional nature of the child, Dell attempts to provide an emotional climate in which the child feels comfortable talking about his stuttering and related matters. Dell may probe from time to time, but he will never force the child to talk about any topic that he does not want to talk about.

In the fourth goal, Dell wants the child to learn to identify what he does when he stutters. Dell wants the child to identify the site of his tension and to feel the difference between when he uses proper tension and when he uses improper tension.

The last goal builds on the previous goals. Dell now teaches the child to reduce the severity of his moments of stuttering by reducing the number of repetitions per stutter or by shortening the length of a prolongation. From his experience with beginning stutterers, Dell believes that, once the beginning stutterer learns what he is doing when he stutters and learns that he has a choice on how he says the word, he will choose the easier way to say it.

Besides working directly with the child, Dell also works with the parents of the beginning stutterer. He attempts to alleviate any guilt they may have over their child's stuttering. He provides them with information about stuttering, and he gives them suggestions as to how they can help facilitate their child's therapy at home. Based upon his experience with the above treatment approach, Dell is optimistic about the outcome of therapy with the beginning stutterer.

HAROLD LUPER AND ROBERT MULDER

Harold Luper and Robert Mulder (1964) in their book, *Stuttering: Therapy for Children*, discuss their treatment for the beginning stutterer, or what they refer to as the "transitional stutterer." They believe it is realistic to have spontaneous or normal fluency as a goal with the beginning stutterer. Luper and Mulder indicate that treatment may involve only parent counseling without direct contact with the child. If the child is seen directly, procedures may or may not involve modifying the child's moments of stuttering. If they see the child directly, their therapy is loosely structured, not programmed instruction. As a general rule, Luper and Mulder prefer less direct procedures, for example parent counseling, before attempting more direct procedures with the child.

In terms of their parent counseling, Luper and Mulder provide the parents with information about speech and language development and about stuttering and its development. Luper and Mulder also encourage the parents to implement a variety of "do's" and "don'ts" with their child. Do's include: providing good fluency models for the child, looking at the child when he talks, and showing interest in what he has to say. Some don'ts include: calling negative attention to the child's stuttering, putting undue pressure on the child for good speech, and interrupting the child.

If the decision is made to involve the child directly in treatment, but not to work on modifying his moments of stuttering, Luper and Mulder recommend some of the following procedures: desensitizing the child to fluency disrupters similar to the way Van Riper does it; providing the child with ample and successful opportunities to talk freely in therapy; allowing the child, if he chooses, to talk about his speech problem; and providing conditions that create fluency for the child, such as speaking in rhythm and choral reading.

If the decision is made to help the child modify his moments of stuttering, Luper and Mulder model "loose contacts" or strategies for producing difficult or hard words by emphasizing relaxation and smooth movements of the speech mechanism.

Summary of Stuttering Modification Therapy

Although all stuttering modification clinicians emphasize teaching the advanced stutterer to modify his moments of stuttering, this is not true for the beginning stutterer. Neither Van Riper nor Bloodstein teach the young child to modify his moments of stuttering. Luper and Mulder recommend teaching the child to use loose contacts to modify his moments of stuttering only if less direct procedures are unsuccessful. Conture and Dell, on the other hand, do appear to employ procedures to teach the beginning stutterer to modify his moments of stuttering.

FLUENCY SHAPING THERAPY

At the beginning of this chapter, we suggested that, in the treatment of the beginning stutterer, the differences between stuttering modification and fluency shaping therapies become less and their similarities become greater. However, before we compare these two therapy approaches at this treatment level, we need to present a representative example of fluency shaping therapy for the beginning stutterer. We have selected Bruce Ryan's programmed therapy for this purpose. Ryan has been doing fluency shaping therapy for many years, and his therapy is a very representative example of this approach. We will also comment upon the clinical procedures of several other fluency shaping clinicians.

Bruce Ryan: Gradual Increase in Length and Complexity of Utterance (GILCU) Program

CLINICIAN'S BELIEFS

Nature of Stuttering

Ryan believes stuttering can be viewed as learned behavior.[2] He thinks it consists of both operant and respondent components or classes of behavior. These components are as follows: a speech act, an attitude, and an anxiety component. The speech act is comprised of words that contain repetitions, prolongations, or struggle behaviors. The attitude consists of verbal statements that the stutterer makes about himself and his speech problem. Both of these components are overt or observable, and Ryan regards them as operant behaviors. The anxiety component is not overt and can be sampled only indirectly through such physiological correlates as palmar sweat. Ryan believes this component is respondent behavior. Since speech behaviors are operant behaviors, Ryan believes they can be modified by operant conditioning procedures. Further, he believes that, by changing speech behaviors, concurrent changes are also made in the attitude and anxiety components of the problem. Thus, he does not target these latter components in therapy. For Ryan, the focus of therapy is on increasing fluent speech and decreasing its reciprocal, stuttered speech. Further, he believes this can be effectively achieved by using operant conditioning and programmed instruction procedures.

---

[2] Sources for Ryan's positions on these clinical issues were Ryan, B. P. (1974). *Programmed therapy of stuttering in children and adults*. Springfield: Charles C. Thomas; Ryan, B. P. (1979). Stuttering therapy in a framework of operant conditioning and programmed learning. In H. H. Gregory (Ed.), *Controversies about stuttering therapy* (pp. 129–173). Baltimore: University Park Press; and Ryan, B. P. (1986). Postscript: Operant therapy for children. In G. H. Shames & H. Rubin (Eds.), *Stuttering: Then and now* (pp. 431–443). Columbus: Charles E. Merrill.

Speech Behaviors Targeted for Therapy

Ryan organizes his therapy into three phases: establishment, transfer, and maintenance. One of his several establishment programs is his Gradual Increase in Length and Complexity of Utterance (GILCU) program. The goal of this GILCU program is to establish or create 5 minutes of fluent conversational speech on the part of the child in the therapy room. To do this, Ryan targets both the beginning stutterer's fluent speech (fluent words) and his stuttered speech (stuttered words). He reinforces, both verbally and with a token, the child's fluent words or utterances, which he gradually and systematically increases in length and complexity from single-word responses all the way up to 5 minutes of conversational speech. During this same time, Ryan verbally punishes any stuttered words the child may have. For example, he tells the child to stop and speak fluently. Once this goal of 5 minutes of fluent conversational speech is attained, Ryan systematically transfers this fluency to the child's natural environment. This is his transfer phase of treatment. It is interesting to note that, except for clinical methods, Ryan's GILCU establishment program is not too dissimilar from Van Riper's procedures for creating a basal level of fluency.

Fluency Goals

What are Ryan's fluency goals for the beginning stutterer? They appear to be either spontaneous fluency or, in a few cases, controlled fluency. He reports that it is very common for these children to develop normal or spontaneous fluency. Ryan also notes that any residual disfluency the child may have following treatment is usually characterized by whole-word or simple part-word repetitions. In his GILCU program, Ryan operationally defines normal fluency as speech that contains 0.5 stuttered words per minute (SW/M) or less and has a rate of 130, ±20, words spoken per minute (WS/M).

Feelings and Attitudes

In his therapy, Ryan does not focus upon any negative feelings and attitudes, such as frustration and concern, that the beginning stutterer may be experiencing because of his speech. Ryan believes that, if he improves the child's fluency, then any negative feelings and attitudes the child may have will also improve.

Maintenance Procedures

As previously mentioned, the last of Ryan's three phases of treatment is maintenance. The goal of this final phase is for the child to maintain his fluency with many different people in many different situations over a 22 month period. Ryan's procedures call for the child and his parents to be seen for 5 rechecks over the 22 month period. The rechecks are scheduled to gradually fade the child from therapy. During each recheck, Ryan obtains a speech sample from the child, and he interviews the child and his parents regarding the child's fluency in his natural environment. If the child has regressed, he is recycled through portions of the treatment program. More will be said later about this maintenance phase of treatment when we discuss Ryan's clinical procedures.

Clinical Methods

All three phases of Ryan's therapy, that is, his GILCU establishment program, his transfer program, and his maintenance program, are very structured approaches to therapy. They all involve the use of behavioral objectives. Each program includes a sequence of steps arranged from easy to difficult. Each step is clearly defined in terms of its antecedent events, its responses, and its consequent events. Ryan measures and records the child's stuttered words, total words spoken, and talking time before, during, and after treatment. From these data, he computes the child's stuttering rate or SW/M and speaking rate or WS/M. He also records the number of hours of treatment and the elapsed calendar time. Criterion levels are specified by Ryan for passing from one step to the next and for completing a program. As it is apparent, a minimum of choices are left to the clinician when using one of Ryan's programs.

CLINICAL PROCEDURES: DIRECT TREATMENT OF THE CHILD

Ryan's first article discussing fluency shaping therapy for children appeared in 1971. More recently, he has described his clinical procedures in his 1974 book, *Programmed Therapy for Stuttering in Children and Adults*, and in a 1984 chapter entitled "Treatment of Stuttering in School Children" in Perkins' *Stuttering Disorders*. These sources served as the primary references for this section, and the reader is referred to them for more detailed information.

As we did with Van Riper, we will first discuss Ryan's direct treatment of the child, and then we will discuss his parent counseling. As noted earlier, Ryan breaks down his direct treatment of the child into three phases: (*a*) establishment, (*b*) transfer, (*c*) and maintenance. We will describe the goals and procedures for each of these phases in turn.

Establishment

Ryan's goal for the beginning stutterer during his GILCU establishment program is for the child to be fluent while conversing with him for 5 minutes in the therapy setting. In this 54 step program, Ryan sequentially takes the child through the modes of reading, monologue, and conversation. In each mode, he begins by having the child produce one word fluently, moves through 18 graduated steps, and ends by having the child produce 5 minutes of fluency. If the child is unable to read, Ryan omits this mode. This would obviously be the case with the preschool beginning stutterer. See Table 9.1 for an outline of Ryan's GILCU program. Now, after this brief introduction, we will discuss the various aspects of the program in more detail.

Before actually beginning the program with the child, Ryan does a number of things. He gives the young stutterer an overview of the program, using language the child can comprehend. He defines stuttering—any word that contains repetitions, prolongations, or struggle behaviors—for the child in terms the child can understand. He explains to the child what the consequences will be when he is fluent on a word and what they will be when he stutters on a word. This will also involve explaining the token reinforcement procedures to the child. We will dis-

Table 9.1   Outline of Gradual Increase in Length and Complexity of Utterance (GILCU) Establishment Program

Antecedent Event	Response	Consequent Event	Criterion
Reading:			
Instructions to read one word fluently.	One fluent word. Stuttering.	"Good" + token. "Stop, read fluently."	0 SW/M.
Instructions to read 2–6 words fluently.	2–6 fluent words.	"	"
Instructions to read one sentence fluently.	One fluent sentence.	"	"
Instructions to read 2–4 sentences fluently.	2–4 fluent sentences.	"	"
Instructions to read for 30 seconds fluently.	30 seconds of fluency.	"	"
Instructions to read for 1–5 minutes fluently.	1–5 minutes of fluency.	"	"
Monologue: Repeat the above sequence.			
Conversation: Repeat the above sequence.			

cuss these consequences and the token reinforcement procedures a little later. Finally, Ryan gives the child a criterion test which consists of 5 minutes of reading, monologue, and conversation.

Let us begin describing the GILCU program itself by discussing the "antecedent events" as they are outlined in Table 9.1. As previously mentioned, Ryan takes the child sequentially through the three modes of reading, monologue, and conversation. Ryan selected these modes because he believes they are the common verbal activities in the child's life. He further believes this sequence is ordered from easy to difficult. Reading is the easiest because the language content is predetermined for the child. This mode is obviously omitted for the child who does not read. Monologue is the next easiest mode because all the young stutterer needs to do is to think of something to say and to say it fluently. Conversation is the most difficult mode because the child must be fluent while answering questions, asking questions, and engaging in all the roles involved in conversation. Ryan notes that, if a child is having difficulty engaging in monologue or conversation, this problem is usually resolved by using pictures, topic ideas, or other such procedures to stimulate the child. Within each mode, the steps or tasks are gradually increased in length and complexity as follows: (*a*) one word, (*b*) 2 words, (*c*) 3 words, (*d*) 4 words, (*e*) 5 words, (*f*) 6 words, (*g*) one sentence, (*h*) 2 sentences, (*i*) 3 sentences, (*j*) 4 sentences, (*k*) 30 seconds, (*l*) one minute, (*m*) 1½ minutes, (*n*) 2 minutes, (*o*) 2½ minutes, (*p*) 3 minutes, (*q*) 4 minutes, and (*r*) 5 minutes. The specific words or content in each step are constantly being varied. Finally, Ryan begins each mode by instructing the child either to "read fluently" or "speak fluently."

The child's "responses" correspond in length and complexity to the antecedent events at each step (see Table 9.1). The child must fluently produce a predetermined number of responses at each step. By going through the 18 steps in each mode, the child progresses from responses of one fluent word to responses of 5 minutes of fluency.

Ryan's "consequent events" consist of both reinforcement and punishment. When the beginning stutterer produces a fluent response, Ryan immediately says "good" and gives the child a token (poker chip, toothpick, mark on a paper, etc.). These tokens are periodically turned in for a tangible reward like a small toy or a piece of candy. Ryan routinely employs token reinforcement in his GILCU program. He reports that the use of token reinforcement increases the child's motivation to come to therapy and also enhances his tendency to attend and respond to the therapy tasks. If the child stutters on a word, Ryan immediately says to the child, "Stop, read fluently," or "Stop, speak fluently," whichever is appropriate.

The term "criterion" refers to a standard or level of performance. In Table 9.1, it refers to the level of performance the child needs to meet to move on to the next step. Ryan's criterion for passing a step is zero SW/M or total fluency. It should be noted, however, that the number of responses this decision is based upon varies with the step. For example, on the first step of each mode, one-word responses, the child must have 10 consecutive fluent responses; whereas, on the last step of each mode, 5 minute responses, the child needs only one fluent response. Still, this last step requires the child to be completely fluent for 5 minutes. Implicit in Ryan's use of criteria for the child's advancement through the program is the principle that the child's responses need to be continuously measured and recorded. Only by doing this, does Ryan have the data to determine if the child is ready to move on to the next step. Thus, Ryan continuously measures and records the child's stuttered words, total words spoken, and talking time throughout each session. From these data, he computes the child's stuttering rate (SW/M) and speaking rate (WS/M).

In the preceding paragraph, we discussed Ryan's criteria for moving the child ahead to the next step. Ryan also has a criterion for "branching." Branching refers to a procedure whereby the child is given additional help or practice on a step on which he is experiencing difficulty. For example, when a young stutterer is having difficulty on a step in the GILCU program, Ryan models the responses for the child. As the child improves in his performance, Ryan gradually fades out the modeling and returns the child to the GILCU program. Ryan's criterion for branching is the child's remaining on a step for 3 sessions or 40 minutes without passing it.

After completing the entire GILCU establishment program, Ryan again gives the child the criterion test. As will be recalled, this consists of 5 minutes each of reading, monologue, and conversation. If the child has 0.5 SW/M or less on this test, he is ready to move on to the transfer phase. If the child has a higher stuttering rate than this, he is recycled through portions of the GILCU program.

Transfer

The goal of this phase of treatment is to transfer the child's fluency from the therapy situation to a wide variety of other settings and other people. Ryan reports that many beginning stutterers begin to spontaneously generalize their fluency even before this phase is begun. Despite the amount of this spontaneous transfer, Ryan still puts the child through a transfer program. The program consists of a number of hierarchies or sequences of speaking situations, arranged from easy to difficult, in which the child practices his fluent reading and conversation. See Table 9.2 for the outline of a transfer program Ryan uses with the beginning stutterer in a school environment. Certain aspects of the program will be different if treatment takes place in a nonschool environment, but the underlying principles will be the same. As can be seen, the program consists of five different hierarchies or situations: physical setting, audience size, home, school, and all day. The last hierarchy is optional depending upon the maturity of the child; many young beginning stutterers will probably not be able to successfully complete it. We will soon discuss all of these hierarchies in more detail, but first, we will make a few general comments about Ryan's procedures during his transfer program.

As in the GILCU establishment program, Ryan instructs the child to either "read fluently" or "speak fluently" in the various settings. The child must read fluently for one minute and converse fluently for 3 minutes in most situations. Ryan or the parents continue to reinforce the child with "good" for fluent responses; however, the token reinforcement is now discontinued. If the child stutters, Ryan or the parents say, "Stop, speak fluently." Either Ryan or the parents also continue to measure and record the child's stuttering. Ryan also maintains a criterion of 0 SW/M for movement from one step to the next. In summary, Ryan's procedures in the transfer program are very similar to his procedures in the GILCU establishment program.

Table 9.2   Outline of Transfer Program

Antecedent Event	Response	Consequent Event	Criterion
Physical Setting: 5 steps with clinician in different physical settings.	One minute of fluent reading. 3 minutes of fluent conversation. Stuttering.	"Good." " "Stop, speak fluently."	0 SW/M.
Audience Size: 3 steps with 3 classmates in therapy room.	"	"	"
Home: 5 steps with parent in therapy room and at home.	"	"	"
School: 4 steps with clinician in school.	"	"	"
All Day: Up to 16 steps (optional).	Up to 16 hours of fluency.	"	"

The first hierarchy in the transfer program is the "physical setting" hierarchy. This involves the child's reading and conversing with only Ryan in five different physical settings, arranged in an easy-to-difficult progression, outside the therapy room. The first step involves being just outside the therapy room door; the last step involves being just outside the young stutterer's classroom.

The next hierarchy is the "audience size" hierarchy. It begins with one of the stutterer's classmates joining the young stutterer and Ryan in the therapy room. The stutterer reads and converses with his classmate. When he meets criterion, the same procedure is repeated with two of his classmates and then with three of his classmates.

The "home" hierarchy comes third. The first step of this hierarchy involves a parent joining Ryan and the child in the therapy room and being trained to carry out the transfer procedures. The parents were informed previously that they would be involved in these and other treatment activities. We will be discussing Ryan's parent counseling procedures later in this chapter. This first step of the hierarchy is now repeated at home. The remaining steps in this hierarchy involve the gradual increase of the audience size in the home environment by the parents. This is done by having other family members and possibly neighbors join the parent and the child as the child reads and converses. After successfully completing the home hierarchy, the child is instructed to speak fluently all the time at home, and the parents are instructed to reinforce his fluency.

The fourth hierarchy is the "school" hierarchy. In the first step of this hierarchy, the child reads and converses with Ryan in the classroom. The last step, and the most difficult one, is a speech that the child gives to his entire class. After completing this hierarchy, the young stutterer is instructed to speak fluently all the time in the classroom, and the teacher is asked to reinforce the child's fluency.

The last hierarchy, the "all day" hierarchy, is optional for the beginning stutterer. It requires maturity on the part of the child and cooperation on the part of the parents and teacher, who must monitor the child. Many young beginning stutterers will not be mature enough to complete this hierarchy, and some parents or teachers may not be cooperative. However, if all the right ingredients are present, the hierarchy goes as follows. The child is instructed to speak fluently for increasingly longer periods of time on each succeeding day. The first day, he is to speak fluently for an hour. On each subsequent day, one hour is added until the child is speaking fluently his entire waking day. The parents and teacher monitor and record the child's consecutive hours of fluency.

After completing the transfer program, Ryan reports that the child is usually speaking fluently in all situations. The child is given the criterion test again, and if he exhibits 0.5 SW/M or less, he moves into the maintenance phase. If the child does not meet this criterion, he is recycled through portions of the transfer program.

Maintenance

The goal of this phase is for the child to maintain his fluency in all situations for a 22 month period following the completion of the transfer phase. Ryan sees the child and his parents on five separate occasions over this period. These rechecks are scheduled in such a manner as to gradually fade the child from therapy. During each recheck, Ryan administers the criterion test to the child and questions the child and his parents regarding the child's fluency at home and at school. If the child has 0.5 SW/M or less on the criterion test and if he is doing well in all other situations, as well, then Ryan schedules the child for the next recheck. If the child has regressed, he is recycled through portions of the treatment program, depending upon the severity of the regression. See Table 9.3 for an outline of this maintenance program. After the child has demonstrated and the parents have reported fluent speech for 22 months, Ryan dismisses the child from treatment.

Clinical Procedures: Parent Counseling

Even before Ryan begins to work with the child in the GILCU establishment program, he is careful to explain the overall treatment to the parents. He wants to enlist their cooperation. He believes they need to understand what their child will be doing in therapy and what they can expect in terms of changes in their child's speech. They also need to know what their role will be in the child's treatment. At this point, Ryan explains to the parents that they will be involved in the "home practice" program, which we have not previously discussed, and the home portions of the transfer phase, which we have previously mentioned.

The home practice program involves the parents helping the child practice being fluent while engaging in reading, monologue, and conversation at home. After the child completes the reading mode of the GILCU program, he is ready to begin to practice reading at home. At this point, Ryan brings the parents into therapy to teach them how to identify stuttered words and how to carry out the treatment procedures at home. They then help the child practice reading 5 minutes daily. After the child completes the monologue mode of the GILCU program, the home practice is modified to include 2 minutes of reading and 5 minutes of monologue. Later, when the child completes the conversation mode, the home practice is again modified to include 2 minutes of reading, 2 minutes of monologue, and 5 minutes of conversation. This daily routine continues until the child begins the home hierarchy of the transfer program.

Inasmuch as we have already discussed the home portions of the transfer program, that is, the home hierarchy and the all day hierarchy, we will conclude

Table 9.3 Outline of Maintenance Program

Antecedent Event	Response	Consequent Event	Criterion
2 weeks.	5 minutes of reading, monologue, and conversation.	—	0.5 SW/M or less.
One month.	"	"	"
3 months.	"	"	"
6 months.	"	"	"
12 months.	"	"	"

our remarks on Ryan's parent counseling by simply referring the reader back to our earlier discussion.

Before concluding our comments on Ryan's GILCU approach, we want to point out that, based upon his data, Ryan reports he has been very successful in treating the beginning stutterer by using operant conditioning and programmed instruction procedures. Though his clinical procedures differ from those of Van Riper, both clinicians report excellent results with the beginning stutterer.

Other Clinicians

As we did during our discussion of stuttering modification therapy, we will now briefly describe the clinical procedures of some other clinicians who are advocates of a fluency shaping approach with the beginning stutterer.

MARTIN ADAMS

Martin Adams has been a productive researcher of stuttering for many years. In a 1980 article, he suggests that beginning stutterers may come from two different etiological backgrounds. One group is a motor-impaired group, which has problems starting or sustaining phonation, and the other group is a language-impaired group, which has problems encoding language. Interestingly, he recommends a similar treatment program for both groups. His therapy for both groups includes rate reduction by prolongation of sounds and the principles embedded in Ryan's GILCU program. Adams believes these two strategies are helpful for both groups, but for different reasons.

Like many fluency shaping clinicians, Adams is a strong supporter of operant conditioning principles in the treatment of stuttering. For example, in this 1980 article, he emphasizes four aspects of reinforcement to which the clinician should give careful attention. First, he stresses the fact that the reinforcer needs to be something the child "really wants." Second, he suggests that, besides reinforcing the child, the clinician also tell the child "why" he is being reinforced. Third, he emphasizes the importance of the latency of the reinforcement; that is, the reinforcer should be applied as soon as possible after the correct response. And fourth, Adams discusses the effect various schedules of reinforcement have upon the rate and permanence of the learning.

In this article, Adams also provides helpful suggestions for transfer and maintenance activities. For example, he recommends that the clinician obtain from the child's parents a "hierarchy of speech-related stimuli" to use in transferring the fluency from the clinic to the child's environment. Items on this hierarchy should be consistently associated with stuttering on the part of the child. Adams concludes this article with a discussion of the importance of measuring treatment effects.

JANIS COSTELLO

Janis Costello (1980, 1983) is a leading advocate of operant conditioning and programmed instruction procedures in the treatment of the beginning stutterer. Costello refers to her "basic" program as an Extended Length of Utterance (ELU) program. This program is similar to Ryan's GILCU program. A detailed description of her ELU program is provided in the 1983 reference noted above. We will be referring to Costello's basic program again in our next chapter, along with its "additives" that we believe Costello would use with the intermediate stutterer. For now, however, we will only be describing Costello's basic ELU program. Costello also discusses procedures for the generalization of fluency to everyday speaking situations.

Costello's ELU program begins with the child producing fluent responses that consist of single monosyllabic words. After 20 graduated steps, it ends with the child conversing fluently for 5 minutes in the therapy setting. Throughout the program, Costello reinforces the child's fluent responses both socially and with tokens that are periodically redeemed for backup reinforcers. She also punishes or gives the child feedback for his stuttered responses. Costello observes and records each response, and she uses predetermined criterion levels to decide when to move the child from one step to the next.

After the child completes the ELU program, and if he has not spontaneously generalized his fluency to his natural environment, Costello engages the child in activities similar to those Ryan uses in his transfer phase. In other words, she brings persons from the child's natural environment into the therapy setting, and she also goes with the child into his real world.

Like most of the other authors we have discussed so far in this chapter, Costello is very optimistic about the chances of improving the fluency of the beginning stutterer.

GEORGE SHAMES AND CHERI FLORANCE

In Chapter 7, we described George Shames and Cheri Florance's (1980) "stutter-free speech" program for the adult or advanced stutterer. We indicated that Shames and Florance divide their adult therapy program into five phases: (*a*) volitional control, (*b*) self reinforcement, (*c*) transfer, (*d*) training in unmonitored speech, and (*e*) follow-up. The child's or beginning stutterer's program is quite similar to the adult's, except the child's program omits phase 4, training in unmonitored speech. Shames and Florance report that children begin to use unmonitored stutter-free speech or spontaneous fluency by themselves. The child's program is also accompanied by a parent-training program.

The goal of the first phase is met if the child gains volitional control over his speech. To do this, Shames and Florance use the DAF machine to help the child learn two important skills, namely, control of rate and continuous phonation. They begin with the DAF machine set at its maximum delay and instruct the child in the use of rate control and continuous phonation to produce a slow, prolonged, stutter-free speech. They then gradually increase the child's speaking rate by systematically reducing the delay times on the DAF machine. By the end of this phase, the child is producing stutter-free speech at a near normal rate while still on the DAF machine. Data are recorded and a token reinforcement is used throughout this phase.

As in the adult program, the goal of the self reinforcement phase is to teach the young stutterer to monitor, evaluate, and reinforce himself for using stutter-free speech while off the DAF machine. The child is systematically withdrawn from the DAF machine, and reinforcement is gradually shifted from the clinician to the child. In the adult program, the self reinforcement is the opportunity for the stutterer to use brief units of unmonitored speech; in the child's program, the self reinforcement is a token.

The child's parents become involved in the transfer phase. They meet with the child and the clinician to plan the home transfer program. This involves designing the transfer situations and the reinforcement system. At first, these transfer situations are similar to activities used in therapy. Later, the parents, clinician, and child develop a contract plan to expand the child's use of his stutter-free speech into other speaking situations. The token reinforcement continues to be employed in the early stages of this transfer phase, but it is gradually replaced with social reinforcement.

Following the completion of the transfer phase, the child is enrolled in the 5 year follow-up program.

Richard Shine

Richard Shine (1980) is another clinician who advocates a fluency shaping approach for the beginning stutterer. He refers to his therapy as "systematic fluency training." Throughout his program, he employs operant conditioning and programmed instruction principles. Shine includes the following five phases in his program: (*a*) picture identification prestep, (*b*) development of speaking variables compatible with fluency, (*c*) fluency training during highly structured activities, (*d*) fluency training during conversational speech and generalization to other environments, and (*e*) maintenance involving periodically scheduled evaluations for at least one year.

During the first phase, Shine selects, from a larger number of pictures, 50 to 60 pictures of items that the child can readily identify and say fluently.

The goal of the second phase is to train the child to use an "easy speaking voice." This involves teaching the child to speak fluently by talking in a manner in which the rate and intensity are significantly reduced. The pictures selected in the first phase are employed during this phase.

During the third phase, Shine's goal is to help the child to become normally fluent while conversing in the therapy setting. Shine uses the following four activities during this phase: picture identification, storybook activity, language lotto, and surprise box activity. In each of these activities, the length and complexity of the child's utterances are systematically increased from easy to difficult. During these activities the child's use of the easy speaking voice is gradually faded out and replaced by a normal manner of speaking. Shine also involves significant others in these activities to facilitate the generalization of the child's fluency to his natural environment.

With regard to the fourth phase, Shine reports that the preschool beginning stutterer usually transfers his fluency to home without any specific transfer activities other than those mentioned above. For the older beginning stutterer, Shine uses transfer activities similar to Ryan's.

The fifth phase involves a gradual fading out of the child from the treatment program. Based upon his experience and data, Shine believes that the beginning stutterer responds well to treatment.

Summary of Fluency Shaping Therapy

In their treatment of the beginning stutterer, all of the fluency shaping clinicians we reviewed in this section initially established fluency in the child in the therapy setting. Then, if the fluency did not automatically generalize, they took steps to systematically transfer this fluency to the child's environment.

COMPARISON OF THE TWO APPROACHES

At the onset of this chapter, we suggested that the differences between stuttering modification and fluency shaping therapies become less and their similarities become greater on a number of issues as one moves to the treatment of the beginning stutterer. This trend is apparent as we compare stuttering modification and fluency therapies for the beginning stutterer on the following five issues: (*a*) speech behaviors targeted for therapy, (*b*) fluency goals, (*c*) attention given to feelings and attitudes, (*d*) maintenance procedures, and (*e*) clinical methods. See Table 9.4 for an overview of the similarities and differences between these two therapy approaches for the beginning stutterer.

With regard to the speech behaviors targeted for therapy, it seems to us that both Van Riper's stuttering modification therapy and Ryan's fluency shaping therapy target the child's fluent responses. More specifically, they both attempt to create or establish a basal level of fluent conversational speech on the part of the child in the therapy setting. It should be noted, however, that not all stuttering modification clinicians agree with Van Riper on this point. For example, Dell

Table 9.4   Similarities and Differences between Stuttering Modification and Fluency Shaping Therapy for the Beginning Stutterer

Clinical Issue	Therapy Approach	
	Stuttering Modification Therapy	Fluency Shaping Therapy
Speech behaviors targeted for therapy.	Fluent responses or moment of stuttering.	Fluent responses.
Fluency goals.	Spontaneous fluency.	Spontaneous fluency or controlled fluency.
Feelings and attitudes.	Little attention given to changing negative feelings and attitudes.	No attention given to changing negative feelings and attitudes.
Maintenance procedures.	Little emphasis given to maintenance procedures.	Some emphasis given to maintenance procedures or periodic rechecks.
Clinical methods.	Therapy often characterized by loosely structured interaction—play activity.	Therapy often characterized by tightly structured interaction or programmed instruction.
	Little emphasis upon collection of objective data.	Considerable emphasis upon collection of objective data.

teaches the child to stutter easier on his moments of stuttering. The other fluency shaping clinicians are in agreement with Ryan with regard to the speech behaviors targeted for therapy.

By and large, both stuttering modification and fluency shaping clinicians agree that spontaneous fluency is a realistic goal to have with the beginning stutterer. They all agree that the probability of this occurring is very great.

Since the beginning stutterer has not acquired many negative feelings and attitudes about his speech, Van Riper and other stuttering modification clinicians spend only a little time on these in therapy. Ryan and the other fluency shaping clinicians do not target feelings and attitudes in their treatment programs.

On the fourth issue, maintenance procedures, the two therapy approaches are quite similar. Since the beginning stutterer usually does not regress, stuttering modification clinicians do not emphasize maintenance procedures. Fluency shaping clinicians, on the other hand, incorporate maintenance phases into their programs; however, they consist only of periodic rechecks.

On the last issue, clinical methods, the two therapy approaches are the most dissimilar in their treatments of the beginning stutterer. The nature of the interaction between the clinician and the child in stuttering modification therapy is loosely structured, often involving play activities. Fluency shaping therapy, on the other hand, is characterized by programmed instruction. The two approaches differ with regard to data collection, too. Stuttering modification therapy puts little emphasis upon the collection of objective data while fluency shaping therapy places considerable emphasis upon this.

In summary, stuttering modification therapy and fluency shaping therapy are quite similar in their treatment goals for the beginning stutterer. In other words, they often do not significantly differ with regard to the following: (*a*) speech behaviors targeted for therapy, (*b*) fluency goals, (*c*) attention given to feelings and attitudes, and (*d*) maintenance procedures. The greatest difference is in their clinical methods, that is, the structure of therapy and the collection of data. Thus, as it will become apparent in the next chapter, the task of integrating these two approaches for the beginning stutterer is not too difficult.

STUDY QUESTIONS

1/ Describe the following clinical procedures that Van Riper uses to create a basal level of fluency: (a) creating suitable fluency models, (b) integrating and facilitating fluency, and (c) reinforcing fluency.

2/ Describe how Van Riper desensitizes the beginning stutterer to fluency disrupters.

3/ Describe Van Riper's counseling with the parents of the beginning stutterer.

4/ What are the goals for the following phases of Ryan's therapy (a) establishment, (b) transfer, and (c) maintenance?

5/   Describe Ryan's GILCU establishment program. Also describe his transfer and maintenance programs for the beginning stutterer.

6/   Compare stuttering modification therapy and fluency shaping therapy for the beginning stutterer on the following five clinical issues: (a) speech behaviors targeted for therapy, (b) fluency goals, (c) attention given to feelings and attitudes, (d) maintenance procedures, and (e) clinical methods.

7/   Are stuttering modification and fluency shaping therapies more similar with regard to the above clinical issues in their treatment of the beginning stutterer or the advanced stutterer?

Suggested Readings

Ryan, B. P. (1971). Operant procedures applied to stuttering therapy for children. *Journal of Speech and Hearing Disorders, 36,* 264–280.

This is a classic article in which Ryan first discusses his gradual increase in length and complexity of utterance approach to the treatment of stuttering in children.

Shine, R. E. (1980). Direct management of the beginning stutterer. *Seminars in Speech, Language and Hearing, 1,* 339–350.

Shine describes his systematic fluency training approach for the beginning stutterer in this article. This includes teaching the child to use an "easy speaking voice" to enhance his fluency.

Van Riper, C. (1973). Treatment of the beginning stutterer: prevention. In C. Van Riper, *The treatment of stuttering* (pp. 371–425). Englewood Cliffs: Prentice-Hall.

In this chapter, Van Riper discusses his procedures for the beginning stutterer. It is an excellent description of the traditional stuttering modification approach to the beginning stutterer.

10

THE BEGINNING STUTTERER: INTEGRATION OF APPROACHES

In the last chapter, we stated that stuttering modification and fluency shaping therapies often do not differ substantially in their treatment goals for the beginning stutterer. Thus, the integration of these two approaches at this level is relatively easy and straightforward. As it will soon become apparent, our direct treatment of the child is more strongly influenced by fluency shaping therapy, although we do include a few stuttering modification components. Our parent counseling is influenced more strongly by stuttering modification therapy.

Before beginning our discussion of the integration of stuttering modification and fluency shaping therapies for the beginning stutterer, it may be helpful to the reader to review the characteristics of this client. As will be recalled, this child is usually between 2 and 8 years of age. In terms of core behaviors, he may exhibit part-word repetitions produced rapidly and with irregular rhythm. He may have vowel prolongations. Some of these core behaviors may contain excessive tension. He may also exhibit blocks. In terms of secondary behaviors, he may have some escape and starting behaviors. This child may be experiencing some frustration because of his stuttering. Finally, he may have a self-concept of himself as someone who has trouble talking, but he usually is not concerned about this. Let us now discuss the integration of these two major therapy approaches with this child.

OUR APPROACH

Clinician's Beliefs

NATURE OF STUTTERING

Even though we have previously stated our beliefs on the six clinical issues, it seems appropriate to summarize our beliefs here as they pertain to the beginning stutterer. We believe that predisposing physiological factors interact with developmental and environmental influences to produce and/or exacerbate repetitions and prolongations. The young stutterer responds to these early disfluencies with increased tension in an effort to inhibit them. He may also be experiencing some occasional frustration during these disfluencies. Further, as the child attempts to cope with these core behaviors, he may develop a variety of escape and possibly starting behaviors that are instrumentally reinforced. Through classical conditioning, certain speech situations may begin to elicit the tension response, which may lead to more severe, tense stutters. Even though the beginning stutterer is aware of his stuttering, he has little or only occasional concern about it.

We believe that, if we can provide the beginning stutterer with a sufficient number of positive and fluent speaking experiences during treatment, this fluency will generalize to more and more speaking situations. We will describe how we do this when we describe our establishing and transferring fluency hierarchy. This increased fluency will also reduce the opportunities the child has to respond to any remaining disfluencies with tension, frustration, or possibly escape and starting behaviors. The combined effect will be to allow time for the child's physiological system to mature and for normal fluency patterns to become stabilized.

We also believe that it is important to reduce, through parent counseling, any developmental or environmental influences that may be contributing to the child's stuttering.

SPEECH BEHAVIORS TARGETED FOR THERAPY

Which speech behaviors do we target in therapy with the beginning stutterer? Like the fluency shaping clinicians, we primarily target or reinforce the child's fluent responses while using a gradual increase in length and complexity of utterance strategy to establish fluency in the clinical situation. We also model and encourage the child to use a slower speech pattern in the early steps of therapy to facilitate the establishment of fluency. This slower pattern is soon faded out. Once fluency is established in the therapy situation, it is systematically transferred to the child's home environment. Occasionally, if a beginning stutterer is still having hard or tense moments of stuttering on some words in the later stages of therapy, we will teach him to stutter easily on these words. Usually, this is not necessary.

FLUENCY GOALS

We believe that, in most cases, the beginning stutterer will gain or regain spontaneous or normal fluency. This is fortunate because our experience suggests that it is usually unrealistic to expect a young child to consistently monitor and modify his speech by using controlled fluency or acceptable stuttering.

FEELINGS AND ATTITUDES

As we noted earlier, the beginning stutterer is experiencing only occasional frustration and has little or only occasional concern about his talking. He has not yet developed any speech fears or avoidances. Thus, we do not believe it is necessary with the beginning stutterer to focus on his feelings and attitudes in therapy.

We do, however, believe it is beneficial to desensitize the child to any fluency disrupting conditions or stimuli that may remain toward the end of the treatment program, although many times it is not necessary. This involves counterconditioning any remaining tension responses associated with these fluency disrupting stimuli. We achieve this by repeatedly pairing the child's new, fluent speech pattern with these stimuli. In other words, the child is now talking fluently in the presence of these stimuli that previously disrupted his fluency. These positive experiences countercondition the tension responses. More will be said on this topic when we describe our desensitizing the child to fluency disrupters procedures.

MAINTENANCE PROCEDURES

Our experience has indicated that the beginning stutterer usually maintains his new-found fluency very well without having to monitor or modify the way he talks. However, we do believe it is important to periodically reevaluate the child's fluency for a couple of years following the end of therapy. During these reevaluations, we obtain a sample of the child's speech and interview the child and his parents regarding the child's fluency in the "real" world. If possible, we also have the parents record a sample of the child's speech at home. If we find any evidence that the child has regressed, we re-enroll him in therapy until his fluency is regained. The length of time between these reevaluations is systematically increased until the child is completely faded out of therapy.

CLINICAL METHODS

In terms of clinical methods, that is, the structure of therapy and data collection, our procedures with the beginning stutterer are influenced more by fluency shaping therapy than by stuttering modification therapy. However, this is less true with regard to the structure of therapy than it is with regard to data collection. For example, we find that some beginning stutterers respond better to a programmed instruction approach, others respond better to a less structured, more game-orientated approach. Thus, the steps in our establishing and transferring fluency hierarchy can be incorporated into either a programmed instruction format or a game-orientated format. We will expand upon this point in more detail when we discuss our clinical procedures in the next section.

In terms of data collection, however, we believe it is very important to measure the child's frequency of stuttering and rate of speech before the beginning of treatment, during treatment, and after the termination of treatment. Depending upon whether we are using a programmed instruction approach or a game-orientated approach during treatment, we either measure all of the child's responses during the entire session or take a probe, or sampling, of the child's responses at the end of each session. The particular measures that we use will be discussed when we discuss our clinical procedures.

Clinical Procedures: Direct Treatment of the Child

We base our direct treatment of the beginning stutterer substantially upon fluency shaping strategies, but we also include some components of stuttering modification therapy.[1] We typically organize our direct treatment of the child into the following four phases: (*a*) establishing and transferring fluency, (*b*) desensitizing the child to fluency disrupters, (*c*) modifying the moments of stuttering (optional), and (*d*) maintaining improvement. The third phase, modifying the moments of stuttering, is used only if the child is still having some hard or tense moments of stuttering toward the end of the establishing and transferring fluency phase.

ESTABLISHING AND TRANSFERRING FLUENCY

Our goal for this first phase of treatment is to have the child conversing fluently with his parents in the home environment. We have found that, when many beginning stutterers are able to do this, they are already automatically generalizing their fluency to many other speaking situations.

To achieve the above goal, we typically take the child through the 13 steps outlined in the establishing and transferring fluency hierarchy in Table 10.1. We will refer to this hierarchy simply as our fluency hierarchy. The antecedent events, responses, consequent events, and criteria in Table 10.1 suggest a programmed instruction methodology. Our experience indicates that some children respond well to a structured or programmed instruction form of therapy while others do not. These latter children often perform better in a less structured, more game-orientated therapy. When we use a less structured approach, we follow the same sequence of steps outlined in Table 10.1, but we are much less concerned with precisely defining and rigorously implementing the above four components of a programmed instruction methodology. We are also less rigorous in our data collection procedures. We will comment upon both methods or styles of therapy when we discuss our procedures for each step of the fluency hierarchy.

---

[1] For an earlier version of integrating stuttering modification and fluency shaping therapies with the beginning stutterer, the reader is referred to Guitar, B. and Peters, T. J. (1980). The preschool child who stutters. In B. Guitar and T. J. Peters, *Stuttering: An integration of contemporary therapies* (pp. 65–76). Memphis: Speech Foundation of America.

Table 10.1 Outline of Establishing and Transferring Fluency Hierarchy

Antecedent Events	Response	Consequent Event	Criterion
Clinician. Single word. Slow speech. Direct model.	Single word. Fluent, slow speech.	Social. Token (optional). Continuous.	19/20 fluent responses for 5 successive strings of 20.
Clinician. Single word. Slow speech. Indirect model.	"	"	"
Clinician. Carrier phrase + word. Slow speech. Indirect model.	Carrier phrase + word. Fluent, slow speech.	"	"
Clinician. Parent. Carrier phrase + word. Slow speech. Indirect model.	"	"	"
Parent. Carrier phrase + word. Slow speech. Indirect model.	"	"	"
Parent-home. Carrier phrase + word. Slow speech. Indirect model.	"	"	"
Clinician. Sentence. Slow speech. Indirect model.	Sentence. Fluent, slow speech.	"	95% fluent responses for 2 successive sessions.
Clinician. Sentence. Normal speech. Indirect model.	Sentence. Fluent, normal speech.	"	"
Clinician. 2 to 4 sentences. Normal speech. Indirect model.	2 to 4 sentences. Fluent, normal speech.	"	"
Clinician. Conversation. Normal speech. No model.	Conversation. Fluent, normal speech.	Social. Token. (optional). Intermittent.	1 SW/M or less for 2 successive sessions.
Clinician. Parent. Conversation. Normal speech. No model.	"	"	"
Parent. Conversation. Normal speech. No model.	"	"	"
Parent-home. Conversation. Normal speech. No model.	"	"	"

Which of the above methodologies should the clinician use? Should she use programmed instruction, or should she employ a more play-orientated form of therapy? Our suggestion is that she do some trial therapy with the child during the first step of the hierarchy and then use the method that works best with the child.

Before discussing each of the steps of the fluency hierarchy in detail, we will make a few introductory comments about the antecedent events, responses, consequent events, and criteria in Table 10.1. In this more easy to more difficult hierarchy, we systematically and gradually modify the antecedent events. We change the person to whom the child is talking from the clinician to the parent; change the physical setting from the clinic to the home; increase the length and complexity of the linguistic unit from a single word, to a carrier phrase, to a sentence, to 2 to 4 sentences, and finally to conversational speech; modify the speech pattern from slow speech to normal speech; and decrease our modeling from a direct model, to an indirect model, and then to no model at all. All of these terms, which specify the antecedent events in Table 10.1, will be defined when we discuss the procedures involved in each step of the hierarchy.

The responses in Table 10.1 are what the child does in response to the antecedent events we provide. First of all, we want the child's responses to be fluent. Second, we want the child's responses to approximate the antecedent events in terms of the length and complexity of the linguistic unit. Finally, we want the child's speech pattern to resemble the pattern that is modeled. However, all three of the above do not always occur. When we discuss the steps of the hierarchy, we will comment upon the acceptable limits of the child's responses.

The consequent events in Table 10.1 are the stimuli that are presented following the child's responses. We generally ignore any stuttering the child may have as he progresses through the hierarchy. We do, however, reinforce the child's fluent responses. We always use social reinforcement, and we sometimes use token reinforcement. Our experience suggests that token reinforcement is not always necessary. In the early steps of the fluency hierarchy, we typically use a continuous reinforcement schedule. In the later steps, we usually use an intermittent schedule. We will have more to say about the type and schedule of reinforcement later.

By criteria in Table 10.1, we mean how well the child must be doing before we go on to the next more difficult step. As a general rule, we believe it is important for the child to be exhibiting a high percentage of fluent responses on a sufficient number of trials or for an adequate period of time before we move on to the next step. In other words, we want a fairly solid foundation of fluency at one level of difficulty before we go on to the next. Ultimately, when the child completes the fluency hierarchy, we want his responses to contain no more than an occasional easy repetition or prolongation. This is compatible with our fluency goal of spontaneous or normal fluency for the beginning stutterer. We will have more to say on criterion levels when we discuss the various steps of the hierarchy.

Now that we have completed our introductory comments on the fluency hierarchy (Fig. 10.1), we will outline the format for our discussion of our procedures for each step of the hierarchy. In discussing each step, we will share our experiences and our recommendations with regard to the antecedent events, responses, consequent events, and criteria. We will also comment upon data collection procedures. Finally, we will conclude our discussion of each step by describing a typical activity that could be used for that step. Throughout the above discussion, we will be commenting upon how the procedures would vary depending upon whether we were using a programmed instruction approach or a more game-orientated style of therapy.

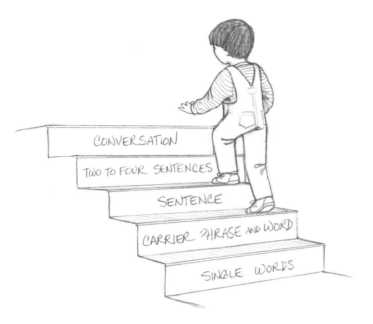

Figure 10.1. Fluency hierarchy.

Clinician, Single Word, Slow Speech, Direct Model. As we suggested earlier, the clinician may want to do some trial therapy during this first step of the fluency hierarchy to determine which structure of therapy to use. In other words, we must discover whether the child will work better in a programmed instruction format or in a less structured, more game-orientated approach. Our experience suggests that, while some children prefer one and some prefer the other, both will work.

In terms of the antecedent events, the first two are easy to define. The term "clinician" indicates that only the clinician is present in the therapy room with the child, and "single word" is self-explanatory.

By "slow speech," we mean speech that is characterized by a slow rate, achieved by slightly prolonging or stretching out all the sounds in the word. A gentle onset of phonation is used to initiate the word, and soft or relaxed articulatory contacts are employed in producing the remainder of the word. This speech pattern is similar to the speech pattern we taught the advanced stutterer in Chapter 8. (See "Using Fluency Enhancing Behaviors" in Chapter 8.) We find this slow speech pattern to be very facilitative of fluency in the beginning stutterer. Besides modeling this slow speech pattern, we instruct the child to say the word as we said it. We encourage him to say the word "slow and smooth" or "slow and easy." We believe slow and smooth seems more appropriate for the child who is having a lot of effortless repetitions, while slow and easy seems more appropriate for the child who is doing more struggling.

We should comment at this time upon our overall speaking pattern during a therapy session. In other words, how do we speak when we are giving the child directions or feedback upon his performance? We speak in a slow and relaxed manner, but not in an abnormal manner. Our rate is a slow, normal rate. In fact, this speaking pattern is the "normal speech" pattern we use in the latter steps of the hierarchy.

A "direct model" consists of our providing the child with both the linguistic unit, in this case a single word, and the speech pattern, in this case slow speech, he is to directly imitate. For example, we would show the child a picture of a car and say "car," using the slow speech pattern. The child is then expected to say "car," using the same slow speech pattern we used.

Responses are what the child does in response to the antecedent events discussed above. With regard to the continuity dimension of fluency, we expect the child's responses to be fluent. But do we expect all of his responses to be fluent? The answer to this question will have to wait until we discuss criteria a little later in this chapter.

There are, however, two other aspects of the child's responses that we need to comment upon here. The first is the linguistic unit produced by the child. As a general rule, we expect the child to produce a linguistic unit that is similar in length and complexity to that produced by ourselves. At this single word level, there is obviously no problem with the child producing a long enough utterance. There is, however, sometimes a problem when the child makes comments between responses. These asides may contain a number of moments of stuttering. Keep in mind we are trying to establish a basal level of fluency; we do not want stuttering mixed in with this fluency. At these times, it is important to instruct the child not to talk between turns. We may even tell him that we will be taking a break soon and that he can then tell us whatever he wishes.

The second aspect of the child's responses that needs commenting upon is the speech pattern produced by the child. We expect the child to imitate our pattern. This is especially true for the slow speech pattern during these early steps of the fluency hierarchy. We have noticed that some children will accurately imitate our slow speech pattern and will be fluent. Other children, however, will not modify their speech pattern, but they will be fluent, anyway. We believe that an effort should be made during these first steps to get the child to modify his speech pattern at least to some degree. For example, we may say to the child, "Don't forget to talk slow and smooth as I am," or "That was smooth, but make it just a little slower next time." We find that, if the child modifies his speech pattern during the early steps of the hierarchy, it seems to facilitate his fluency on the latter steps.

Now, for some comments on the consequent events. As we indicated earlier, we generally ignore any stuttering the child may have. We do, however, reinforce the child's fluent responses. There are two types of reinforcement that we typically use in our approach with the beginning stutterer. We always use social reinforcement, and we sometimes use token reinforcement. When socially reinforcing or praising the child for his fluent responses, we keep varying our choice of words. We will say, "That's great," "You're really doing well," "Good job," and so on. We do not want to keep saying "good" over and over until it loses all its impact or influence upon the child's behavior. We also think it is beneficial to appropriately and frequently incorporate the terms "slow and smooth" or "slow and easy," into our reinforcement or comments to the child. We believe this helps the child become aware of and acquire the appropriate speech pattern more readily.

We do not routinely employ token reinforcement with a beginning stutterer. Our experience suggests it is often not necessary. However, when a child is not motivated to come to and participate in treatment, token reinforcement procedures can be very helpful (Fig. 10.2). The clinician will need to be alert to any motivational problems during these early steps of the hierarchy. We have also found that the more game- or play-orientated the therapy, the less the need is for token reinforcement. In this situation, the motivation is provided by the innately enjoyable activities. Conversely, the more drill-like the therapy, the greater the need for a token reinforcement. In this case, the motivation is provided by the backup reinforcer. Let us now discuss setting up and running a token reinforcement procedure.

First of all, we explain to the child and his parents that the child will earn a token, that is, a chip, bean, or tally mark, for each fluent response or utterance that he produces in therapy. We then discuss with the child and his parents the sorts of things or activities the child enjoys. We go on to explain that, when the child earns a predetermined number of tokens, he will win a favorite object or an opportunity to engage in an enjoyable activity. It is important that the child truly want these "prizes" or backup reinforcers because if he does not, he will not be motivated to work for the tokens. In this case, we would not be providing the needed motivation.

These backup reinforcers do not need to be expensive. We have used pieces of gum, balloons, inexpensive toys and trinkets, opportunities to draw on the blackboard or play a computer game, and so on. Parents often provide us with backup reinforcers.

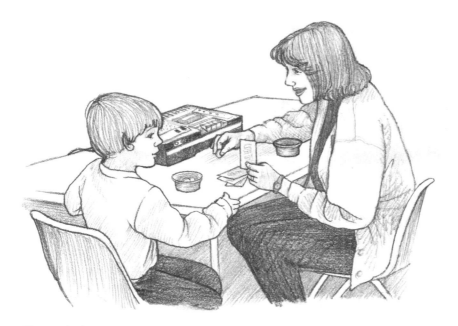

Figure 10.2.   Token reinforcement procedures can be very helpful at times.

Once a "menu" of backup reinforcers has been established, we determine a "price" or number of tokens needed to win each item. With the younger beginning stutterer, we find it effective to set the price at a level where the child can win a prize every session. This maintains his interest and motivation in therapy. With the older beginning stutterer, the price can probably be set higher because this child usually does not need to receive a backup reinforcer as frequently to maintain his interest in earning tokens. It also enhances motivation if the child receives continual feedback regarding the number of tokens he still needs to win his prize. Such techniques as transferring tokens from one cup to another help the child visualize this situation.

With regard to the schedule of reinforcement, we typically employ continuous reinforcement in these early steps of the hierarchy. In other words, we reinforce every fluent response.

If we are using a programmed instruction format, we will typically use a criterion level of 19 fluent responses out of 20 responses for 5 successive strings of 20 responses. In this case, we will need to record every response to determine whether or not the child meets the criterion. A somewhat less rigorous procedure we sometimes use is to score a probe of 20 responses at the end of the therapy session. In this case, if the child has 19 fluent responses out of 20 responses, we go on to the next step. If we are not using a programmed instruction approach, we will expect the child to have no more than 4 or 5 stuttered responses during an entire therapy session. We can keep track of these in our head. Our experience indicates that most beginning stutterers can meet any of the above criteria within 1 or 2 therapy sessions.

A typical activity for this step is "picture identification." In terms of materials, this only requires a stack of picture cards. These picture cards should depict objects that can be named by a single word. They should also represent all the word-initial phonemes in the language. We name a picture, using slow speech, and the child is to name the same picture, using slow, fluent speech. If the child does this, we enthusiastically reinforce him. We let him know that his response is either "slow and smooth" or "slow and easy," depending upon the term we decided to use with the child. If we determine that the child needs token reinforcement for motivational purposes, we also give him a token. Depending upon whether we use a programmed instruction therapy or a less structured form of therapy, we count and record the child's responses, more or less rigorously, to determine if he is meeting criteria. This is an example of the kind of activity we use for this step. In fact, we usually use three or four different activities like this during each therapy session. This helps maintain the child's interest and involvement in therapy. We typically use a variety of clinician-made and commercially available objects, pictures, parts of articulation and language kits, and children's games.

Clinician, Single Word, Slow Speech, Indirect Model.   This step differs from the first step in only one aspect, the model that is provided for the child. We now provide the child with an "indirect model," rather than a direct model. An indirect model involves our providing the child with the speech pattern he is to reproduce but not the exact linguistic unit he is to reproduce. For example, in this case, we may name an object, using a slow speech pattern. The child then names a different object, but he is expected to use our slow speech pattern. With the indirect model, the child hears the slow speech pattern between each of his responses. All the other antecedent events remain the same.

The responses, consequent events, and criteria that were used in the first step also continue to be employed here. Likewise, the same methods, structure of therapy, and data collection procedures that were used in the first step continue to be used in this step. In other words, we are beginning to gradually move up our more easy to more difficult hierarchy by modifying one antecedent event at a time. This same strategy will continue to be employed, with only one exception, as we progress from step to step in the hierarchy.

A representative activity for this step is "surprise box." The material required for this activity is a box with various objects in it. We close our eyes, pick an object out of the box, and name the object, using slow speech. We then ask the child to close his eyes, pick a different object out of the box, and name it, using slow, fluent speech. If the child says the word, using slow, fluent speech, we reinforce him along the lines previously determined. If the child is fluent on the word but does not use the slow speech pattern, we tell him, "That is good and smooth, but remember to talk slow as I am on the next word." If the child stutters on the word, we either ignore his response, or we may remind him to talk slow and smooth or slow and easy on the next word. Again, depending upon which structure of therapy worked best for the child, we implement this surprise box activity in either a programmed instruction format or in a less structured, more game-orientated style of interaction with the child. The typical beginning stutterer usually completes this step in a therapy session or two.

Clinician, Carrier Phrase + Word, Slow Speech, Indirect Model. We now begin to increase the difficulty of the task by expecting the child to say something longer and a little more complex. We now use a "carrier phrase + word." By a carrier phrase + word, we mean a predetermined sequence of words preceding the stimulus word. For example, "I see the _____," or "I think this is a _____." All the other antecedent events for this step remain the same.

We expect the child's response to be slow, and there should be no stutters in the response. We also want the child's responses to contain the same carrier phrase that we use. However, since we are providing an indirect model, we want the child to use a different stimulus word. The consequent events, criteria, and clinical methods for this step are similar to those of the preceding step.

A good activity for this step is "flashlight." This involves our placing different picture cards around the therapy room. We then turn off the lights. When the child spots a picture card with the flashlight, we say, "I see the _____," using slow speech. Then the child shines a different picture card and says, "I see the _____," using slow, fluent speech. We use several activities like this in a typical therapy session. We offer one word of caution at this point. In selecting carrier phrases to go with the activities, it is important to continually vary the carrier phrases. We have seen some children's fluency become associated with specific carrier phrases. By varying the carrier phrases, this problem can be avoided. Most beginning stutterers can meet our criteria for this step in one or two therapy sessions.

Clinician and Parent, Carrier Phrase + Word, Slow Speech, Indirect Model. We now begin transferring the child's fluency to a "parent." We do this by having one of the parents join the child and us in the therapy room. Everything else about this step, that is, the other antecedent events, the responses, the consequent events, and the criteria, is similar to the previous step.

We believe it is beneficial to begin transferring or generalizing the child's use of slow, fluent speech to the home early in the hierarchy, rather than waiting to do so until the child is fluent at the conversational level with the clinician. Our experience suggests that this facilitates the transfer process in the long run. It also has some additional benefits for the parent counseling process. First, it gets the parents directly involved early in their child's treatment. Second, when the parents have to use the slow speech pattern while interacting with their child in therapy, they begin to appreciate how difficult it can be to change the way we talk. This provides them with some insight into what their child is going through.

When the parent joins the child and us in therapy, there are a couple of tasks we need to initially accomplish. First, we need to teach the parent to use the slow speech pattern. If she or he has been observing our therapy sessions up to this point, this task will be much easier. If not, then we will need to spend some time explaining and modeling the slow speech pattern. We have found it very beneficial to have the child help us teach and evaluate their parent in the use of slow speech. Children love to teach their parents how to do something! Second, we need to teach the parent to correctly evaluate, reinforce, and record her or his child's responses. This will also involve some explaining and modeling on our part. During the first session or two with the parent in the therapy room, we take the lead to accomplish the above tasks. But then, over the next session or so, we gradually turn the responsibility for the session over to the parent. That is, the parent provides the slow speech model and reinforces and records the child's responses. We remain a participant in the therapy activity, but the parent is now functioning as the clinician.

A typical activity that we use at this point in therapy is the game "concentration." This involves placing a set of matched picture cards face down on a table. The parent turns over two cards, one at a time, and before turning over each card says, using slow speech, "I think this is a _____." If the two cards match, the parent keeps the pair. If they don't, the cards are placed face down again on the table. Either we or the child then take our respective turns, using slow, fluent speech. As on other steps, three or four such activities are used during a therapy session. Once the parent has helped the child meet the predetermined criterion level, we move on to the next step.

Parent, Carrier Phrase + Word, Slow Speech, Indirect Model. The only change we make in this step of the hierarchy is to physically remove ourselves from the therapy situation. Everything else remains the same as the preceding step. We will now sit back and observe as the parent conducts therapy with the child. In our work environments, we have the ability to observe this interaction through a one-way mirror. If these facilities are not available to the clinician, it would be possible to observe the parent doing therapy with the child by sitting back quietly in a corner of the therapy room.

There are a couple of reasons we include this step in the fluency hierarchy. First, we want to make sure that the child continues to be fluent when we are not present. Second, we want to make sure that the parent is reinforcing fluent responses and counting stuttered responses in accordance with the methods we have been using with the child up to this point in therapy. In other words, we want the parent to be able to carry out, without our being present, the same clinical methods we have been employing with the child. These issues will be very important for the successful implementation of the next step of the hierarchy.

Good activities for this step include children's games like "Go Fish" and "Old Maid." These games require the players to use some carrier phrase when taking their turn. These games are also readily available, and most parents and children are familiar with them.

Once the child has met the criterion for this step and we feel the parent is doing well in their role as clinician, we simultaneously move on to the next two steps. The next step, "parent-home, carrier phrase + word, slow speech, indirect model," involves only the parent and the child at home. It does not directly involve the clinician. Thus, we are free to move on to the following step, "clinician, sentence, slow speech, indirect model."

Parent-Home, Carrier Phrase + Word, Slow Speech, Indirect Model. With two exceptions, this step is the same as the previous one. The first exception is that the parent now conducts the therapy sessions at home, rather than in the therapy room. The other antecedent events stay the same, as do the consequent events. For example, the parent continues to engage in the same activities and games, or similar ones, which were used in the three previous steps. If the child has been receiving token reinforcement, this continues; and the tokens that the child earns at home are added to the tokens he earns with the clinician to buy backup reinforcers.

The second exception is that the criterion on this step is applied differently. We expect the child to exhibit the same level of fluency he has been exhibiting up to this point in therapy, but the child does not move on to another step when he meets this criterion level. Rather, he continues to stay on this same step at home until he reaches the last step of the hierarchy, namely, "parent-home, conversation, normal speech, no model." This present step could be regarded as an additional practice step. More specifically, we ask the parent to engage in these transfer activities with their child for 10 or 15 minutes a day, 4 or 5 days a week, until the child reaches the last step of the hierarchy or the point where he is able to engage in fluent conversation with his parents at home.

We believe this weekly practice is beneficial to the outcome of the treatment program and reasonable from the point of view of time. In our experience, it does not become a burden for either the parents or the child. We regularly check with the parents to see if they are having any problems and if the child is continuing to be fluent during these practice sessions. After these sessions have been going well for a while, some parents will ask us if the other parent could be involved in the activities. This is fine if the child continues to be fluent.

Clinician, Sentence, Slow Speech, Indirect Model. In this step, we continue to move up our hierarchy by increasing the length, complexity, and spontaneity of the linguistic unit. We now move to the "sentence" level. This task requires the child to make up his own sentences in response to objects, pictures, or questions. In accordance with our strategy of changing only one antecedent event at a time, all the other antecedent events of this step remain the same.

In terms of the child's responses, we count a sentence as being fluent only when it contains no moments of stuttering. In other words, sentences must be completely fluent to be fluent. We would also like the child to generate grammatically complete sentences. However, if the child does not give us a grammatically complete sentence, we will not make an issue of it. Our prime goal is a fluent sentence.

Sometimes, we have a problem with a child's responses when he gets stuck in a linguistic rut and repeatedly produces sentences that are similar in grammatical form. We do not want the child's fluency associated with only one form. It is as if the child is stuck back at the carrier phrase level and is continuously repeating the same grammatical form in each sentence. For example, the child may say, "I see the ball," "I see the car," "I see the house," etc. If this occurs, we have found that, by giving the child some suggestions for other types of responses and by using a variety of sentences as examples in our indirect modeling, we can get the child out of this rut.

At this step, we still stay with a continuous reinforcement schedule for the child's fluent responses. However, we do make some changes in the criteria. Our experience suggests that it is more difficult for children to be fluent while generating their own sentences than while they are saying carrier phrases + words. For this reason, we think it is important for our criteria to be more rigorous on this step. In other words, we think the child needs more practice at this level. Thus, we now want the child to maintain a high level of fluency for at least two sessions before we move on to the next step. If we are using a programmed instruction approach, we usually require the child to have 95% fluent responses for 2 successive therapy sessions. This requires us to score and record each sentence so that we can compute the percentage of correct responses for the session. If we are just taking a probe towards the end of each session, we may score only 10 or 20 sentences and compute the percentage of correct responses from these. In this case, we still want the child to be successful for at least two days. If we are using a less structured form of therapy, we may expect the child to have only four or five sentences containing moments of stuttering during a therapy session. These we can note in our head. Again, we still want at least two days of successful fluency.

"Barrier games" are good activities to use during this step. Barrier games require a barrier, such as a piece of cardboard, between the clinician and the child. This barrier only needs to be large enough so that the clinician and the child can not see the sheet of paper each has on the table in front of her or him. When we use a barrier game, we give the child instructions to draw something somewhere on his sheet. For example, we may say, "Draw a horse in the bottom right corner of your page." We then draw the same thing in the same location on our sheet. Next, the child tells us to draw something somewhere on our sheet of paper; and at the same time, he draws the same item in the same spot on his sheet. After we each have taken a number of turns, we take the barrier down and compare our pictures. In this activity, the child is still hearing us model (indirect model) slow speech during our turns, but he is generating his own sentences.

Clinician, Sentence, Normal Speech, Indirect Model.   It is now time to fade out the slow speech pattern and begin to model a "normal speech" pattern for the child's responses. As we indicated earlier, normal speech denotes speech that is relaxed and is characterized by a slow, normal rate. Besides modeling (indirect model) normal speech for the child, we also tell him he can talk just a little bit faster now. We tell him to listen carefully to our speech. Usually, we have no problem getting the child to change his speech pattern from slow speech to normal speech. In fact, many children may already have increased their rate somewhat over the last few steps of the hierarchy. Besides doing the above things, we also remind the child to continue to talk "smooth" or "easy", whichever term we have been using with him. All the other antecedent events, consequent events, and criteria for this step remain the same as for the preceding one.

An activity we sometimes use on this step is "scrapbook." Here, the child and the clinician make scrapbooks with pictures in them of things we like. We may make just one scrapbook for the two of us, or we may each have our own scrapbook. We begin by cutting a picture out of a magazine and saying a sentence about the picture, modeling normal speech. Then we glue the picture in the scrapbook. The child then cuts out a different picture; makes up a sentence, using fluent, normal speech; and glues his picture in the scrapbook. If necessary, we give the child instructions to slightly increase his speaking rate, and we reinforce his responses if they contain fluent, normal speech. This activity may continue for 10 to 20 minutes. As usual, this activity may be only one of several activities that we use during a given therapy session.

Clinician, Two to Four Sentences, Normal Speech, Indirect Model.   It is time again to increase the length and complexity of the linguistic unit. We now go to the "2 to 4 sentences" level. At this level, the clinician generates 2 to 4 sentences in response to pictures or objects, and then the child produces 2 to 4 sentences in response to different pictures or stimuli. Thus, the clinician is still providing an indirect model of the normal speech pattern for the child between each of the child's responses. On this step, we want the child to produce a response that is longer than just one sentence, but we do not want him to go on talking forever. This is a transitional step, which immediately precedes the move to conversation. As in the past, all the other aspects of this step remain the same as the last step.

A very good activity for this step is "sequencing cards." This involves the use of sequencing cards, which are found in many commercially available language kits. We begin by arranging a set of cards, usually three to five, in sequence and then telling a two to four sentence story based on the cards. By doing this, we are still providing the child with an indirect model of fluent, normal speech. The child then takes the next set of cards and arranges them in sequence. He tells a story, using fluent, normal speech. At this point, to be reinforced for a fluent response, the child needs to produce two to four fluent sentences. This is a long way from the first step of the hierarchy, when he was getting reinforced for each fluent word. Once the child meets the criterion for this step, we move on to conversation.

Clinician, Conversation, Normal Speech, No Model.   Unlike all of the preceding steps, we change two antecedent events on this step. First, with regard to the linguistic task, we go to "conversation." This involves spontaneous interaction with the child while engaging in games or play activities. Second, with regard to the level of modeling, we provide the child with "no model." We continue to speak at a slow, normal rate and in a relaxed manner, but we are no longer taking turns while interacting with the child. Thus, the child does not necessarily hear us model the normal speech pattern between each of his responses.

At the conversation step, we begin to use intermittent reinforcement. We now reinforce the child after he is fluent on half a dozen or so utterances or sentences. It is important to present this reinforcement during pauses in the conversation so that we do not interrupt the child while he is engaging in speaking. As the child experiences more and more success on this conversation step, we gradually increase the amount of fluency required before he gets reinforced. In other words, we are beginning to fade out our reinforcement of the child's fluency.

We also change the type of measurement used in the criterion on this step. We go from using percentage of fluent responses to using stuttered words per minute (SW/M). We do this because computing SW/M is much easier at the conversational level. All one needs to do to compute the SW/M is to count the number of stuttered words the child has during a therapy session, measure his talking time with a stopwatch during the session, and divide the stuttered words by the time. If we are using a programmed instruction approach, we typically use 1 SW/M or less for two successive sessions as our criterion. If we choose not to measure his fluency over the entire session, we may take probes of his fluency during the last 5 or 10 minutes of each therapy session and determine his SW/M for these periods. In this case, we still want him to exhibit 1 SW/M or less during these probes for two successive therapy sessions. If we choose not to measure the child's talking time during the therapy sessions, we probably expect him to have not more than 5 or 10 stuttered words per session for 2 successive therapy sessions.

At this point in our discussion of the fluency hierarchy, it seems appropriate to comment upon our fluency goals for the typical beginning stutterer. As will be recalled, we said that, in most cases, the beginning stutterer will gain or regain spontaneous or normal fluency. We further stated that we think it is unrealistic to expect a child this young to consistently monitor and modify his speech to use controlled fluency. This is what we begin to observe around this point in the hierarchy. The child usually has a lot of spontaneous fluency. Sometimes, he seems to be monitoring his speech in order to use his fluent, smooth or easy speech pattern, but quite often, he is not monitoring; he is just being spontaneously fluent.

We sometimes use "art projects" as one of our activities during this step of the hierarchy. We engage the child in conversation while we are working on these art projects together. These projects are often related to a central theme, such as holidays, seasons of the year, etc. We find it very easy to reinforce and measure the child's fluency while doing these activities.

Clinician and Parent, Conversation, Normal Speech, No Model.   For awhile now, one of the parents and the child have been practicing fluent, slow speech in carrier phrases + words at home. Now, it is time to transfer fluent, normal conversational speech to the parent. At this point, we bring the parent back into the therapy room. This is the only aspect of this step that differs from the preceding step.

When we bring the parent back into therapy, we must familiarize her or him with the new, normal speech pattern. Again, if the parent has been observing the therapy, this will usually be a relatively easy task. If the parent has not been observing the sessions, this may require some explaining and modeling. Usually, getting the parent to use a slow, normal rate and a relaxed manner of speaking is not a big problem. The only trouble comes when the parent seems to be an innately rapid speaker. In these cases, we most likely have already been discussing this problem with the parent during the parent counseling sessions. With these fast-talking parents, we also find it helpful to have the child critique his parent's speech rate during therapy. Children love this role, and parents usually respond well to it. We must also spend some time with the parent explaining the new, intermittent reinforcement schedule and the new criterion level. They will need practice in implementing these, too.

Activities that seem to work well in therapy at this time include open-ended conversations with the child regarding what he did at school that day or what he plans to do that evening; spontaneous conversations that arise while playing children's games, such as Candyland™ or checkers; or conversations that develop while playing with toy farm sets, doll houses, computer games, etc.

Parent, Conversation, Normal Speech, No Model. As we did earlier when we transferred fluent, slow speech in carrier phrases + words to the parent, we now remove ourselves from the therapy situation. We do this by observing the parent and child through a one-way mirror or from the corner of the therapy room. All the other components of this step are identical to the previous step.

As before, we believe this step is important for two reasons. One, we want to make sure that the child maintains his fluency when we are no longer present. Two, we want to make sure the parent is reinforcing and evaluating the child's fluency accurately. To evaluate these two sets of behaviors, we observe the interaction between the parent and the child in the type of conversational activities described in the two previous steps. We reinforce the parent for the things that are going well and give suggestions for improving the things that may not be going well.

Once the child meets the criterion for this step and the parent is working well as the clinician, we simultaneously move on to the last step of the hierarchy, "parent-home, conversation, normal speech, no model," as well as to the next phase of our direct treatment of the child, "desensitizing the child to fluency disrupters." We will first discuss the last step of the hierarchy, and then we will describe how we desensitize the child to fluency disrupters.

Parent-Home, Conversation, Normal Speech, No Model. This step is similar to the previous step, except that the parent is now engaging the child in conversation at home, not in the therapy room. As we did earlier during the "parent-home, carrier phrase + word, slow speech, indirect model" step, we now ask the parent to engage in this transfer step with the child for 10 or 15 minutes a day, 4 or 5 days a week. This present step replaces the earlier step in terms of the daily practice sessions at home. Besides using some of the conversational activities that were used in the preceding steps, many parents simply set aside a specific period each day for their child to practice using his smooth or easy speech. Typical practice periods include the times after school, after dinner, or before bed. We want the child to maintain the same level of fluency during these periods that he was having in therapy, and we regularly check with the parent to see if he is doing so. As on the earlier practice step, some parents gradually get the other parent involved in these activities. The parents continue with these practice sessions at home until the child is into the "maintaining improvement" phase of therapy.

As we stated at the beginning of this section on the establishing and transferring fluency hierarchy, we find that many beginning stutterers, when they reach this point in treatment, are already transferring their fluency, usually spontaneous fluency, to many other speaking situations. Thus, many times just completing this hierarchy is all that is necessary.

However, in other cases where the child's fluency does not automatically transfer to all situations, additional steps may be needed. These steps may involve bringing siblings or playmates to the therapy sessions, having the child's teacher attend several sessions, bringing grandparents to therapy, or conducting therapy in other physical settings, such as the child's favorite fast-food restaurant. These additional steps will vary for each child. During these additional steps, the clinician and the child meet with the other persons or in the other physical settings, and the child practices using his smooth or easy speech. The other persons involved should be aware of the purpose of the sessions. In other words, the child's fluency should be treated openly and matter-of-factly. The activities used during these sessions should be something that would be appropriate for the situation. For example, if one of the child's playmates comes to a therapy session, it is appropriate for everyone to play a game that the children enjoy. During the game, the beginning stutterer is practicing his smooth or easy speech, and the clinician is reinforcing this fluency. By going through these additional steps, the child's fluency, in most cases spontaneous fluency, continues to generalize to speaking situations throughout his speaking day. This establishing and transferring fluency phase of therapy comes to an end when the child is exhibiting spontaneous fluency or controlled fluency, but usually spontaneous fluency, in all speaking situations.

DESENSITIZING THE CHILD TO FLUENCY DISRUPTERS

As we indicated before, once the child completes the "parent, conversation, normal speech, no model" step of the fluency hierarchy, we usually begin this phase of our direct treatment of the child. With some children, it is not necessary. Our goal here is to desensitize the child to any remaining fluency disrupting stimuli that may still precipitate stuttering for him. Many of the child's fluency disrupters have already been eliminated or significantly reduced as part of our parent counseling, and we will be talking about this process soon. However, some fluency disrupters, because of their nature, cannot be totally eliminated from a child's life. The child needs to live with them. For example, some parents report at this time that, when their child gets excited, he still has some stuttering. Other parents report other conditions that still tend to disrupt their child's fluency. It varies with the child. We believe these children need to be desensitized to these remaining fluency disrupters.

Our procedures are similar to Van Riper's, but with some variations. As will be recalled, Van Riper created a basal level of fluency or a few minutes of fluent speech by providing simple fluency models for the child, by engaging the child in rhythm or timing activities, and by reinforcing the child for fluency without him being aware of it. We, on the other hand, by taking the child through our fluency hierarchy, already have the child conversing fluently with us for an entire therapy session. This is our basal level of fluency.

Suppose a child's fluency does break down when he becomes excited. How do we desensitize him to this excitement? We are very open with the child regarding our goal. We tell him that we are going to try to get him excited and his job is to practice using his smooth or easy speech in spite of this. We then engage the child in some activity that excites him. For example, one of the authors remembers playing "basketball" with a young stutterer in a therapy room that had been emptied of all its furniture except a wastebasket. It was the basket, and a foam rubber ball was the basketball. In the beginning, the tempo of the game was slow. The child was told to use his smooth or easy speech. When the child was fluent, he was reinforced for his fluency; he was praised for using his smooth or easy speech. If he had some stutters in his speech, he was reminded to use his smooth or easy speech. If the excitement seemed too great for him to monitor his speech, the basketball game was slowed down. The clinician did not want to push the child beyond his fluency breaking point. When the child was being fluent, the tempo of the game was gradually picked up. Finally, after a number of therapy sessions like this, arms and legs and balls were flying all over the therapy room, and still the child remained fluent. The excitement no longer disrupted his fluency. We were on the way to desensitizing the child to excitement.

We are confident that the clinician will be able to think of other, and possibly more appropriate, activities for desensitizing her beginning stutterer to his fluency disrupters. Whatever the activity, the important things to do are the following: let the child know you are going to be introducing the fluency disrupter, tell the child he is to use his smooth or easy speech, reinforce him for using his smooth or easy speech, and gradually and systematically expose him to stronger and stronger dosages of the fluency disrupter. Be careful not to overexpose him to the fluency disrupter; we do not want his fluency to substantially break down. This desensitization process continues until the child is in the "maintaining improvement" phase of treatment or until there are no more fluency disrupters.

MODIFYING THE MOMENTS OF STUTTERING (OPTIONAL)

Modifying the moments of stuttering is an optional phase to our treatment program for the beginning stutterer. Most beginning stutterers respond well to the fluency hierarchy previously described and do not need this phase. A few children, however, may still have some tense moments of stuttering remaining during the later steps of the hierarchy. These residual stutters are not as hard or as tense as they were originally, but there is still some tension present. They are milder versions of the original stuttering. We believe it is important to give these children a tool for coping with these remaining stutters. Thus, we take time to teach them how to stutter easy. During the therapy sessions, we alternate teaching the child to stutter easy and working on the remaining steps of the hierarchy. Once the child has learned to stutter easy, we can work on a step of the hierarchy and easy stuttering at the same time. In other words, the child can be practicing his fluent, easy speech pattern; and if he happens to have a tense moment of stuttering, he can stutter easy on it.

How do we teach these children to stutter easy on these residual stutters? To do this, we adopt some of Van Riper's (1973) and Dell's (1979) ideas for treating the intermediate stutterer, whom Van Riper calls the young, confirmed stutterer and Dell calls the confirmed stutterer. We explain to the child that there are two ways of stuttering on a word. There is the "hard way," and the "easy way." We model both ways for the child. The hard way resembles the child's typical, tense, residual moments of stuttering; this may vary from child to child. The easy way consists of saying the word slowly by slightly stretching out all the sounds of the word. A gentle onset of phonation is used to initiate the word, and soft articulatory contacts are used throughout the remainder of the word. We remind the child of the "slow and easy"[2] speech we used in the early steps of the fluency hierarchy. We point out to the child that the slow and easy speech, which we used earlier, is similar to the easy way of stuttering about which we are talking, now.

Once the child understands what we mean by the hard way and the easy way of stuttering, we engage the child in some fun activities during which we repeatedly put easy stuttering into our speech. We also encourage the child to use voluntary, easy stuttering frequently in his own speech. At first, we do this while we are using single words or short utterances; later, it is beneficial to do this while we are engaging in conversational speech. We want the child to develop the ability to use these slow movements, gentle onsets, and soft articulatory contacts on individual words in connected speech. We also want him to feel comfortable producing words in this manner. During these activities, we strongly reinforce the child for using voluntary easy stuttering. Sometimes, when children develop the ability to use these forms of voluntary easy stuttering, they begin to automatically replace their tense moments of stuttering with these easy moments of stuttering. If this does not occur, we will then need to teach the child to modify his moments of stuttering as he is experiencing them. To do this, we suggest the following progression of procedures.

First, we need to model for the child how this modification will look and sound. We begin to stutter, simulating the child's typical, residual moment of stuttering. Then we come out of this stutter with a slow, relaxed movement. We provide this model for the child many times. In essence, this is a Van Riper pull-out. However, we do not call it by this name when talking with the child; we call it the easy way of stuttering.

Second, we have the child join us as we simulate his stuttering and ease out of it with slow, relaxed movements. In other words, we are easy stuttering in unison with the child. We want the child to feel what it is like to turn a hard stutter into an easy stutter. We give the child lots of support and reinforcement for doing

---

[2] Since this child still has some mild, tense, residual stutters, the chances are good that he had some tense struggle behaviors in the beginning of therapy; and thus, we probably used the term "slow and easy" with him, instead of "slow and smooth."

this with us; it is not always easy for a child to deal directly with his moments of stuttering in this manner.

Third, we want to help the child catch himself in a moment of stuttering and then to ease out of the stutter and through the rest of the word, using slow, relaxed movements. It is often helpful to squeeze the child's arm when he gets caught in a moment of stuttering. When we squeeze his arm, he is to hang on to his stutter. Then, when we release our grip on his arm, he is to ease out of the moment of stuttering and complete the rest of the word, using slow and relaxed articulatory movements. We may even join the child at this time and lead him out of his stutter. We give the child a lot of support and reinforcement during this procedure. It takes time and practice to develop this skill, but once the child learns to do this, he is well on his way to learning easy stuttering.

MAINTAINING IMPROVEMENT

Once the child has reached the point where he is exhibiting spontaneous fluency or controlled fluency, usually spontaneous fluency, in all speaking situations, we move into the maintaining improvement phase of therapy. We do not dismiss the child at this point; rather, we gradually fade him out of active treatment. We begin this process by scheduling therapy sessions weekly for a month and then biweekly for a month or two. If things continue to go well, we then begin to see him for a series of reevaluations.

During these reevaluations, we obtain a sample of the child's speaking and interview the child and his parents regarding how things have been going since the last appointment. We begin by having monthly reevaluations for several months, then every other month for several months, then, finally, once a semester for a year, after which we dismiss the child. Many times, we have the parents bring in a recorded sample of the child's talking at home. If, at any point in this process, the child seems to be regressing, we will bring him back into active, more intensive treatment. The nature of this treatment will depend upon what the problem seems to be, but it will usually involve spending more time in one or more of the three phases of treatment the child has previously completed. The typical beginning stutterer will spend approximately two years in this last phase of treatment.

Clinical Procedures: Parent Counseling

We have a number of goals in mind when we counsel the parents of the beginning stutterer. These include (*a*) explaining the treatment program and the parents' role in it, (*b*) explaining the possible causes of stuttering, (*c*) identifying and reducing fluency disrupters, and (*d*) identifying and increasing fluency enhancing situations.

We may begin to respond to some of these goals, for example, the first two, during the initial evaluation. We usually focus upon the other goals in later counseling sessions. These goals are not always worked on in the sequence listed above; we will take our cues from the parents' concerns and questions. Further, we find that we usually discuss a given topic a number of times over several sessions. As we learn more about the child and his family and as the parents learn more about stuttering and its treatment, old issues are revisited from new points of view. For example, we may feel the need to further explore some aspect of the child's life, or the parents may possibly have more questions about a given topic. In other words, counseling the parents of the beginning stutterer is not a step-by-step set of procedures; it is an ongoing, dynamic process (Fig. 10.3).

Explaining the Treatment Program and the Parents' Role in It

Most parents want to know the nature of the treatment program. They want to know what we are going to be doing to them and their child. They also want to know how long it is going to take. We believe it is very important that they have a good idea of what is involved. After all, this is going to have a considerable impact upon their time and activities for the next year or two. At this point, we explain the fluency hierarchy and, in particular, their role in the transfer steps. We also briefly comment upon their role in identifying and reducing fluency disrupters, which we will be discussing shortly. Usually, we do not explain the desensitizing the child to fluency disrupters and the modifying the moments of stuttering phases at this time. If it becomes necessary, we will explain these phases at the appropriate point. In terms of time commitment, we tell the parents that it is best if we see their child 2 or 3 times a week for 30 to 45 minutes each time. We tell the parents that often the therapy program takes anywhere from 6 months to 2 years. We are careful to answer any questions they may have.

Parents will often ask what they should tell their child about coming to speech therapy. Many times, these parents have been told or have read that they should not mention their child's stuttering to him. It has been "hush-hush." We

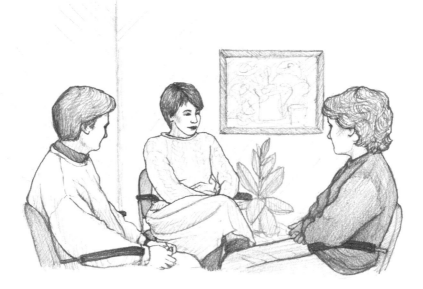

Figure 10.3. Parent counseling is an ongoing process.

believe this is a unwise approach. From our experience, most of these children know that they have problems talking. They are not embarrassed by it or ashamed of it, but they know they have trouble getting words out upon occasion. In fact, they often know they "stutter!" If the significant adults in their lives can't talk about this matter, children often begin to think that what they have must be so terrible that even mother and father can not talk about it. This is an awful message to give a child. We believe that it is much wiser to talk openly about the stuttering. Thus, we suggest to the parents that they tell their child something along the following line. We suggest they tell him he will be going to speech school to get help with his stuttering or talking. Usually, we will use the word stuttering; it is a commonly used and descriptive word. Occasionally, we may not use the word stuttering if the child is very young and seems unaware of the term. Furthermore, we suggest that the parents tell the child that quite a few young children need help in learning to talk smoothly and this is what he is going to do at speech school. We also suggest that they tell the child that, with this help, he will grow up talking as fluently as everybody else, and this is most likely true.

Another question that parents often ask is, "What should I do when my child is having many episodes of hard stuttering and seems upset by it?" Again, we recommend that they talk openly about the stuttering. We point out to them that, if their child came into the house with a bloody nose, they would not ignore it; rather, they would acknowledge it and help the child. Thus, we suggest to the parents that, when their child seems to be having a difficult time with his stuttering, they should acknowledge it and be reassuring. Some statement like, "Boy, that was a hard one, wasn't it; at speech school you will learn to say those easily." This is only an example. The parents will need to express these thoughts and feelings in a way with which they feel comfortable.

One additional bit of information about stuttering, which we share with the parents, is the research data relative to spontaneous recovery. This material was presented in Chapter 1. As will be recalled, of the children who begin to stutter, between 50 and 80% of them will recover without any formal treatment. We tell the parents that, with treatment, these percentages go up substantially. Whereas we can not guarantee success with every beginning stutterer, this information is very reassuring for most parents. We tell them that they have good reason to be hopeful!

EXPLAINING THE POSSIBLE CAUSES OF STUTTERING

We believe it is very important for the parents of the beginning stutterer to be given an explanation of the possible causes of the disorder, and we share with them our interpretation of the current theoretical and research literature. In some cases, parents have no information about the causes of stuttering. If they are going to participate in their child's treatment, and we want them to, they need to understand the rationale for our treatment program. In many other cases, parents feel guilty because of some outdated or inaccurate information they may have. They may have been exposed to a theory that is no longer valid, or they may have been given some erroneous information by a well-meaning, but misinformed, friend or relative. These parents then blame themselves for some supposed misdeed on their part. They need good, current information about the nature of stuttering. Often, just supplying this information relieves the parents of their guilt. We have found the following material to be helpful supplements to our parent counseling: Eugene Cooper's (1979) pamphlet, *Understanding Stuttering: Information for Parents*, and the Speech Foundation of America's booklets (Conture and Fraser, 1989), *Stuttering and Your Child: Questions and Answers*, and (Guitar and Conture, undated), *If You Think Your Child Is Stuttering*.

What do we tell the parents of the beginning stutterer about the possible causes of the disorder? We share with them, in language appropriate to their background, the type of information we discussed in Section I of this book. We tell them that we believe that predisposing physiological factors interact with developmental and environmental influences to produce and/or exacerbate the initial repetitions and prolongations. The child responds to these disfluencies with increased tension in an effort to inhibit them. The child also learns a variety of escape and, possibly, starting behaviors to cope with these repetitions and prolongations. We go on to suggest that the predisposing physiological factors are most likely neurological in nature and are related to the child's ability, or rather lack of ability, in the area of speech production. We suggest the child has problems in timing the fine motor movements required for fluent speech. We also suggest that, in many cases, the predisposing physiological factors are probably genetic in origin. Thus, the child brought something to this problem, too.

We also explore with the parents the developmental and environmental influences that may be interacting with the predisposing physiological factors to cause the child to stutter. These were reviewed in Chapter 3. In some cases, we do not identify any developmental or environmental factors that seem to be contributing to the problem. However, when we do identify some possible factor, we attempt to lessen its influence. For example, if we learn that the child's stuttering got worse soon after the birth of a baby sister or brother, we suggest to the parents that this factor may be contributing to the problem. We point out how none of us function well when we are under stress and how their child's speech may be especially vulnerable to it. We note that, when he is under stress, his fine timing or coordination of his speech mechanism tends to break down. We then explore with the parents ways to reduce the disrupting influence of this new rival for their love and attention. For example, it would be especially important for the parents to give the beginning stutterer much love during this time. After the parents have explored other options with us, they will usually come up with many other things they can do to reassure their child during this transition period. Our experience suggests, in most cases, that the solution to reducing the impact of these developmental and environmental influences is fairly straightforward. In a few cases, it is more difficult. In these cases, we have found that referral for counseling to a private psychotherapist or mental health agency is necessary.

IDENTIFYING AND REDUCING FLUENCY DISRUPTERS

We believe, along with many other clinicians, that it is important to explore with the parents one special group of environmental influences that often interact with the child's physiological predisposition to exacerbate the stuttering.

Broadly speaking, these are variables present in the child's speech and language environment. They include the parents' speech and language patterns as well as the conditions under which the child attempts to speak. As we discussed in Chapter 3, there are a number of these conditions that seem to disrupt children's fluency. We refer to these as fluency disrupters. These conditions include: improper speech and language models, unrealistic speech and language expectations, calling negative attention to the stuttering, competition for the floor, interruptions, listener loss, demand speech, time pressures, display speech, excitement, and other emotionally disturbing situations. These conditions were discussed in Chapter 3, and the reader may wish to refresh her understanding of them. It is important, though, that the clinician and the parent identify these fluency disrupters and explore ways to reduce them. How do we do this?

We begin by explaining to the parents what we mean by fluency disrupters. That is, we explain to the parents that, quite often, certain situations in a child's speech and language environment seem to cause him to be more disfluent. We then discuss with the parents the most common fluency disrupters. If the parents' speech rate appears to be too rapid or if their language usage is too sophisticated to provide a good fluency model for their child, we work with them on slowing their rate or simplifying their language patterns around their child. We then ask the parents to carefully observe their child for the next week or so and to note those situations that seem to cause more stuttering for him. Then, when we get together with the parents for our next counseling session, we search with them to determine if there are any patterns to these situations. Sometimes, the parents come to the next session having already figured out what type of situations seems to give their child the most trouble. Other times, it may take several weeks of observation and brainstorming with us to identify any patterns. In some cases, there does not appear to be a pattern to the type of situations that disrupt the child's fluency.

Once a pattern, or patterns, has been determined, we explain to the parents that our goal is to reduce, as much as realistically possible, the fluency disrupters in their child's life. We don't have any specific set of recommendations on how to do this; rather, we explore with the parents possible ways they can do this. After all, the parents are the ones who are going to make the modifications in their child's speech and language environment. We can only give suggestions and help them consider possible alternatives. Once the parents decide how they are going to modify a given situation, we support and encourage them in their efforts. We also monitor, on a regular basis, their progress in changing the child's environment and their observation of the effect this change is having upon the child's fluency. Two examples may be helpful here.

The first example involves a father who had unrealistic speech and language expectations for his four-year-old son. This father was an engineer and was well educated in the physical sciences. He believed that it was important for his son to know the physical laws of nature. Unfortunately, even though this father was well-intentioned, he was not well-informed in child development. This became apparent when we were discussing the situations in which his son was most disfluent. For example, the father reported that on the previous night his son had been very disfluent when they had been discussing the law of gravity. The father reported that the son had said, "I-I-I-Is gra-gra-gravity the rea-rea-rea-son I ca-ca-ca-can ju-ju-jump higher on the-the-the moo-moo-moo-moon tha-than I ca-ca-can on earth?" This, and many other examples, soon illustrated that this father was attempting to teach his son scientific concepts that were well beyond his son's capabilities. When this was pointed out to the father, he replied, "I just wanted my son to be ready for kindergarten." To relieve his concern, we evaluated the boy on several tests of cognitive and language development. As we expected, he performed a year or two above his chronological age on each of them. When the father learned this, he no longer felt it was necessary to teach his son these difficult concepts at this time. The father modified the nature of his interaction with his son, and the son's fluency soon began to improve.

The next example involves a mother who was constantly, but unknowingly, interrupting her six-year-old son. She also tended to interrupt everybody else, including ourselves. When we asked her to look for situations at home where her son was most disfluent, she was unable to identify any situations. We then asked her to tape-record a conversation with her son at home and bring it back to our next counseling session. When she brought it back, we listened to it together. Her son was quite disfluent on the tape, and she was interrupting him every third sentence or so. She began talking before he was done with his sentences, she asked him questions while he was still in the middle of his sentences, and, at times, she even interrupted and corrected the content of his messages. After listening to about half the tape she said, "Do I always do that? I'm constantly interrupting him!" She was obviously unaware of this behavior on her part. Once she became aware of it, she tried very hard to change. It was difficult for her, but she did improve. So did her son, and we believe this change on her part contributed to his improvement.

These two examples also illustrate another point we want to make. Our experience suggests that the vast majority of parents want to help their children improve their fluency. Neither this father nor this mother were engaging in these behaviors to be mean or spiteful; they were simply unaware of the influence their behaviors were probably having upon their child. When it was suggested that they change, they did their best to do so. Accordingly, we do not want to make these parents feel guilty for these past mistakes. We tell them that we know they love their child, that this was an understandable mistake, and that we know they want to help their child. We accept their past errors and encourage them to change in the future.

IDENTIFYING AND INCREASING FLUENCY ENHANCING SITUATIONS

We not only want to identify and reduce fluency disrupting situations, but we also want to identify and increase fluency enhancing situations. Most beginning stutterers have some situations in which they are usually fluent. These are often relaxed, one-on-one situations with a parent. It may be while sharing a story with mother before going to bed or while working on a quiet project with father. Just as we have the parents identify fluency disrupting situations, we also have the parents identify those situations in which the child is often fluent. Once these situations are identified, we encourage the parents to engage their child in these activities as often as possible, at least on a daily basis. The more practice the child has at being fluent, the more solid his fluency will become.

We also talk with the parents about the fact that beginning stuttering is often cyclic in nature. Beginning stutterers often have "good days" and "bad days." On the child's good days, we encourage the parents to engage the child in a lot of talking. We want him to experience his fluency. On the child's bad days, we suggest to the parents that they attempt to find more quiet activities for him to do. We do not want the child to experience the struggle and possible frustration involved in this stuttering. We realize the parents will not be able to apply these suggestions perfectly, but to the degree they are able to have their child experience a lot of fluency on his good days and experience less stuttering on his bad days, we believe their efforts will be helpful.

This concludes our integration of stuttering modification and fluency shaping therapies for the beginning stutterer. Now, let us look at how some other clinicians integrate these two approaches.

OTHER CLINICIANS

Hugo Gregory and Diane Hill

Hugo Gregory and Diane Hill (Gregory, 1984a, 1986a; Gregory & Hill, 1980) believe that stuttering develops from an interaction between the child and environmental variables. They include five treatment objectives for the beginning stutterer or the child who is "atypically disfluent with or without complicating speech, language, or behavioral factors." These objective are (*a*) to avoid increasing the child's awareness of his stuttering, (*b*) to increase the amount of the child's fluency, (*c*) to increase the child's tolerance for fluency disrupters, (*d*) to help the child gain competence in areas, such as articulation or syntactic development, that may interfere with his fluency development, and (*e*) to increase the child's self-acceptance. The fourth objective will be discussed in the next section of this chapter when we consider the treatment of concomitant speech and language problems. Gregory and Hill also recommend that the child's parents be involved in a parent counseling program.

With regard to the first objective, Gregory and Hill will not call attention to the child's stuttering; however, if the child brings it up, they will acknowledge it. At these times, Gregory and Hill will make some reassuring statement to the child.

To increase the amount of the child's fluency, Gregory and Hill model an "easy, relaxed speech" for the child. This speech is characterized by "smooth movements into and between words." The child's dependence upon this modeling is systematically reduced through the following hierarchy: direct model, delayed model, intervening model, no model, and question model. At the same time, the length and complexity of the child's utterances are increased from single-word responses, to phrases, to sentences, and finally, to conversation. Also concurrent with the above procedures, the child's use of easy, relaxed speech is systematically generalized to other physical settings and other people. Gregory and Hill typically generalize the use of easy, relaxed speech at a given linguistic level to other physical and social conditions before moving on to longer and more complex linguistic utterances. Gregory and Hill reinforce easy, relaxed speech responses and employ criterion levels to move on to more difficult steps.

To increase the child's tolerance for fluency disrupters, Gregory and Hill employ desensitization procedures similar to Van Riper's. These desensitization procedures are applied at the various length of response levels.

To meet the last objective, increasing the child's self-acceptance, Gregory and Hill may engage the child in art projects and deliberately make mistakes. They are then very accepting of these mistakes.

Among Gregory and Hill's goals for the parents during parent counseling are the following: to provide the parents with information on how stuttering may develop, to help the parents identify moments of stuttering, to help the parents identify factors that increase their child's stuttering, and to help the parents develop a problem-solving approach to reducing those factors that increase their child's stuttering.

Meryl Wall and Florence Myers

Meryl Wall and Florence Myers (1984) believe that stuttering results from a lack of synergism between psycholinguistic, physiological, and psychosocial factors in children. They state that their therapy is "eclectic" and argue that all three factors—psycholinguistic, physiological, and psychosocial—need to be taken into account in both the direct treatment of the child and in the parent counseling.

With regard to psycholinguistic factors, Wall and Myers state that their therapy has a "language-based orientation," regardless of whether the child has a concomitant speech and language disorder or not. In their basic approach to therapy for all children who stutter, Wall and Myers interact with the child in a loosely structured activity while, at the same time, controlling the length and semantic-syntactic complexity of the child's utterances. They usually begin by eliciting one- or two-word utterances from the child. They do this in a variety of ways, such as using imitation, having the child name objects or pictures, or asking questions. When the child is fluent at this level, they gradually begin to work on longer and more complex linguistic tasks. They will go through the following sequence: two- and three-word phrases, simple sentences, complex sentences, picture descriptions, storytelling, and conversation. Throughout all of these tasks, the clinician is gradually putting greater linguistic demands upon the child. The child needs to be fluent at one level before the clinician moves on to the next one. We will discuss Wall and Myers' views on dealing with concomitant speech and language problems in the next section of this chapter.

In terms of physiological factors, Wall and Myers provide the child with an "easy speech" model to facilitate fluency during the language-based tasks described above. Easy speech is characterized by a slow-normal rate, relaxed articulation, gentle voice onset, and slightly reduced volume. If the child still has blocks on some words, Wall and Myers will give the child techniques, such as Van Riper pull-outs, to modify these stutters.

Among the things that Wall and Myers do to deal with psychosocial factors are the following: share information about stuttering with the parents, help the parents talk with their child about his stuttering, help the parents reduce fluency disrupters in the child's environment, and help the child deal with any teasing he may be experiencing. In summary, this is a brief description of how Wall and Myers integrate the above three factors in their treatment of the beginning stutterer.

SUMMARY OF INTEGRATION OF APPROACHES

Earlier in this chapter we stated that stuttering modification and fluency shaping therapies are quite similar in their treatment of the beginning stutterer. Some stuttering modification clinicians teach the child to modify his moments of stuttering, but others reinforce fluency in ways similar to those of fluency shaping clinicians. Stuttering modification clinicians also tend to give a little attention to the child's feelings and attitudes about his speech, whereas fluency shaping clinicians tend not to do this at all. From the discussion of our clinical procedures and from the descriptions of Gregory and Hill's and Wall and Myers' clinical procedures, the reader should recognize that it is possible to incorporate some work on modifying the moment of stuttering and some work on attending to feelings and attitudes with a basic fluency shaping program in the treatment of the beginning stutterer.

TREATMENT OF CONCOMITANT SPEECH AND LANGUAGE PROBLEMS

One of the clinical issues we discussed in Chapter 5 was the clinical management of concomitant speech and language problems in the beginning stutterer. We noted that the research indicated that some of these children are delayed in their speech and language development, especially in their articulation development. We further noted that recently a number of clinicians have recommended the treatment of these concomitant speech and language problems in the beginning stutterer, and we strongly supported these new developments. We will discuss the recent contributions of Gregory and Hill, Wall and Myers, and Riley and Riley.

In discussing the contributions of these clinicians, we will limit our remarks primarily to these clinicians' views on the clinical management of the concomitant speech and language problems as they interface with the treatment of the stuttering, not on these clinicians' overall treatment approach to stuttering. We have already discussed Gregory and Hill's and Wall and Myers' procedures for the beginning stutterer earlier in this chapter. We will present enough information about Riley and Riley's overall treatment program so that the reader can understand how their work on the child's speech and language problems relates to their work on the child's stuttering. We will conclude this section with a discussion of our own experiences integrating the treatment of stuttering with the treatment of concomitant speech and language problems.

Hugo Gregory and Diane Hill

Hugo Gregory and Diane Hill (Gregory, 1984a, 1986a; Gregory & Hill, 1980) believe that concomitant speech and language problems can contribute to maintaining or increasing stuttering in the young stutterer. Thus, in their treatment of the "child atypically disfluent with complicating speech, language, or behavioral factors," they believe it is important to target these problems in therapy.

As will be recalled, one of their objectives was "to increase the amount of the child's fluency." As part of their procedures to do this, they systematically increased the length and complexity of the child's utterances from single-word responses, to phrases, to sentences, and finally, to conversation. Gregory and Hill suggest this strategy lends itself very readily to working on syntactic or articulation errors. For example, Gregory and Hill point out that, depending upon the developmental level of the child's language, various syntactic structures can be practiced at the same time the child is practicing his fluency. In other words, by using the appropriate instructions and materials, the clinician can have the child practice both a specific syntactic structure and easy, relaxed speech at the same time. Gregory and Hill also indicate that this applies equally well to articulation therapy. Depending upon where the child is in articulation therapy, he could be practicing his new phoneme in a response of a given length and complexity at the same time he is practicing his fluency.

Gregory and Hill report that a significant percentage of the young stutterers they see have word retrieval problems. To help these children, Gregory and Hill have two goals. The first goal is to help the child feel comfortable with pauses in his speech. To accomplish this, they model delays in their responses to naming tasks and then say something like, "I can't think of what that is called; everybody has problems like this sometimes." They also give the child ample time to recall words. Their second goal is to give the child a strategy for retrieving words. To do this, Gregory and Hill help the child learn to build associations between objects and their semantic attributes, such as function, size, shape, color, etc. Then they create situations to give the child practice in using this strategy to retrieve words.

Gregory and Hill also work with the parents to improve the speech and language models to which the child is exposed at home. For example, if the parents speak too rapidly, ask too many questions too fast, or do not listen to the child, Gregory and Hill will instruct and model for the parents during therapy more appropriate speech and language behaviors for them to use around the child.

Glyndon and Jeanna Riley

Glyndon and Jeanna Riley (1983, 1984) advocate a "component model" of treatment for the child at their "intervention level II: chronic stuttering." By treating the underlying and maintaining components of the stuttering, Riley and Riley report that the child, in most cases, regains normal fluency. In other words, at this intervention level, Riley and Riley neither modify the child's moments of stuttering nor reinforce his fluent responses; they only treat the underlying and maintaining components of the stuttering.

There are nine components in their model; four are "neurogenic" components, and five are "traditional" components. The neurogenic components are: attending disorders, auditory processing disorders, sentence formulation disorders, and oral motor disorders. The five traditional components are: disruptive communicative environment, unrealistic parental expectations, abnormal parental need for child to stutter, high self-expectations by the child, and manipulative stuttering. It seems to us that three of these components are directly related to the treatment of concomitant speech and language problems. They are auditory processing disorders, sentence formulation disorders, and disruptive communicative environment.

Riley and Riley report that approximately 27% of their young stutterers have auditory processing disorders. By auditory processing disorders, they mean the child has problems receiving and manipulating auditory information. The child may have any of the following problems: retaining auditory images, making figure-ground distinctions, or selecting meaningful from nonmeaningful auditory signals. Treatment goals depend upon the child's particular auditory processing problem. Typical goals may include increasing the child's auditory memory or increasing his ability to follow directions. Riley and Riley recommend a number of commercially available and published programs for improving children's receptive language abilities.

Among sentence formulation disorders, Riley and Riley include the following types of disorders: word retrieval problems; word order problems, involving reversals and transpositions; and formulation problems, involving incomplete and fragmented sentences. They report approximately 30% of their young stutterers have these types of problems. Treatment goals depend upon the child's particular problems, and again, Riley and Riley recommend a number of commercially available and published materials for treating these expressive language difficulties. However, they recommend programs based upon generative grammar, not those based simply on length of utterances. Riley and Riley also stress the importance of a careful analysis of the child's syntax so that the treatment program is targeted at the child's level of language ability.

Riley and Riley report 53% of their young stutterers come from disruptive communicative environments. By this, they are referring to fluency disrupters in the child's environment, such as the child having difficulty getting the parents' attention, the child being interrupted while talking, and the child being rushed while speaking. Riley and Riley counsel the parents regarding the importance of reducing these fluency disrupters.

Meryl Wall and Florence Myers

Meryl Wall and Florence Myers (1984) note that some clinicians are reluctant to work on a young stutterer's concomitant speech or language problem because they fear that calling attention to the child's speech and language will exacerbate the stuttering. Wall and Myers believe that, for the most part, this fear is unjustified.

As will be recalled, Wall and Myers' (1984) basic approach to therapy for all children who stutter is a "language-based orientation" approach. In this approach, they control the length and semantic-syntactic complexity of the child's utterances. They typically go through the following sequence: two- and three-word phrases, simple sentences, complex sentences, picture descriptions, story-telling, and conversation. Wall and Myers suggest that this method of sequencing linguistic tasks assures that the length and semantic-syntactic complexity of the therapy activities can be kept within the child's capacity. They suggest that, in the early stages of therapy, the vocabulary should consist of words already in the child's repertoire. In the later stages of therapy, new words can be added to the child's lexicon. In a similar manner, in the early stages of treatment syntactic structures already in the child's repertoire should be used. Later on, new grammatical structures can be gradually introduced. However, Wall and Myers recommend that the clinician follow the normal developmental sequence in introducing new sentence structures. Wall and Myers recommend that, as the clinician moves the child through this sequence of linguistic tasks, work on easy speech or pull-outs can be incorporated with work on new vocabulary or new syntactic structures.

What about the child with a phonological or articulation disorder? Wall and Myers recommend that, if the child's disability is mild and not interfering with intelligibility, the problem should be treated after the fluency has been stabilized. However, if the disability is severe and interfering with intelligibility, the problem should be dealt with immediately because it could be adding considerable stress to the child's communicative attempts. If treatment of a phonological or articulation disorder is begun, Wall and Myers recommend that the phoneme or phoneme group selected for treatment be the one that is the easiest for the child to produce. Words and syntactic structures selected for practice material should be ones with which the child can easily cope. Wall and Myers further suggest that work on sound production can be integrated with work on fluency; for example, practice of the new sound in a word can be integrated with practice of easy speech.

Wall and Myers also have suggestions for the parents of a child with both a beginning stuttering problem and a delayed speech and language problem. If the parents talk fast, they are asked to talk more slowly around their child. If the parents use language that is way beyond the child's semantic-syntactic level, they are asked to simplify their language when talking to their child. To help the parents make these changes in their speech and language and, thereby, be better fluency models for their child, they are encouraged to watch the clinician work with their child and observe how she modifies her rate and language to enhance the child's fluency.

Besides improving the fluency models the parents present to the child, Wall and Myers also discuss with the parents other ways they can use language at home to enhance their child's fluency. They point out that asking close-ended questions, which require short responses, will usually elicit more fluency in the child than asking open-ended questions, which require longer and more complex answers. For example, "Did you have fun at Doug's birthday party?" will usually elicit a shorter and more fluent response than "What did you do at Doug's birthday party?" By employing the above and other strategies, Wall and Myers help the parents provide the child with a linguistic environment that is more conducive to fluency.

Our Experience

We believe it is important to treat the beginning stutterer's concomitant speech and/or language problem. We believe that, as the child gains more competence and confidence in speaking ability, the result is a positive effect upon his fluency. Further, we have not had any experiences where we felt treating the other speech or language problem exacerbated the stuttering.

The most frequent concomitant speech and language problems we find in beginning stutterers are phonological and/or syntactic disorders. We integrate our treatment of the child's fluency with treatment of these other problems much as Gregory and Hill and Wall and Myers do. That is, as we move up our fluency hierarchy, we target both the child's fluent responses and his phonological and/or syntactic responses. In other words, as we go up the hierarchy, we often have the child practice both smooth, fluent speech and correct phonemes and/or syntactic structures at the same time. However, there are two issues that we typically encounter as we integrate this work on the child's fluency with work on these other speech and language problems. One issue deals with sequencing, and the other deals with terminology. Let us first discuss the issue of sequencing.

In most cases, the children we see are referred to us because someone, usually the parents, are concerned about the child's stuttering. Thus, we usually begin our treatment program by responding to this concern. That is, we begin by increasing the child's fluency by use of our fluency hierarchy. After we successfully complete several steps of this hierarchy, we then begin work on a concomitant speech or language problem. However, the child often can not be successful working on this concomitant problem at his present level of linguistic difficulty in the fluency hierarchy. For example, if the child is at the "carrier phrase + word" level in the fluency hierarchy when we begin working on a misarticulated phoneme, it is quite possible that he will not be able to correctly use this phoneme at the carrier phrase + word level. We may need to begin teaching this phoneme at the nonsense syllable or word level. At this point, the child is not practicing fluency and correct articulation at the same time in the same response. Rather, part of each therapy session is spent practicing fluency in the fluency hierarchy, and part of each session is spent practicing correct articulation. Only when the child is able to be successful at a given linguistic level with both his fluency and his articulation are they worked on together in the same response. These same principles apply when we integrate therapy for fluency with therapy for syntactic problems. Thus, in terms of the linguistic unit, work on fluency sometimes coincides with work on the other concomitant speech and language problems, and sometimes one precedes the other.

Now, let us consider the issue of terminology. As we mentioned before, we use verbal reinforcers, such as "that's great" or "good job," when the child produces a fluent response. We also refer to these fluent responses as being "smooth" or "easy." Now what do we do when we are working on both fluency and a concomitant speech or language problem at the same time? Suppose we are working with a child on both fluency and a specific syntactic structure, and he produces a response that is fluent but not syntactically correct; what do we say? If we say "good" we are reinforcing fluency, but we are also reinforcing a response that is syntactically incorrect. We do not want to do this. We find that, if we label the target responses differently, we usually do not have significant problems. For example, we worked with one four-year-old beginning stutterer who had both phonological and syntactic problems. When we worked on both fluent and correct syntactic responses at the same time, we referred to a fluent response as being "smooth" and a syntactically correct response as being "a good sentence." Besides using this verbal feedback, we also used token reinforcement with the boy. On any given response, he could earn two, one, or zero tokens, depending upon whether his response was both fluent and syntactically correct, either fluent or syntactically correct, or neither fluent nor syntactically correct. When we targeted both fluent and correct phonological responses at the same time, the procedures were the same but we referred to a phonologically correct response as "having the good sound." We found that, by using the above procedures with this boy, he did not have any problem keeping things straight.

Like the other clinicians we have discussed in this section, we believe it is important to work with the parents of the young stutterer to improve, when necessary, the speech and language models to which the child is exposed at home.

Summary of Treatment of Concomitant Speech and Language Problems

In summary, there appears to be support for integrating work on the beginning stutterer's fluency and his other speech and/or language problems. None of the above clinicians reported adverse effects upon the child's stuttering. Further, it appears that this integration can be successfully accomplished by employing a strategy that gradually and systematically increases the length and complexity of the child's responses.

TREATMENT OF THE BORDERLINE STUTTERER

At times, a child is referred for an evaluation, and he turns out not to be a beginning stutterer; rather, he turns out to be a borderline stutterer. We will conclude this chapter with a few brief comments about the clinical management of this child.

As will be recalled, the borderline stutterer usually has more disfluencies than the normal child. He often has more than 10 disfluencies per 100 words. He is likely to have more part-word repetitions and prolongations in his speech than revisions and interjections, and his part-word repetitions may exhibit more than 2 repetitions per instance of disfluency. At the same time, however, the borderline stutterer's disfluencies differ from the beginning stutterer's. They are loose and relaxed; they do not exhibit tension. The borderline stutterer also does not exhibit any secondary behaviors. Further, he has little or no awareness of his speaking difficulty. Only rarely will he express surprise or frustration about it.

As we previously suggested, we believe that many borderline stutterers have a physiological predisposition to stutter. Consequently, we believe that they will benefit from environmental changes that will help them compensate for this predisposition. We believe that, in most cases, if the communicative and emotional stresses in the child's environment can be reduced, the child will go on to develop normal fluency patterns. Thus, we do not work directly with this child. Instead, we counsel the parents of the borderline stutterer along lines similar to those we use for the beginning stutterer. More specifically, our goals with these parents include (*a*) explaining the possible causes of stuttering, (*b*) identifying and reducing fluency disrupters, and (*c*) identifying and increasing fluency enhancing situations. Readers are referred to an earlier section of this chapter, during which we discussed counseling the parents of the beginning stutterer, to refresh their memories regarding the clinical procedures associated with each of these goals. What we said there applies equally well to our counseling of the parents of the borderline stutterer.

Besides meeting with these parents a number of times to discuss and help them implement the above goals, we monitor the child's fluency on a monthly basis. This involves seeing the child and obtaining a sample of his speech. It also involves interviewing the parents regarding the child's fluency at home. It is common for the child to regain normal fluency within 3 to 6 months. If the child does not, we then enroll him in therapy as a beginning stutterer.

STUDY QUESTIONS

1/ List the 4 phases of Peters and Guitar's therapy for the beginning stutterer. What is the goal for each of these phases?

2/ Briefly, describe Peters and Guitar's establishing and transferring fluency hierarchy.

3/ Describe Peters and Guitar's procedures for the following phases of treatment: (a) desensitizing the child to fluency disrupters, (b) modifying the moments of stuttering, and (c) maintaining improvement.

4/ Describe Peters and Guitar's counseling with the parents of the beginning stutterer.

5/ Based upon Gregory and Hill's, Wall and Myers', and Peters and Guitar's experiences, describe how the treatment of beginning stuttering and other speech and language disorders can be integrated.

6/ What suggestions do Peters and Guitar have for the treatment of the borderline stutterer?

Suggested Readings

Gregory, H. H. & Hill, D. (1980). Stuttering therapy for children. *Seminars in Speech, Language and Hearing, 1*, 351–363.

In this excellent article, Gregory and Hill discuss the importance of concomitant speech and language problems in maintaining or increasing disfluencies in young stutterers. They also give suggestions for working with these problems.

Riley, G. D. & Riley, J. (1984). A component model for treating stuttering in children. In M. Peins (Ed.), *Contemporary approaches in stuttering therapy* (pp. 123–171). Boston: Little, Brown & Company.

Over the last several years, the Rileys (husband and wife) have been developing a rather unique approach to the treatment of beginning stuttering in children. Rather than treat the stuttering behavior, they treat the underlying and maintaining components of the stuttering problem. A "must" article for serious students of stuttering in children.

Wall, M. J. & Myers, F. L. (1984). Therapy for the child stutterer. In M. J. Wall & F. L. Myers, *Clinical management of childhood stuttering* (pp. 179–227). Baltimore: University Park Press.

In this excellent chapter, Wall and Myers describe their language-based approach to therapy. In this approach, they integrate stuttering modification and fluency shaping therapies along with work on the child's concomitant speech and language problems.

11

THE INTERMEDIATE STUTTERER: STUTTERING MODIFICATION AND FLUENCY SHAPING THERAPIES

Now that we have completed the discussions of the treatment procedures for both the advanced and the beginning stutterer, we will discuss the treatment of the intermediate stutterer. Most often, the clinical procedures for the intermediate stutterer are a combination or a modification of procedures for the advanced and the beginning stutterer. This is true for both stuttering modification and fluency shaping therapies. Thus, understanding the treatment of the intermediate stutterer is easier if one first understands the treatment of the other two treatment levels.

When we discussed the advanced stutterer, we noted that stuttering modification and fluency shaping therapies substantially differ on a number of clinical issues. These issues include (*a*) speech behaviors targeted for therapy, (*b*) fluency goals, (*c*) attention given to feelings and attitudes, (*d*) maintenance procedures, and (*e*) clinical methods. Later, when we discussed the beginning stutterer, we indicated that the differences between these two therapies on a number of these clinical issues become substantially less at this developmental/treatment level. With the intermediate stutterer, the reader will find that stuttering modification and fluency shaping therapies are *more* similar than they are for the advanced stutterer but *less* similar than they are for the beginning stutterer.

Before discussing stuttering modification therapy, fluency shaping therapy, and the integration of these two approaches for the intermediate stutterer, we will review the characteristics of the intermediate stutterer. As will be recalled, the intermediate stutterer is usually between 6 and 13 years of age. Thus, he is typically in elementary school. The older intermediate stutterers, however, will be in junior high school.

In terms of core behaviors, the intermediate stutterer may exhibit part-word or monosyllabic word repetitions that contain excessive tension, vowel prolongations that exhibit tension, and blocks. His secondary behaviors may include escape behaviors, starting behaviors, and for the first time, avoidance behaviors. These avoidance behaviors may include word substitutions, circumlocutions, and avoidance of speaking situations. In terms of the feelings and attitudes associated with his stuttering, the intermediate stutterer is experiencing frustration and embarrassment; and he is beginning to experience fear. Finally, he has a definite self-concept as a stutterer. Now, let us turn to the treatment of the intermediate stutterer.

STUTTERING MODIFICATION THERAPY

As we have done for the other two treatment levels, we will use Charles Van Riper's therapy to illustrate a stuttering modification approach to this treatment level. We will describe Van Riper's therapy for the intermediate stutterer in detail, and we will then comment briefly upon the therapies of a number of other stuttering modification clinicians.

Charles Van Riper: Easy Stuttering

CLINICIAN'S BELIEFS

Nature of Stuttering

As previously discussed, Charles Van Riper (1982) views stuttering as a disorder of timing. When the child stutters, there are disruptions in the timing and sequencing of the movements involved in speech production. These mistimings or disruptions account for the core behaviors. Van Riper suggests these mistimings may be due to an organic predisposition, to a faulty feedback system, or to communicative or emotional stress. Van Riper also believes the intermediate stutterer's secondary behaviors, such as escape, starting, and avoidance behaviors, and the negative feelings and attitudes associated with the stuttering are learned. Thus, they can be unlearned in therapy.

Speech Behaviors Targeted for Therapy

As with the advanced stutterer, Van Riper believes it is important to teach the intermediate stutterer to modify his moments of stuttering. To do this, Van Riper teaches the young stutterer to stutter in an "easy" manner.[1] This involves prolonging all the sounds in the stuttered word. It also involves slow, smooth transitions from sound to sound. By teaching the child to stutter in this easy manner, Van Riper is helping the child unlearn the struggle and secondary behaviors associated with his moments of stuttering. Van Riper is also helping the child learn how to cope with the mistimings in his speech.

Fluency Goals

What are Van Riper's fluency goals for the intermediate stutterer? Van Riper states that the disorder often "melts away" once the child begins to use easy stuttering. This implies that the child develops spontaneous fluency or becomes a normal speaker. With other children, however, it appears that Van Riper's fluency goal is controlled fluency or acceptable stuttering. Van Riper expects these latter children to be using easy stutterings whenever they are experiencing some difficulty.

Feelings and Attitudes

As will be recalled, we stated that the intermediate stutterer is experiencing some embarrassment over his stuttering. We also said that he is beginning to develop some situation and word fears. Van Riper basically agrees with this definition of the intermediate stutterer. Consequently, even though these feelings are not as strong or as well established as they are in the advanced stutterer, Van Riper believes it is important to target these negative feelings in therapy. As we will soon see, Van Riper suggests a number of clinical procedures to reduce the intensity of, or to help the intermediate stutterer cope with, these negative feelings.

Maintenance Procedures

Van Riper believes that, in contrast to the advanced stutterer, the intermediate stutterer requires much less stabilization of his new speech pattern. In this regard, the intermediate stutterer is similar to the beginning stutterer. Van Riper notes that, usually, all that is required to maintain the child's improved fluency is an occasional booster session, during which the child practices a lot of easy stutters. Van Riper also observes, as we stated, that the problem often "melts away" once the intermediate stutterer begins to use the new, easy stutters in his everyday speech.

---

[1] The reference for Van Riper's belief on this and the remaining clinical issues is Van Riper, C. (1973). *The treatment of stuttering*. Englewood Cliffs: Prentice-Hall.

Clinical Methods

As with the other two treatment levels, Van Riper's therapy with the intermediate stutterer is loosely structured. In fact, his therapy with this child often occurs within the context of a game. Even though Van Riper has definite goals for each therapy session, his therapy could never be described as a programmed instruction approach. As with the other treatment levels, Van Riper does not discuss the issue of data collection.

CLINICAL PROCEDURES: DIRECT TREATMENT OF THE CHILD

Van Riper's therapy for the intermediate stutterer is a combination of his therapies for the advanced and the beginning stutterer. As with the advanced stutterer, Van Riper organizes his direct therapy for the intermediate stutterer into four phases: namely, (*a*) identification, (*b*) desensitization, (*c*) modification, and (*d*) stabilization. And, as with the beginning stutterer, Van Riper believes it is important to counsel the parents of the intermediate stutterer. Van Riper also believes it is important to counsel the child's classroom teacher as part of the overall treatment program. Van Riper (1973) discusses all of these clinical procedures in his chapter on the "young confirmed stutterer" in his book, *The Treatment of Stuttering*. We will begin by discussing his direct treatment of the child.

Identification Phase

Van Riper's goal for this phase of treatment is to get the child to identify the components of his stuttering problem; however, he does not attempt to do this with the specificity he does with the advanced stutterer. Van Riper also believes it is extremely important, even more than with the advanced stutterer, to establish a warm, close relationship with the intermediate stutterer. This is crucial to the success of therapy. Furthermore, Van Riper believes that it is essential that the clinician shows, through her behavior, that stuttering does not bother her.

Van Riper begins the identification process by helping the child identify his avoidance, postponement, and starter behaviors. Van Riper believes most intermediate stutterers are aware of these "tricks" and use them voluntarily rather than automatically or habitually. To help the child identify these behaviors, Van Riper plays "catch me" games in which he and the child take turns catching one another using these behaviors.

In contrast to his approach to the advanced stutterer, Van Riper does not attempt to get the intermediate stutterer to confront and identify the struggle associated with his core and escape behaviors. Van Riper believes that many children find this too painful. What Van Riper does, instead, is to have the child learn to differentiate between "hard" and "easy" stutters. Again, he uses "catch me" games for this purpose.

With regard to situation fears, Van Riper helps the child identify and talk about these speaking fears. He believes this helps the child to become more comfortable with these situations. However, Van Riper believes it is unwise to have the child identify sound and word fears because they are still unstable in the intermediate stutterer, and he does not want the child to become more sound or word conscious than he already is.

Desensitization Phase

During this phase of treatment, Van Riper does a number of things to reduce the child's fears and other negative emotions associated with his stuttering. Though this goal is similar to that for the advanced stutterer, Van Riper's procedures for the intermediate stutterer are quite different. For example, since one way to reduce the child's negative feelings about his stuttering is to reduce the amount of the child's stuttering, Van Riper attempts to increase the child's fluency in the therapy situation. To do this, Van Riper employs procedures that he uses with the beginning stutterer, that is, he attempts to create a basal level of fluency by providing simple fluency models, by engaging in rhythm or timing activities, and by reinforcing fluency. It may be helpful to reread those sections of Chapter 9 to refresh one's memory on these procedures.

Van Riper also desensitizes the intermediate stutterer to various fluency disrupters. He does this by first establishing a basal level of fluency and then, gradually, introducing the child's fluency disrupters into the situation. Again, the reader is referred to Chapter 9 for a discussion of Van Riper's procedures for desensitizing the beginning stutterer to fluency disrupters. The only difference in the case of the intermediate stutterer is the fact that Van Riper informs the child of the purpose of the activity and encourages the child to resist the fluency disrupter.

Van Riper believes that it is important for the intermediate stutterer to stop avoiding feared speaking situations and feared words, if he happens to be aware of these feared words. Van Riper tells the child that, the more he runs away from his stuttering, the more he will be afraid of it. To help the child understand this principle, Van Riper tells stories to the child about people who run away from their fears and, consequently, become more fearful. Conversely, he shares stories about people who confront their fears and overcome them.

If the young stutterer is being teased about his stuttering, Van Riper believes it is important that the teasing be stopped. To do this, he talks to the teaser privately about it. He tells the teaser that this will cause the child's stuttering to get worse, and therefore, he must stop teasing. He then follows up to make sure that this happens. Van Riper also believes it is important to give the young stutterer some defenses against teasing. He suggests the best defense is acceptance rather than fighting or running away. If the child can say, "I know I stutter, so what?," most teasers will lose interest in teasing.

Van Riper believes it is helpful to provide some basic information about stuttering at an appropriate level to the intermediate stutterer. This reduces some of the confusion and unpleasantness associated with the problem. For example, he tells the child that, just as there are some children who find it difficult to swim or draw pictures well, other children find it difficult to talk smoothly. He tells the child that he is not the only one with this problem; rather, there are over 2 million people with this problem in our country. Van Riper then explains to the child that his problem is one of learning how to say words easy and that he will learn how to do this in speech class. Along these same lines, he attempts to remove any stigma from the word "stuttering." He points out to the child that everybody stutters at times, especially when they are confused, hurried, or upset. Van Riper then explains that there are two kinds of stuttering, easy stuttering and hard stuttering, and that easy stuttering usually goes away by itself.

Finally, Van Riper attempts to reduce the unpleasantness of stuttering by modeling easy, relaxed, unhurried stuttering in his own speech. He shows the child that he can stutter and still remain calm. He shows the child that he can stumble on his words and still not struggle on them. He suggests that many children learn from this modeling that they, too, can remain calm and not struggle when they stutter on a word. With other children, however, Van Riper suggests that it may be necessary to have the child voluntarily put these unforced and unhurried stutters into his own speech. To do this, he engages the child in games during which they both put these easy stutters into their speech. Van Riper believes, that by experiencing these easy, relaxed, unhurried stutters while engaged in a pleasurable activity with a supportive clinician, the child loses much of his unpleasant feelings associated with the act of stuttering.

Modification Phase

The goal of the modification phase is to teach the child to stutter in an "easy" manner. By this, Van Riper means the child is to say the stuttered word by prolonging the whole word rather than by prolonging any one sound in the word. There should also be slow, smooth transitions from sound to sound.

Van Riper begins by attempting to get the child to substitute this new, easy stuttering pattern for his old, hard stuttering. He suggests that these young stutterers, unlike advanced stutterers, are often able to substitute this easy stuttering for hard stuttering with surprising ease. To help the child do this, he fills his own speech with a lot of easy stutters. In other words, he is providing the child with this easy model over and over again. Van Riper also stutters along with the child in this new way when the child is experiencing one of his old, hard stutters. Van Riper reports that, by repeatedly providing these easy models for the child, the child often begins to use them in his own speech. When this happens, Van Riper strongly reinforces these new behaviors. To further strengthen the use of these new, easy stutters, Van Riper attempts to get the child to cancel or erase his old, hard stutters by pausing and saying the word over again, using an easy stutter. He admits, however, that he is often unable to get the intermediate stutterer to use these cancellations. Despite this, Van Riper indicates that it is not difficult to get the intermediate stutterer to use his new, easy stutters in place of his old, hard ones.

Even though Van Riper believes that it is often easier for intermediate stutterers to replace their hard stutters with easy ones, he sometimes finds it beneficial for these children to learn how to modify their hard stutters by using pull-outs. To show the child how to do this, Van Riper begins by simulating the child's hard stuttering and then modeling how to ease out of the block with a slow, smooth movement. After ample modeling of these releases or pull-outs for the child, he then joins the child, stuttering in unison with him, while the child is still caught in a hard stutter. While the child is still struggling, Van Riper shifts into a slow, smooth release to complete the word. Van Riper reports that, by modeling pull-outs for the child in these ways, he soon teaches the child to use them in his own speech.

Van Riper does not teach intermediate stutterers to use preparatory sets. He reports that these children react negatively to having to constantly scan ahead for difficult sounds and words. Besides, he believes that, by teaching them to do so, it only increases their sound and word fears. Instead, Van Riper relies on the natural tendency for the easy stutters and pull-outs to move forward in the word to become automatic preparatory sets. He reports this occurs without any formal therapy.

Stabilization Phase

The goal of this last phase of treatment is to stabilize the child's use of his new, easy way of stuttering. In contrast to the advanced stutterer, Van Riper reports that the intermediate stutterer does not require much stabilization of his new form of stuttering. Van Riper suggests that, once the child begins to use easy stuttering, the disorder dissipates.

During this stabilization phase, Van Riper gradually fades the child out of therapy. One of the few things he does in therapy during this period is to have the child talk with him, deliberately using numerous easy stutters. Van Riper also makes himself available to the child whenever the child wants to talk to him about any problems he may be having with his speech. Finally, Van Riper will schedule some extra booster sessions, if it becomes necessary. Van Riper concludes his discussion of the direct treatment of the intermediate stutterer by stating that he believes the prognosis for this child is excellent.

CLINICAL PROCEDURES: PARENT COUNSELING

Van Riper believes it is important to provide the intermediate stutterer with a home environment that is conducive to fluency. In our discussion of Van Riper's parent counseling for the beginning stutterer in Chapter 9, we described what he does to create such an environment. We indicated that, among other things, Van Riper provides the parents with some basic information about stuttering, advises the parents not to call negative attention to their child's speech, helps them identify and decrease situations that disrupt their child's fluency, and helps them identify and increase situations that increase the child's fluency. Van Riper believes these goals are equally important for the intermediate stutterer; however, there is no need to repeat the discussion of these procedures here. The reader is referred to Chapter 9 for this discussion.

Van Riper does suggest, though, that there are two major differences between counseling the parents of the beginning stutterer and counseling the parents of the intermediate stutterer. First, the parents of the intermediate stutterer should have open, frank discussions with their child about his stuttering and his therapy. The child knows he stutters. He is going to therapy for his stuttering. Van Riper suggests that it would be very unwise for the parents not to talk about the problem with their child at this time. Van Riper reports that, once he models for the parents how to discuss their child's stuttering with him and they are able to do this, both the child and his parents are much relieved.

Second, Van Riper enlists the parents as co-therapists. He wants them to be observers and reinforcers. He carefully explains and models for them the responses he is attempting to teach the child. Van Riper needs them to report changes in their child's speech behaviors at home. He also wants them to positively reinforce at home the behaviors, such as easy stutters, that he is teaching the child to use in therapy.

CLINICAL PROCEDURES: CLASSROOM TEACHER COUNSELING

Van Riper believes the classroom teacher plays a very important role in the treatment of the intermediate stutterer. After all, she is the one who determines the qualities of the classroom environment for the child. Van Riper believes the teacher's attitudes toward the stuttering child and her policies on classroom recitation are crucial in the child's recovery.

First of all, Van Riper recommends that the classroom teacher talk privately with the child about his stuttering. Van Riper suggests that the teacher let the child know that she is aware of his stuttering and wants to help him. He suggests that she let the child know that she will not hurry, interrupt, or say the word for him when he stutters; rather, she will listen patiently while he is speaking. Van Riper believes that this type of listening on the teacher's part will also provide an excellent model for the other children in the classroom to employ when they are interacting with the stutterer.

Secondly, Van Riper believes that the classroom teacher's oral participation policies are very important. Van Riper notes that calling on children in alphabetical order, demanding long oral reports, or excusing the child from all oral recitation can be detrimental to the child's recovery. Besides discouraging these practices, Van Riper also advises the classroom teacher to talk with the child about his oral participation. Van Riper suggests to the teacher that she ask the child for his input on how he would like to orally participate in the class. If the child does not have any thoughts on this matter, the teacher can offer him alternatives. For example, she can ask him if he would rather be called on early or late in the class period. She can ask him if he would prefer to play a part or sing in the chorus in a Christmas play. In deciding these matters, Van Riper believes the teacher should be guided by the principle that it is important for the child to orally participate in the class, but at the same time, it is important for the child to feel comfortable in this participation.

Other Clinicians

To complete our discussion of stuttering modification therapy for the intermediate stutterer, let us now consider what some other stuttering modification clinicians do to treat these children.

OLIVER BLOODSTEIN

Oliver Bloodstein (1975) discusses his treatment for the intermediate or "phase 3" stutterer in his chapter in Eisenson's *Stuttering: A Second Symposium*. It is a combination of his treatments for the beginning and the advanced stutterer. From his treatment for the beginning stutterer, Bloodstein borrows the following two components: (*a*) general speech improvement and (*b*) personal development. The goal of both of these components is to combat the child's concept of himself as a defective speaker. This is in line with his anticipatory struggle view of stuttering. From his treatment for the advanced stutterer, he takes the symptom modification component. Bloodstein suggests that this last component, symptom modification, receive the most emphasis in the treatment for the intermediate stutterer. The reader is referred to Chapters 7 and 9 for a review of Bloodstein's treatment procedures for the beginning and the advanced stutterer.

As may be recalled, the goal of the general speech improvement component is to improve the child's self-confidence as a communicator, and the goal of the personal development component is to increase the child's sense of personal worth. Bloodstein believes that both of these components will help the child overcome his belief that he is a defective speaker and that he must struggle to speak adequately.

The goal of the symptom modification component is to teach the child to modify his moments of stuttering. Bloodstein helps the child reduce the tension and fragmentation in his speech. Rather than struggle on a word, Bloodstein teaches the child to move forward through a stuttered word in a deliberate and unhurried manner.

CARL DELL

In his booklet, *Treating the School Age Stutterer: A Guide for Clinicians*, Carl Dell (1979) discusses his treatment procedures for the intermediate or "confirmed" stutterer. His direct treatment of the child is organized into a number of phases. They include: (*a*) saying the words in three ways, (*b*) locating tension, (*c*) cancelling, (*d*) changing stuttering to a milder form, (*e*) inserting easy stuttering into real speech, (*f*) changing hard stutterings during real speech, (*g*) building fluency, and (*h*) building independence. Dell also recommends counseling the child's parents and his classroom teacher.

Dell begins by explaining to the child that there are three ways of saying words: the regular or fluent way, the hard stuttering way, and the easy stuttering way. The hard way is characterized by a typical moment of stuttering, and the easy way is characterized by an easy, effortless prolongation or repetition. Dell's first step is to have the child identify these three ways of saying words in the clinician's speech. The next step involves the child producing words in these three different manners. At first, it may be necessary to have the child imitate the clinician, but soon the child is able to produce these three different ways on his own. Putting these pseudostutterings into his own speech is also a very good desensitization activity for the child.

The next phase involves helping the child locate the tension within his speech mechanism when he stutters. Dell wants the child to know what is happening when he is caught in a stutter This identification of tension is first done in pseudostutterings and then in real stutterings.

Dell now teaches the child to cancel his hard stutters. When the child has a hard stutter on a word, he is to say the word over. This time, however, he is to say it using an easy stutter. These cancellations are used only during therapy activities.

In the next phase, Dell teaches the child to turn a hard stutter into an easy stutter. In other words, Dell teaches the child to use Van Riper's pull-outs. These are practiced during therapy activities, using pseudostuttering.

Dell now begins to have the child insert a lot of voluntary, easy stutterings into his speech. Dell engages the child in activities in which they both use a great many of these easy stutters. Besides providing a good model of the final target behavior, easy stuttering, this is an excellent desensitization activity for the child.

Now, Dell is ready to teach the child to change real, hard stutters into easy stutters during running speech. Dell reports that this is often a difficult task for the child to learn, but once he learns to do it, he is well on the way to recovery. One technique that Dell finds helpful is to touch the child when the child gets caught in a real stutter. The child is to hold on to the block until Dell lets go, and at that point, the child is to come out of the block, using an easy stutter.

In the building fluency phase, Dell desensitizes the young stutterer to fluency disrupters in the same way that Van Riper does. The reader is referred to the earlier discussion of these procedures.

Finally, in the building independence phase, Dell gradually fades the child out of therapy. Dell does not believe the child needs to be totally "cured" before he is dropped from therapy. Rather, when the child is doing well, Dell temporarily discontinues him for a period of time to let him continue on his own. If the child regresses a bit, Dell brings him in for a booster session. There will often be a number of these cycles before the child is finally dismissed.

Dell's parent counseling involves providing the parents with information about stuttering, attempting to alleviate any guilt they may have over the child's stuttering, and encouraging them to remind the child to use his easy stuttering at times when he is having a lot of hard stuttering.

Dell's counseling of the classroom teacher involves providing the teacher with information about stuttering, helping her respond more objectively to the child's stuttering in the classroom, and helping her deal more effectively with the difficult issue of the child's oral participation in the class.

HAROLD LUPER AND ROBERT MULDER

Harold Luper and Robert Mulder (1964) refer to the intermediate stutterer as the "confirmed stutterer" in their book, *Stuttering: Therapy for Children*. Their therapy for this child involves direct treatment of the child as well as parent counseling. The direct treatment of the child is broken down into a number of phases.

The first phase has several objectives. During this phase, Luper and Mulder develop a healthy clinical relationship with the child. They help the child understand that he will need to take an active role in changing his speech behaviors and attitudes. They point out to the child that a cure is not the usual outcome of therapy; rather, a gradual reduction in stuttering and fear of talking is much more typical. To help reduce the child's sensitivity to his stuttering, Luper and Mulder explain to the child that he is a normal individual except for his speech problem.

During the second phase of therapy, Luper and Mulder help the child eliminate his unsatisfactory ways of approaching difficult words and situations. First of all, they want the child to eliminate his use of avoidances. To do this, they try to instill in the child a willingness to use his difficult words and to talk in difficult situations. They attempt to convince the child to be "brave" in facing these difficult tasks. In doing this, Luper and Mulder make an analogy between overcoming fear of talking and overcoming some other fear the child has previously overcome, such as fear of going off a diving board. During this phase of treatment, Luper and Mulder also suggest to the child better ways of approaching his difficult words. They show the child how to say these words using reduced tension or "loose contacts," rather than approach these words with excessive tension.

In the next phase of therapy, Luper and Mulder help the child modify his struggles during the actual moments of stuttering. To do this, they use Van Riper's techniques of cancellations and pull-outs. Luper and Mulder also provide some suggestions for modifying specific phonemes.

During the fourth phase of therapy, Luper and Mulder help the child reduce any residual word and situation fears. They begin by discussing with the child why he is afraid of these words or situations. They suggest that gaining some understanding of his fears may help the child to alleviate them. Luper and Mulder also decondition these residual fears by using hierarchies of gradually increasing difficulty. In other words, the child needs to experience his old feared words and situations over and over again under different circumstances until he is no longer afraid of them. Luper and Mulder are careful to ensure that, as the child proceeds through these hierarchies, he has positive speaking experiences.

In the last phase of treatment, Luper and Mulder help the child develop new speech attitudes. They help the child feel free to have a certain amount of "bobbles" in his speech. They also provide the child with a lot of enjoyable speaking experiences.

The thrust of Luper and Mulder's parent counseling is to help the parents reduce stress upon their child and to help them be good listeners to him.

JOSEPH SHEEHAN

In Chapter 7, we discussed Joseph Sheehan's therapy for the advanced stutterer. As will be recalled, we stated that Sheehan views stuttering as an approach-avoidance conflict. The stutterer stutters whenever his tendency to go ahead and talk is equal to his tendency to hold back and avoid talking. Based upon this theory, Sheehan's therapy for the advanced stutterer has twin goals; namely, increasing the stutterer's approach tendencies and decreasing his avoidance tendencies. The emphasis, however, is on reducing the avoidance tendencies. The reader may wish to reread the description of Sheehan's clinical procedures for the advanced stutterer in Chapter 7 at this time. Sheehan recommends going through procedures similar to these with the intermediate stutterer or the "older child stutterer."

More specifically, Sheehan (1975) does the following things with this child. He explains to the child that everybody stumbles on some words, but that the child has gotten into the habit of struggling or stuttering on words to avoid stumbling on them. Sheehan tells the child that, if he accepts the idea that he is going to stumble on some words, then he will not struggle so hard against doing it. Sheehan then explains to the child that, if he is going to stumble on some words anyway, he may as well learn to say these words smoothly and easily. In other words, Sheehan shows the child that he has a choice in how he stutters. Finally, Sheehan explains to the child that it is unwise to substitute words or avoid certain speaking situations. Sheehan tells the child that it is much better in the long run to go ahead and say what he wants to say.

Sheehan also believes that it is important to counsel the parents of all children who stutter. Sheehan believes that children who stutter have too many demands placed upon them by their parents. At the same time, they receive insufficient support. These demands often revolve around such issues as academic performance, music lessons, tidiness, etc. As part of his therapy for the child who stutters, Sheehan counsels the child's parents to be less demanding and more supportive of their child. Sheehan's capacities and demands perspective was discussed in Chapter 3.

Summary of Stuttering Modification Therapy

All of the stuttering modification clinicians we discussed in this section believe that it is important to teach the intermediate stutterer to modify his moments of stuttering. Further, to some degree, they all believe it is important to target the child's feelings about his stuttering and attempt to eliminate his use of avoidance behaviors. Thus, with regard to these clinical issues, these clinicians' goals for the intermediate stutterer are quite similar to their goals for the advanced stutterer. However, their clinical procedures for these two treatment levels are obviously somewhat different. Finally, all of these clinicians believe it is important to counsel the parents of the intermediate stutterer.

FLUENCY SHAPING THERAPY

To illustrate a fluency shaping approach for the intermediate stutterer, we will describe Bruce Ryan's therapy in detail. We will also comment briefly upon the therapies of a number of other fluency shaping clinicians.

Bruce Ryan: Delayed Auditory Feedback (DAF) Program

CLINICIAN'S BELIEFS

Nature of Stuttering

As we discussed earlier in Chapter 9, Ryan views stuttering as learned behavior.[2] He sees stuttering as having three components, namely, a speech act, an attitude, and anxiety. The speech act consists of words that contain repetitions, prolongations, or struggle behaviors. Ryan believes these are operant behaviors. The attitude component consists of verbal statements the child makes about himself, and Ryan also believes these are operant behaviors. Finally, the anxiety com-

---

[2] References for Ryan's positions on these clinical issues are Ryan, B. P. (1974). *Programmed therapy of stuttering in children and adults*. Springfield, IL: Charles C Thomas, and Ryan, B. P. (1984). Treatment of stuttering in school children. In W. H. Perkins (Ed.), *Stuttering disorders* (pp. 95–105). New York: Thieme-Stratton.

ponent consists of various physiological responses the child may have related to his stuttering, and Ryan believes these are respondent behaviors. Since the speech behaviors are operant behaviors, Ryan believes they can be modified by using operant conditioning and programmed instruction procedures. Thus, the focus of his therapy is on increasing fluent speech behaviors and decreasing stuttering behaviors. Further, he believes that, by changing speech behaviors, concurrent changes are also made in the child's attitude and anxiety components of his problem.

Speech Behaviors Targeted for Therapy

As will be recalled, Ryan organizes his treatment into three phases: establishment, transfer, and maintenance. One of his several establishment programs is his delayed auditory feedback (DAF) program. Ryan uses this program with the child who exhibits "severe stuttering." The goal of this DAF program is to establish 5 minutes of fluent conversational speech with the clinician in the therapy room. With the DAF machine set on its maximum delay, the child is taught to speak in a slow, prolonged, fluent pattern. This fluent pattern is reinforced and moments of stuttering are punished. The DAF is then systematically faded out, and the child's fluent speech pattern is gradually increased in rate. These procedures will be described in more detail when we discuss Ryan's clinical procedures in the next section of this chapter. After the child has attained 5 minutes of fluent conversational speech with the clinician in the therapy room, Ryan systematically transfers this fluency to the child's natural environment.

Fluency Goals

Ryan's fluency goals for the intermediate stutterer appear to be either spontaneous fluency or controlled fluency. To pass Ryan's criterion test and ultimately be dismissed from the program, the child must exhibit 0.5 stuttered words per minute (SW/M) or less. Ryan regards this as "normal-sounding speech."

Feelings and Attitudes

How much attention does Ryan give to changing the child's feelings and attitudes about his speech? Quite simply, he believes that, if he improves the child's fluency, then the negative feelings and attitudes the child may have will also improve.

Maintenance Procedures

As we previously mentioned, one of Ryan's three phases of treatment is the maintenance phase. The goal of this phase is for the child to maintain his fluency over a 22 month period. During this period, the child's speech is sampled, and the child, his parents, and his teacher are interviewed regarding the child's fluency in the natural environment. If the child regresses, he is recycled through parts of the establishment or transfer phases of the treatment program.

Clinical Methods

As will be recalled from our discussion of Ryan's treatment for the beginning stutterer in Chapter 9, his therapy is based very heavily upon operant conditioning and programmed instruction principles. In other words, it is very structured and a great deal of emphasis is placed upon data collection. This is equally true for his DAF program for the intermediate stutterer.

CLINICAL PROCEDURES: DIRECT TREATMENT OF THE CHILD

In his 1984 chapter, "Treatment of Stuttering in School Children," Ryan discusses his treatment procedures for the intermediate stutterer, whom he refers to as the child who exhibits "severe stuttering." This is our primary reference for this section. The reader may also wish to refer to Ryan's 1974 book, *Programmed Therapy of Stuttering in Children and Adults*, for additional information. We will begin by discussing Ryan's direct treatment of the child, which involves the establishment, transfer, and maintenance phases. We will then describe his procedures for counseling the child's parents and his classroom teacher.

Establishment

Ryan uses his delayed auditory feedback (DAF) establishment program with the intermediate stutterer (Fig. 11.1). This is also the establishment program he typically uses with the advanced stutterer. The goal of this program is to have the child speaking fluently with the clinician for 5 minutes in the clinical setting. However, before beginning the program, Ryan does a number of things. He gives the child an overview of the program. He defines stuttering for the child—any word that contains a repetition, prolongation, or other struggle behavior. He explains to the child that he will be reinforced for fluent speech and punished for stuttering. The reinforcement involves social reinforcement and, possibly, token reinforcement; the punishment is social punishment. Ryan also gives the child a criterion test, which consists of 5 minutes of reading, monologue, and conversation.

The DAF establishment program is a 26-step program that begins by

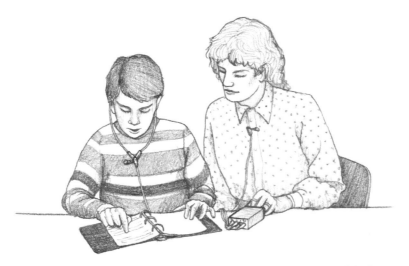

Figure 11.1. Use of delayed auditory feedback (DAF) to establish fluency.

teaching the child to use a "slow, prolonged, fluent pattern of speech." This pattern training part of the program starts with Ryan's reading sentences with the child and ends with the child's reading in a slow, prolonged, fluent pattern for 5 consecutive minutes. See Table 11.1 for an outline of Ryan's DAF program.

The DAF machine is now introduced at 250 msec delay, and the child is told to use his slow, prolonged, fluent speech pattern while he is orally reading. When he does, this speech pattern is socially reinforced. If the child stutters or speeds up, he is reminded to use his slow, prolonged, fluent speech. The child needs to have 5 consecutive minutes of fluent, oral reading at this delay. That is, he needs to meet a criterion of 0 stuttered words per minute (0 SW/M) for 5 consecutive minutes. When he does, the DAF is reduced by 50 msec; and the child is now to obtain another 5 consecutive minutes of fluent, oral reading at this new delay. In this manner, the DAF is systematically faded out in 50 msec steps until the child is reading without the aid of the machine. In this fading out process, the child is required to have 5 consecutive minutes of fluent, oral reading at each of the 6 delay times (250, 200, 150, 100, 50, and 0 msec) and also 5 consecutive minutes of fluent, oral reading off the DAF machine. As the delay time is reduced, the child's speaking rate is gradually increased. Eventually, the child is reading fluently without the aid of the DAF machine at a slightly below normal, oral reading rate.

After the child completes the reading component of the DAF establishment program, he goes on to the monologue and conversation parts of the program. These components replicate the steps involved in the reading component, except that the child now engages in either monologue or conversation. Everything else, that is, the reinforcement, punishment, criterion, etc., remain the same. Ryan reports that most children complete the establishment program speaking fluently at a slightly less than normal speaking rate.

Table 11.1   Outline of Delayed Auditory Feedback (DAF) Establishment Program

Antecedent Events	Response	Consequent Event	Criterion
Pattern Training in Reading			
Instructions to read in a slow, prolonged pattern.	Slow, prolonged, fluent reading.	"Good."	0 SW/M.
Reading:			
Instructions to read. DAF: 250 msec.	Slow, prolonged, fluent reading.	"Good."	0 SW/M.
	Stuttering	"Stop, use your slow, prolonged, fluent pattern."	
Instructions to read. DAF: 200 msec.	"	"	"
Instructions to read. DAF: 150 msec.	"	"	"
Instructions to read. DAF: 100 msec.	"	"	"
Instructions to read. DAF: 50 msec.	"	"	"
Instructions to read. DAF: 0 msec.	"	"	"
Instructions to read.	Fluent reading.	"	"
Monologue: Repeat the above sequence.			
Conversation: Repeat the above sequence.			

After completing the DAF establishment program, Ryan gives the child the criterion test. As will be recalled, this consists of 5 minutes of reading, monologue, and conversation. If the child has 0.5 SW/M or less, he goes on to the transfer phase; otherwise, he is recycled through portions of the establishment program.

Transfer

As will be recalled, the goal of Ryan's transfer phase is to transfer the child's fluency from the therapy room to a wide variety of other settings and other people. To do this, Ryan uses a number of hierarchies or sequences of speaking situations, arranged from easy to difficult, in which the child practices his fluent reading and fluent conversation. During these activities, Ryan instructs the child to speak fluently. He continues to socially reinforce the child's fluency and to remind the child to speak fluently if he stutters. The child must continue to meet the criterion of 0 SW/M for certain periods of time to pass each step.

The transfer program that Ryan uses with the intermediate stutterer is very similar to the transfer program he uses with the beginning stutterer. The only difference between these two programs is that Ryan typically uses a few more hierarchies with the older, intermediate stutterer than he uses with the younger, beginning stutterer. With the beginning stutterer, Ryan uses the physical setting, audience size, home, school, and all day hierarchies; and the reader is referred to Chapter 9 for a description of these hierarchies. We will not repeat that material here. In addition to these hierarchies, Ryan uses the telephone and strangers hierarchies with the intermediate stutterer. We will shortly describe these hierarchies. See Table 11.2 for an outline of Ryan's entire transfer program for the intermediate stutterer.

The "telephone" hierarchy is an 11-step program. It begins with the child saying, "Hello" and "Goodbye" to a dead telephone, and it ends with the child engaging in 3 consecutive minutes of fluent conversation on the telephone with a friend or stranger.

The "stranger" hierarchy begins with the child conversing with people around the school, such as the school secretary or principal, and ends with the child talking with complete strangers in local businesses. At each of the 4 steps the child needs to maintain 3 consecutive minutes of fluent conversation.

Ryan reports that, by the end of this transfer phase, the child is usually speaking fluently in all speaking situations. He has also increased his speaking rate to a normal rate. Ryan again gives the child the criterion test. If the child passes (0.5 SW/M or less), he goes on to the maintenance phase. If the child does not pass, he is recycled through portions of the transfer phase.

Maintenance

As we indicated in Chapter 9, the goal of Ryan's maintenance phase is for the child to maintain his fluency in all situations over a 22-month period following the completion of the transfer phase. This involves gradually fading the child out of therapy. At the end of this phase, the child is dismissed from treatment. Since Ryan's maintenance procedures for the intermediate stutterer are identical to his

Table 11.2   Outline of Transfer Program

Antecedent Event	Response	Consequent Event	Criterion
Physical Setting:			
5 steps with clinician in different physical settings.	One minute of fluent reading.	"Good"	0 SW/M
	3 minutes of fluent conversation.	"Good"	
	Stuttering.	"Stop, speak fluently."	
Audience Size:			
3 steps with 3 classmates in therapy room.	"	"	"
Home:			
5 steps with parent in therapy room and at home.	"	"	"
School:			
4 steps with clinician in school.	"	"	"
Telephone:			
11 steps on the telephone.	3 minutes of fluent conversation.	"	"
Strangers:			
4 steps with strangers.	"	"	"
All Day:			
Up to 16 steps (optional).	Up to 16 hours of fluency.	"	"

procedures for the beginning stutterer, the reader is referred to Chapter 9 for a description of these procedures.

CLINICAL PROCEDURES: PARENT COUNSELING

Ryan's parent counseling for the intermediate stutterer is very similar to his parent counseling for the beginning stutterer. Before Ryan begins the DAF program with the child, he explains this DAF program and the overall treatment plan to the parents. He wants them to understand what their child will be doing in therapy and what they can expect in terms of improvement in their child's speech. Ryan also wants to enlist the parents' cooperation with the "home practice" program and the "home" and "all day" hierarchies of the transfer phase. These three latter procedures were described when we discussed Ryan's parent counseling procedures for the beginning stutterer in Chapter 9. Since they are identical for the intermediate stutterer, the reader is referred to the previous discussion.

CLINICAL PROCEDURES: CLASSROOM TEACHER COUNSELING

Before the child's treatment begins, Ryan explains the overall treatment plan to the classroom teacher. He also enlists her aid in the "school" hierarchy of the transfer phase. Finally, Ryan explains to the teacher that she may observe improvement in the child's speech at any time during the treatment program.

Other Clinicians

We will conclude our discussion of fluency shaping therapy for the intermediate stutterer with a brief description of the clinical procedures of some other fluency shaping clinicians.

JANIS COSTELLO

In the preceding chapter on the beginning stutterer, we described Janis Costello's Extended Length of Utterance (ELU) program. We indicated that this program is similar to Ryan's Gradual Increase in Length and Complexity of Utterance (GILCU) program. Costello (1983) regards this as her "basic" program for all children who stutter. She does, however, suggest that if this basic program produces "less-than-satisfactory" results with a child, she will consider using "additives" with the basic program. The additives she considers using are rate control, gentle onset, linguistic simplification, and attitude modification.

Rate control is the first additive she considers using with her ELU program. This is especially true if her assessment data indicate the child speaks too rapidly. Costello believes it is not necessary to use delayed auditory feedback to control the child's speaking rate. She prefers to simply instruct the child to talk slower during the ELU program. She then only reinforces the child's responses that are both fluent and within a given speaking rate limit. Costello may also, at times, model the desired rate for the child. As the child progresses through the ELU program, his speaking rate is allowed to gradually increase, as long as fluency is maintained, until a normal speaking rate is attained.

The next additive that Costello considers using with her ELU program is gentle onset of phonation. She believes this is most appropriate for a child who exhibits hard blocks. Costello instructs the child to use these gentle onsets during the ELU program. As the child moves through the program, the use of gentle onsets is faded out.

Costello's third additive is linguistic simplification. Costello states that she considers employing this strategy, along with her ELU program, only when the child has documented deficiencies in such areas as word retrieval or the use of syntactic rules.

The last additive that Costello discusses is attitude modification. By and large, Costello believes that most children who stutter do not have attitudinal problems because of their stuttering. Her recommendation is that, unless there is reason to suspect that a child has a serious attitude problem, it is best to just use her basic ELU program.

WILLIAM PERKINS

In Chapter 7, we described William Perkins' "replacement of stuttering with normal speech" program for the advanced stutterer. In this program, Perkins teaches the advanced stutterer to use a number of fluency skills to facilitate the coordination of his speech mechanism, and thereby, enhance his fluency. As will be recalled, these fluency skills include the following: rate, phrasing, phrase initiation, soft contact, breathy voice, blending, and rhythm. The reader is referred to

Chapter 7 for a description of these skills and a review of Perkins' clinical procedures for the advanced stutterer.

With the intermediate stutterer or the stutterer "of school age whose stuttering has become an established problem," Perkins (1979) uses a modification of his program for the advanced stutterer. His goal is to teach the young stutterer to use the above fluency skills. Perkins not only teaches these skills in the clinical setting, but he also teaches these skills within the context of the family. Besides teaching the child to use these fluency skills, Perkins also teaches the child's parents, and occasionally siblings, to use them. The parents then model these skills for the child and also monitor the child's use of them. The child also monitors his parents, in addition to being monitored by them. Thus, the child is a member of a group in which everyone is participating equally in the use of fluency skills.

GEORGE SHAMES AND CHERI FLORANCE

We described George Shames and Cheri Florance's (1980) "stutter-free speech" programs for the adult stutterer and the child stutterer in Chapters 7 and 9, respectively. These are Shames and Florance's two treatment programs. The reader may wish to review the previous descriptions of these two programs. We need only briefly review these programs here before we discuss what Shames and Florance suggest for the intermediate stutterer.

As will be recalled, the adult program is divided into five phases: (*a*) volitional control, (*b*) self reinforcement, (*c*) transfer, (*d*) training in unmonitored speech, and (*e*) follow-up. The child program, which is for children approximately 3 to 8 years of age, is quite similar to the adult program, except for the omission from the child program of phase 4, training in unmonitored speech. Shames and Florance indicate that phase 4 is not necessary with young children because they begin to use unmonitored stutter-free speech or spontaneous fluency by themselves. Another difference in the two programs is the major involvement of the parents in the transfer phase of the child program.

Since the adult program is for adults and the child program is for children approximately 3 to 8 years of age, what do Shames and Florance do with the intermediate stutterer who is usually between 6 and 13 years of age? Shames and Florance suggest the adolescent intermediate stutterer, who is demonstrating a need to be independent from his parents, will probably do better in the adult program, while the younger intermediate stutterer will probably do better in the child program. Shames and Florance do admit, however, that at times it is difficult to determine when a child is too old for the child program. They suggest that, as the child moves through the volitional control and self reinforcement phases of the program, the clinician will get to know the child well enough to determine which path to take in the remaining phases of the program.

RONALD WEBSTER

We discussed Ronald Webster's "precision fluency shaping program" in Chapter 7 when we discussed the treatment of the advanced stutterer. As will be recalled, the goal of this program is to teach the advanced stutterer to use certain fluency-generating target behaviors. When the stutterer uses these target behaviors, he will be fluent. The two most important target behaviors are slightly increased syllable duration and gentle voice onset. For a review of these target behaviors and Webster's entire program, the reader is referred to our previous discussion in Chapter 7.

With children between 5 and 12 years of age, Webster (1979) modifies his precision fluency shaping program to use simplified instructions and therapy materials appropriate to the child's language abilities. Webster stresses the importance of giving the child a great deal of positive feedback when he is working on his target behaviors. Webster also requires that one of the child's parents attend a number of therapy sessions so that the parent can learn how to provide support for the child as he is acquiring the use of target behaviors. Webster reports that children in this age range develop the use of fluency-generating target behaviors quite readily.

Summary of Fluency Shaping Therapy

All of the fluency shaping clinicians discussed in this section employ procedures to first establish fluency in the clinical setting and then generalize this fluency to the intermediate stutterer's everyday speaking environment. In all cases, their clinical procedures are procedures or modification of procedures that they use with either the beginning or the advanced stutterer.

COMPARISON OF THE TWO APPROACHES

At the beginning of this chapter, we suggested that stuttering modification and fluency shaping therapies for the intermediate stutterer are more similar than they are for the advanced stutterer but less similar than they are for the beginning stutterer. Let us now compare these two therapy approaches for the intermediate stutterer on the following clinical issues: (a) speech behaviors targeted for therapy, (b) fluency goals, (c) attention given to feelings and attitudes, (d) maintenance procedures, and (e) clinical methods. See Table 11.3 for an overview of the similarities and differences between these two approaches for the intermediate stutterer.

With regard to the first issue, speech behaviors targeted for therapy, all of the stuttering modification clinicians we reviewed in this chapter teach the intermediate stutterer to modify his moments of stuttering. All of the fluency shaping clinicians, on the other hand, target fluent responses or fluency skills. With regard to this issue, these two therapy approaches differ substantially, much as they did for the advanced stutterer.

On the second issue, fluency goals, both stuttering modification and fluency shaping clinicians have spontaneous fluency and controlled fluency as goals for the intermediate stutterer. Stuttering modification clinicians, however, include acceptable stuttering as a reasonable goal; whereas, fluency shaping clinicians do not.

Stuttering modification and fluency shaping clinicians differ with regard

Table 11.3   Similarities and Differences between Stuttering Modification and Fluency Shaping Therapies for the Intermediate Stutterer

Clinical Issue	Therapy Approach	
	Stuttering Modification Therapy	Fluency Shaping Therapy
Speech behaviors targeted for therapy.	Moments of stuttering.	Fluent responses or fluency skills
Fluency goals.	Spontaneous fluency, controlled fluency, or acceptable stuttering.	Spontaneous fluency or controlled fluency.
Feelings and attitudes.	Some attention given to reducing negative feelings and attitudes.	No attention given to reducing negative feelings and attitudes.
Maintenance procedures.	Minimal emphasis given to maintenance procedures.	Minimal emphasis given to maintenance procedures.
Clinical methods.	Therapy often characterized by loosely structured interaction—play activity.	Therapy often characterized by tightly structured interaction or programmed instruction.
	Little emphasis upon collection of objective data.	Considerable emphasis upon collection of objective data.

to the attention they give to reducing the negative feelings and attitudes of the intermediate stutterer. They do not, however, differ as much on this issue as they do in the case of the advanced stutterer. With the advanced stutterer, stuttering modification clinicians pay considerable attention to reducing the stutterer's negative feelings and attitudes. In contrast, with the intermediate stutterer, these clinicians pay somewhat less attention to changing these feelings and attitudes. Fluency shaping clinicians, on the other hand, do not target these feelings and attitudes with either the advanced or the intermediate stutterer.

On the fourth issue, maintenance procedures, stuttering modification and fluency shaping therapies are quite similar. Both give minimal attention to the issue.

As has been the case at the other two treatment levels, stuttering modification and fluency shaping therapies usually differ with regard to clinical methods. Stuttering modification therapy is usually characterized by a loosely structured interaction between the clinician and the child. Fluency shaping therapy, on the other hand, is usually characterized by a programmed instruction approach. Further, stuttering modification therapy usually puts little emphasis upon data collection; fluency shaping therapy puts considerable emphasis upon it.

In summary, stuttering modification and fluency shaping therapies for the intermediate stutterer are more similar than they are for the advanced stutterer but less similar than they are for the beginning stutterer. The greatest difference, excluding clinical methods, is in the speech behaviors targeted for therapy, and to a lesser degree, the approaches differ in the attention they give to reducing negative feelings and attitudes.

STUDY QUESTIONS

1/   What are Van Riper's goals for the intermediate stutterer during each of the following four phases of treatment: (a) identification phase, (b) desensitization phase, (c) modification phase, and (d) stabilization phase?

2/   Briefly, describe at least three clinical procedures Van Riper employs during his desensitization phase with the intermediate stutterer.

3/   How does Van Riper teach the intermediate stutterer to substitute an easy stutter for his hard stutter?

4/   What are Ryan's goals for the intermediate stutterer during each of the following three phases of treatment: (a) establishment phase, (b) transfer phase, and (c) maintenance phase?

5/   Describe Ryan's delayed auditory feedback (DAF) program for the intermediate stutterer.

6/   Briefly describe Ryan's transfer procedures for the intermediate stutterer.

7/   Compare stuttering modification and fluency shaping therapies for the intermediate stutterer on the following five clinical issues: (a) speech behaviors targeted for therapy, (b) fluency goals, (c) attention given to feelings and attitudes, (d) maintenance procedures, and (e) clinical methods.

Suggested Readings

Ryan, B. P. (1984). Treatment of stuttering in school children. In W. H. Perkins (Ed.), *Stuttering disorders* (pp. 95–105). New York: Thieme-Stratton.

   In this relatively brief chapter, Ryan describes his fluency shaping procedures for the school age child.

Van Riper, C. (1973). Treatment of the young confirmed stutterer. In *The treatment of stuttering* (pp. 426–451). Englewood Cliffs: Prentice-Hall.

   In this chapter, Van Riper provides a comprehensive discussion of a classic stuttering modification approach to the treatment of the intermediate stutterer.

12

THE INTERMEDIATE STUTTERER: INTEGRATION OF APPROACHES

In the previous chapter, we indicated that stuttering modification and fluency shaping therapies for the intermediate stutterer are more similar than they are for the advanced stutterer but less similar than they are for the beginning stutterer. We also pointed out that both stuttering modification and fluency shaping clinicians combine or modify their respective therapies for the advanced and/or the beginning stutterer when they work with the intermediate stutterer. In other words, these clinicians usually do not have a unique therapy for the intermediate stutterer; rather, they use a combination or modification of their therapies for the other two treatment levels. As the reader will soon see, this is also true for clinicians who integrate stuttering modification and fluency shaping therapies with this treatment level. Before we begin discussing the integration of these two approaches, however, it may be helpful to briefly review the characteristics of the intermediate stutterer.

As will be recalled, the intermediate stutterer is usually between 6 and 13 years of age. Thus, he is typically in elementary or junior high school. He is exhibiting part-word and monosyllabic word repetitions and vowel prolongations that contain excessive tension. He is also exhibiting blocks. In terms of secondary behaviors, he is exhibiting escape, starting, and avoidance behaviors. The avoidance behaviors may include word substitutions, circumlocutions, and avoidance of certain speaking situations. This child is also experiencing frustration, embarrassment, and the beginning of fear related to his stuttering. Finally, he has a definite concept of himself as a stutterer. Let us now turn to the integration of stuttering modification and fluency shaping therapies for this child.

In the last chapter, we suggested that the greatest difference, excluding clinical methods, between stuttering modification and fluency shaping therapies for the intermediate stutterer is the speech behaviors targeted for therapy. To a lesser degree, we suggested that these two approaches also differ with regard to the attention they give to reducing negative feelings and attitudes. Therefore, in our integration of these two approaches, we will concentrate our efforts on integrating these two aspects of therapy. As it will become apparent, our direct treatment of this child contains elements of both stuttering modification and fluency shaping therapies. Our parent counseling and classroom teacher counseling are influenced more strongly by stuttering modification therapy.

As we have done previously, we will first discuss our own approach to integrating stuttering modification and fluency shaping therapies for the intermediate stutterer. We will then describe the clinical procedures of other clinicians who integrate these two approaches with this treatment level.

OUR APPROACH

Clinician's Beliefs

NATURE OF STUTTERING

As we have previously stated, we believe that predisposing physiological factors interact with developmental and environmental factors to produce and/or exacerbate the core behaviors or repetitions and prolongations. The child responds to these disfluencies with increased tension in an effort to inhibit them. This tension increases the severity of struggle behavior. Further, as the young stutterer attempts to cope with these core behaviors, he develops a variety of escape and starting behaviors. We believe these behaviors are operantly reinforced. Then, in the early elementary school years, frustration and some embarrassment are associated with the stuttering, and fear begins to become associated with it. These negative emotions generalize through classical conditioning to more and more words and speaking situations. Finally, the child begins to avoid these feared words and situations. We believe that these avoidance behaviors are reinforced through avoidance conditioning. With the onset of these avoidance behaviors, the child has become an intermediate stutterer. By this time, the child has also developed a definite concept of himself as a stutterer.

Since the tension response, the escape, starting, and avoidance behaviors, and the negative feelings and attitudes are learned, we believe they can be unlearned or modified. Furthermore, since these learned components are not as well established as they are in the advanced stutterer, they are easier to change. We believe that, if we can provide the intermediate stutterer with a sufficient number of fluent and emotionally positive speaking experiences in therapy, this fluency and the positive feelings associated with speaking will generalize to other environments. We use operant and classical conditioning principles to do this. Further, since predisposing physiological factors may be contributing to the core behaviors or physiological disruptions in the speech of many intermediate stutterers, we believe it is also important to help these children cope more effectively with these disruptions in their speech.

In implementing the above beliefs about the nature of stuttering in the intermediate stutterer, we need to keep in mind that this client is younger than the advanced stutterer. This needs to be taken into consideration in the selection of our clinical procedures.

Finally, we believe it is important to reduce developmental and environmental influences that may be contributing to the child's stuttering. We do this by counseling the child's parents and his classroom teacher.

SPEECH BEHAVIORS TARGETED FOR THERAPY

We believe it is beneficial to combine fluency shaping and stuttering modification strategies for the intermediate stutterer. In terms of fluency shaping procedures, we use either our delayed auditory feedback program, which we use with the advanced stutterer, or our establishing and transferring fluency hierarchy, which we use with the beginning stutterer. These procedures were described in Chapters 8 and 10, respectively. The procedure we use will depend upon the age of the child and the results of some trial therapy.

We have two goals in mind when we use either of the above two procedures. First, we want to establish fluency in the clinical setting. Often, this fluency contains a great deal of spontaneous fluency. Second, we want the child to learn to use the following fluency enhancing skills: slower rate, gentle onsets, and soft contacts. Once this fluency, which is usually a combination of spontaneous and controlled fluency, is established in the clinical situation, it is then transferred to other speaking situations.

Finally, we think that it is important for the intermediate stutterer to learn to modify his moments of stuttering. To do this, we use procedures similar to those we described in Chapter 10 as optional procedures for the beginning stutterer. We believe that both these stuttering modification skills and the fluency enhancing skills mentioned above will help the intermediate stutterer cope more effectively with any physiological mistimings that disrupt his speech.

FLUENCY GOALS

Which fluency goals are realistic for the intermediate stutterer? Some intermediate stutterers may become normal or spontaneously fluent speakers. This is more true for the younger than the older intermediate stutterer. More typically, this child will need to use a controlled fluency to sound normal. This is often a difficult task for a youngster to do on a consistent basis. Although he may use a controlled fluency in a given situation, a child this age often does not have the motivation or the self-discipline to use a controlled fluency throughout his daily talking. Thus, we believe that a realistic fluency goal for many intermediate stutterers is acceptable stuttering, that is, fluency characterized by mild or very mild stuttering.

Feelings and Attitudes

How much attention should be given to the intermediate stutterer's feelings and attitudes about his speech? Since this child is experiencing some frustration and embarrassment and is beginning to experience some fear related to his speech, we believe it is important to reduce these negative feelings. Furthermore, since this child is beginning to avoid certain words and avoid speaking in certain situations, we also believe it is important to eliminate or reduce these avoidances. Even though these negative feelings and avoidance behaviors are not as pronounced or as well established in the intermediate stutterer as they are in the advanced stutterer, we believe that, for effective treatment to occur, these aspects of the problem must be given some attention in therapy.

In selecting clinical procedures to reduce the intermediate stutterer's negative feelings about his speech and to eliminate or reduce his avoidance behaviors, it is important to keep in mind that this client is younger than the advanced stutterer. Thus, the clinical procedures for the advanced stutterer that were discussed in Chapter 8 would not be appropriate for this younger client. Different or modified procedures are needed.

Maintenance Procedures

The typical intermediate stutterer may need some help in maintaining his improvement. He will certainly not need the extensive help required by the advanced stutterer, but he may need more than the minimal help required by the beginning stutterer.

To help the intermediate stutterer maintain his improvement, we believe it is very important to periodically reevaluate his fluency. During these reevaluations, we obtain a sample of his speech and interview him regarding his talking in everyday speaking situations. We also interview the child's parents and his classroom teacher regarding his fluency. If we find there has been a regression, we reenroll the child in therapy for a month or two. Our experience indicates that some of these children may have one or two mild regressions before their fluency finally stabilizes. In time, the regressions and our reevaluations become further apart. The day then comes to dismiss the child from treatment. We have found that these procedures are usually adequate for helping the intermediate stutterer maintain his improved fluency.

Clinical Methods

The clinical methods we employ for the intermediate stutterer, that is, our structure of therapy and our data collection procedures, are influenced by both stuttering modification and fluency shaping therapies. In terms of the structure of therapy, we may employ a loosely structured type of interaction between the clinician and the child. For example, with the younger intermediate stutterer, we may use a game-orientated approach. With the older intermediate stutterer, we may employ a teaching/counseling type of interaction. Both of these types of interactions are loosely structured. On the other hand, we may decide to use a highly structured, programmed instruction approach with both the younger and the older intermediate stutterer. The type of interaction that we decide to use will depend upon the outcome of some trial therapy.

In terms of data collection, we believe it is important to measure the child's stuttering and his rate of speech before, during, and after the treatment program. If we use a game-orientated or teaching/counseling type of approach, we will take a probe or sampling of the child's speech at the end of each therapy session. If we use a programmed instruction approach, we will measure all of the child's responses during each therapy session.

Clinical Procedures: Direct Treatment of the Child

Both of us have been combining or integrating aspects of stuttering modification and fluency shaping therapies for the intermediate stutterer for a number of years.[1] Our direct treatment for this child consists of components of both approaches. Based upon our current beliefs, we believe it is important to include the following in our treatment of the intermediate stutterer: (a) understanding stuttering, (b) using fluency enhancing skills and modifying the moments of stuttering, (c) reducing negative feelings and attitudes and eliminating avoidances, and (d) maintaining improvement. As the reader may recall, these are the same components that were involved in our treatment of the advanced stutterer. In other words, the overall goals for these two treatment levels are fairly similar. The specific clinical procedures, however, are quite different. The procedures for the intermediate stutterer are designed for a younger client whose stuttering is not as fully developed. Now, let us discuss the specific clinical procedures that we use in our direct work with this child.

UNDERSTANDING STUTTERING

In this phase of treatment, we have a number of goals. First, we help the child to identify his moments of stuttering and the "tricks" he uses to hide them. Second, we give the child, at an appropriate level, an explanation for his stuttering. And third, we give the child an overview of what he will be doing in therapy. We will discuss each of these goals separately, but in actual practice, these goals are often interwoven into the same therapy sessions.

Identifying Moments of Stuttering and the Tricks Used to Hide Them. When we first meet the child, we believe it is very important to establish a good rapport with him. During the first several therapy sessions, we spend considerable time getting to know the child. We show interest in him and what he has to say. We are warm and friendly. We also demonstrate through our behavior that we are comfortable with and accepting of his stuttering. This relationship continues to develop as we work with the child throughout the next two phases of therapy. That is, while we are teaching the child to use fluency enhancing behaviors and to modify his moments of stuttering and while we are helping the child reduce his negative

---

[1] The reader is referred to Guitar, B., & Peters, T. J. (1980). The elementary school child who stutters. In B. Guitar & T. J. Peters, *Stuttering: An integration of contemporary therapies* (pp. 51–62). Memphis: Speech Foundation of America for an earlier version of integrating stuttering modification and fluency shaping therapies with the intermediate stutterer.

feelings and attitudes and eliminate his avoidance behaviors, we continue to convey to the child our interest in and acceptance of him and his stuttering. We also demonstrate our belief in and support of his ability to improve his speech. We believe that this type of accepting and supporting relationship is necessary if the child's beginning speech fears are going to become deconditioned. We also believe this rapport is mandatory if the child is going to take our advice to attempt to change his manner of speaking and to risk giving up his avoidance behaviors.

After we get to know the child and he feels comfortable with us, we begin to broach the topic of stuttering with him. We want the child to be able to identify his moments of stuttering and the tricks he uses to hide them. A good way to begin is to simply acknowledge to the child that he is coming to therapy for help with his stuttering and to ask him if he is aware of when he stutters. Some children will say "yes" and some will say "no." Regardless of the child's answer, we usually have the child first identify stutters in our speech. This is less threatening to the child. We then insert stutters into our speech and ask the child to signal when he hears one. At first, our stutters are mild ones; later, they may more closely resemble the child's typical moments of stuttering. If the child is able to identify our stutters, we praise him for his ability. If he is unable or unwilling to identify our stutters, we point them out to him or make them a little more obvious. With a little practice along these lines, the child is soon able to identify the stutters in our speech. These identification activities can take place while we are conversing with the child on some topic of interest or while we are playing some age-appropriate game. It is essential, however, that we interact with the child in a relaxed and accepting manner.

The next step is to help the child identify his own moments of stuttering. Some children will be able and willing to do this immediately; others may be unable or reluctant to do so. With this latter child, we often need an intermediate step in which we signal the child when we hear him stutter. We find that, with patience, encouragement, and a little practice, children are soon able to identify most of their stutters. Again, these identification activities can occur while conversing or playing games with the child. We also find Van Riper's "catch me" games helpful here.

We now ask the child if he is aware of any "tricks" he uses to hide his stuttering. We are interested in having him identify his starters, postponements, and word and situation avoidances. It is important to identify these behaviors because we are going to encourage the child not to use these tricks in later phases of treatment. We begin this process by giving the child examples of starting, postponing, and avoiding behaviors we have seen in other children. We tell the child about other children we know who use "well" or "um" before difficult words. We describe how some children do not talk in their classrooms because they are afraid they might stutter, or we tell the child about children who substitute easy words for hard ones. By sharing these and other examples with the child and by asking if any of these apply to him, we make it easier for the child to be open with us about the tricks he uses. By this time, many children are able and willing to share their tricks with us. In other cases, however, it may be necessary to point these behaviors out to the child. To help the child become more aware of these tricks, we use "catch me" games in which we and the child take turns catching one another using these tricks.

Besides identifying the tricks that the child uses to hide his stuttering, we also probe for the reasons that he uses these tricks. In our experience, though, many of these children are unwilling and/or unable to discuss in much detail their feelings of embarrassment or fear associated with their stuttering. We do not push the child on this point, but we do let him know that these sorts of feelings are very understandable and very natural. We encourage expression of these feelings and reinforce any comments of this nature.

By now, the child has shared his moments of stuttering and the tricks he uses to hide them with us, and he has found us to be understanding and accepting listeners. Some deconditioning of his speech fears has already occurred. The child has also learned some of the terms we will be using in the remaining phases of therapy. Thus, some basic groundwork has been laid for the following phases of treatment.

Explaining Stuttering.   We believe it is important for the intermediate stutterer to be given some explanation for his stuttering. He knows he stutters. He knows he has been stuttering, probably for a number of years. At some level, this child needs to be given some explanation for why he talks differently from his friends. What do we say to this child?

We tell this child that he stutters because he has a "speech machine" that has a tendency to be more disfluent or bumpy than that of his peers. We may even suggest that he was born this way. We do not want this child to believe that he did or did not do anything to cause his speech problem. We do not want him to feel guilty because of his stuttering. We are careful to explain that this tendency to be disfluent has nothing to do with his intelligence or his personality. In other words, his tendency to be disfluent is specifically related to his ability, or lack of ability, to say his words smoothly. We point out that many other children have problems in other areas. For example, some children have problems in learning to read, or some children have a hard time at sports. We go on to explain to the child that this tendency to be disfluent only accounts for the individual moments of stuttering or what we call the core behaviors.

We then go on to explain to the child that the tricks he uses to hide his stuttering are things he has learned to do. In a sense, these are habits he has learned to hide his stuttering. We point out to the child that these tricks have been reinforced or learned because they have temporarily gotten him out of embarrassing or uncomfortable speaking experiences.

We also believe it is beneficial for the intermediate stutterer to know that a lot of children stutter. In other words, he is not the only person in the world who stutters. Often this child may not know any other children who stutter. He may believe that he is only one of a very few who have this problem. We tell the child that about 1 in 100 children stutter. We tell him that there are over 2 million people in the United States of America who share this problem with him. We believe this sort of information helps the child feel less unique and less isolated because of his stuttering.

Giving an Overview of Therapy.   Finally, we believe it is important for the intermediate stutterer to have an overview of his treatment program. We explain to the child that we will help him learn to talk more fluently and to stutter more easily on his remaining moments of stuttering. To help him understand how he will do this, we model fluency enhancing behaviors and stuttering modification techniques. We also tell the child that we will help him become more comfortable with his stuttering and overcome his habit of using tricks to hide it. We point out that these tricks are learned and that they can be unlearned. Finally, we explain to the child that it is going to take some time and effort, but by working together we can lick this problem.

USING FLUENCY ENHANCING BEHAVIORS AND MODIFYING THE MOMENTS OF STUTTERING

When we discussed the treatment of the advanced stutterer in Chapter 8, we had the "reducing negative feelings and attitudes and eliminating avoidances" phase precede the "using fluency enhancing behaviors and modifying the moments of stuttering" phase. We did say, however, that with some advanced stutterers, we found it beneficial to have this order reversed. We stated that this was especially true for those stutterers who found it very difficult to confront their speech fears. Because of their young age, we believe this situation applies to most intermediate stutterers. Thus, with intermediate stutterers, we typically have the "using fluency enhancing behaviors and modifying the moments of stuttering" phase precede the "reducing negative feelings and attitudes and eliminating avoidances" phase. We find that intermediate stutterers can deal with their speech fears and avoidance behaviors much more easily after they have increased their fluency.

To increase the intermediate stutterer's fluency, we begin by teaching him to use fluency enhancing behaviors. To do this, we have two options. The first is to follow procedures like those we described for the advanced stutterer. This involves the "using fluency enhancing behaviors" procedures that we described in Chapter 8. As will be recalled, this includes the use of a DAF program. The second option is to follow procedures similar to those for the beginning stutterer. This involves the "establishing and transferring fluency" procedures that we discussed in Chapter 10. These procedures include the 13-step hierarchy we use in establishing and transferring the child's fluency. Regardless of which of the above fluency shaping procedures we use, we then follow it by teaching the child to modify any residual stutters. To do this, we use the "modifying the moments of stuttering" procedures we use with the beginning stutterer. These procedures were described in Chapter 10.

How do we decide which fluency shaping procedure to use? The age of the child and some trial therapy helps us to determine which option to use. We find that older intermediate stutterers, aged 11 to 13 years, usually can learn to use some fluency enhancing behaviors by going through the DAF program that we use with the advanced stutterer. On the other hand, we find that younger intermediate stutterers, aged 6 to 8 years, usually do not relate well to the DAF machine and work better by going through the establishing and transferring fluency hierarchy or fluency hierarchy that we use with the beginning stutterer.

In addition to considering the age of the intermediate stutterer, we also do some trial therapy to see how the child responds to these two different fluency shaping procedures. First, this involves determining how the child responds during reading, if he can read, or how he responds during conversation with the DAF machine set at 250 msec delay. Besides using the DAF to enhance the child's fluency, we also model a speech pattern that is characterized by a slow rate, gentle onsets, and soft contacts for the child to imitate. Second, this involves determining how the child responds to typical activities from the fluency hierarchy. We see how the child responds when we engage him in the following four tasks from the hierarchy: (*a*) single word, slow speech, and direct model, (*b*) single word, slow speech, and indirect model, (*c*) carrier phrase + word, slow speech, and indirect model, and (*d*) sentence, slow speech, and indirect model. Here again, we model, either directly or indirectly, a speech pattern that is characterized by a slow rate, gentle onsets, and soft contacts for the child to imitate. Readers may want to refer to Chapter 10 to refresh their memories of these steps.

In doing this trial therapy, we want to see how the child responds to the early steps of each of the two fluency shaping procedures. We are interested in answering two questions. First, how effective is the procedure in increasing the child's fluency, and second, how comfortable is the child with the procedure? In the final analysis, we want to use the fluency shaping procedure that appears to be the most effective in increasing the child's fluency while, at the same time, using a procedure with which the child is comfortable.

Using Fluency Enhancing Behaviors. Let us assume that the child is an older intermediate stutterer and finds it easy to talk in a slow, fluent manner during the DAF trial therapy, and further, that he is comfortable while talking on the DAF machine. We will begin by discussing the application of this fluency shaping procedure to the intermediate stutterer. Later, we will discuss the application of the fluency hierarchy with an intermediate stutterer. Since our DAF fluency shaping procedures—that is, our procedures for "using fluency enhancing behaviors"—were thoroughly described during the discussion of our treatment of the advanced stutterer in Chapter 8, we will only briefly review these procedures here. The reader is referred to the earlier discussion for more specific information. We will comment here, though, upon the differences between applying these procedures with the intermediate stutterer and with the advanced stutterer.

As will be recalled, we asked the advanced stutterer to read a handout which described the following fluency enhancing behaviors (FEBS): slower rate, gentle onsets, and soft contacts. We usually do not use this handout with the intermediate stutterer; rather, we describe and model these FEBS for him. We also explain how the DAF machine will help him use these FEBS. Since most of the intermediate stutterers with whom we use this procedure are able to read, we typically begin with oral reading. With the DAF set at 250 msec delay, we spend some time teaching the child how to use FEBS appropriately. We then begin working our way through the program. That is, we explain to the child that he needs to obtain 30 minutes of fluency with no more than one stuttered word per minute at each of the following delay times: 250, 200, 150, 100, 50 and 0 msec. We reinforce the child's use of FEBS and his fluency. If he is not using FEBS to be fluent, we give him appropriate feedback. This may involve the use of reminders, additional instructions, or more modeling. After the child completes the above sequence of steps while orally reading, we then have him go through the same sequence again while conversing with us. We continue to reinforce his fluency and remind him to use his FEBS when he is not fluent. When the child completes this establishment program, he is conversing very fluently. This fluency is usually a combination of a great deal of spontaneous fluency and some controlled fluency. Typically, intermediate stutterers do not use, or fortunately, do not need to use, FEBS as conscientiously as advanced stutterers to be fluent.

It is now time to transfer this fluency from us to significant other people in the child's life and from the therapy room to other physical settings. As the reader will remember, we used four hierarchies with the advanced stutterer. These hierarchies included speaking situations inside the clinic with the clinician, outside the clinic with the clinician, outside the clinic without the clinician, and on the telephone. We do not use these rather structured hierarchies with the intermediate stutterer, for two reasons. First, the intermediate stutterer's fluency typically generalizes more readily than that of the advanced stutterer; therefore, these hierarchies are not needed. Second, since the intermediate stutterer is still a child, it is unrealistic to expect him to carry out many of these transfer activities outside of the therapy situation, especially those that require him to do them by himself. So what do we do to generalize the child's fluency to significant other people in his life?

We begin by having one of the child's parents join the child and us in the therapy room. Our goal is to have the child using his FEBS and maintaining his fluency with this parent and us at the same level that he did with just us in the therapy room. By now, we have explained FEBS to the parents during one of our counseling sessions. It is also possible that the parent has observed the child using FEBS during some therapy sessions. Thus, the parent is already familiar with what the child is supposed to be doing. Besides transferring the child's fluency to the parent, we also want the parent to learn how to appropriately reinforce the child for his new fluency. Thus, over a few therapy sessions, we gradually turn the role of clinician over to the parent. When things are going well, we remove ourselves from the therapy session and observe the parent and child interact. Once we feel that the child is maintaining his fluency with his parent and the parent is appropriately reinforcing the child, we ask them to have sessions like these at home on a regular basis. We want them to have at least one 15 or 20 minute fluent or "good" talking period at home 4 or 5 times a week.

Besides being fluent with this parent, we also want the child to experience his new fluency with the other parent. We have the second parent join the child and the first parent in the their good talking times at home. We also encourage the second parent to reinforce the child's fluency. If the transfer of fluency to this other parent does not go well at home, we have that parent join us and the child in therapy. Usually, this is not necessary.

Besides transferring the child's fluency skills to his parents in the home, we also want to transfer the fluency to other significant people in his life and to other physical settings. We have the child's siblings and friends join us in therapy for a number of sessions. We may have the child's grandparents or his classroom teacher come to therapy, if it can be arranged. If the child is having particular difficulty in a specific physical setting, we will conduct therapy there. For example, we have had therapy with a child and his friend at the child's favorite fast-food restaurant. The people and, possibly, the physical settings will vary with each child, depending upon with whom and where he is still having trouble. During these sessions, the other persons are made aware of the purpose of the sessions. They are told that the client is to be using his FEBS to be more fluent. In other words, the child's fluency and his use of FEBS are treated matter-of-factly. We reinforce the child's fluency and his use of FEBS and remind him to use them if he is being disfluent. We do not want these other persons to become surrogate clinicians like the parents, but we do want the young stutterer to have the experience of using his FEBS and being fluent with these other important people in his life. We find that these experiences facilitate the generalization of the child's new fluency.

Establishing and Transferring Fluency. Now, let us assume the child is a younger intermediate stutterer and neither does well on nor likes the DAF machine. With this child, we use the fluency hierarchy that we used with the beginning stutterer. Since these procedures were thoroughly discussed in Chapter 10, we will only briefly review them here. The reader is referred to the earlier discussion for more detailed information. We will comment, however, on some modifications we often make in this fluency hierarchy when we use it with an intermediate stutterer.

As will be recalled, the fluency hierarchy consists of a 13-step program that begins with the child imitating the clinician as she says a single word, using slow, prolonged speech, gentle onsets of phonation, and relaxed articulatory contacts. The program ends with the child conversing fluently at a normal rate with a parent at home. In this more easy to more difficult hierarchy, we gradually change the length and complexity of the linguistic unit from a single word, to a carrier phrase + a word, to a sentence, to 2 to 4 sentences, and finally, to conversation; change the speech pattern from slow speech to normal speech; change the modeling from a direct model, to an indirect model, and then to no model at all; change the person to whom the child is talking from the clinician to the parent; and change the physical setting from the therapy room to the child's home. Throughout this program, the child's fluent speech is being reinforced. This is the basic program. What modifications do we sometimes make with the intermediate stutterer?

First, if the child responds well to the trial therapy, we may skip one or two of the early steps in the program. For example, if the child uses the slow speech pattern well and is fluent on the "carrier phrase + word" level, we often skip the "single word" level steps. We find that the intermediate stutterer, being older than the beginning stutterer, often thinks these beginning steps of the hierarchy are "too easy" and gets "bored" with them.

Second, we do not expect the beginning stutterer to use fluency enhancing behaviors to increase his fluency after the termination of therapy; rather, this child is usually spontaneously fluent. We do, however, expect the intermediate stutterer to use FEBS after the termination of therapy to occasionally increase his fluency. Thus, as we progress through the fluency hierarchy with the intermediate stutterer, we encourage him to use a slightly slower speaking rate, gentle onsets, and relaxed articulatory contacts to increase his fluency. We reinforce these behaviors. We explain to the child that these will be skills he will be able to use in situations in which he wants to sound more fluent. In other words, we put more emphasis upon teaching FEBS to the intermediate stutterer than we did with the beginning stutterer.

The third modification involves the transfer or generalization of the child's fluency. When we discussed the beginning stutterer we stated that, by the completion of the fluency hierarchy, many beginning stutterers are already automatically generalizing their fluency to other speaking situations. We do not find this happening so readily with many intermediate stutterers. We usually find it necessary to go through the same transfer procedures we described earlier in this chapter when we talked about transferring the child's fluency following the DAF program. The reader is referred to that discussion for those procedures.

There is, however, one slight difference in the above procedures if the child completes the establishing and transferring fluency hierarchy, rather than the DAF program. As will be recalled, the last step of the fluency hierarchy involves the child talking fluently with a parent at home. Thus, in this case, the initial step of the above transfer procedures is already completed.

By this time, it becomes apparent whether or not the child has any tense or hard residual stutters left in his speech. This is true whether he has gone through the DAF program or the fluency hierarchy. If he does have any of these hard stutters left, we believe it is important to give him some tools to cope with these moments of stuttering. Let us now consider how we do this.

Modifying the Moments of Stuttering.   When we discussed our treatment of the beginning stutterer in Chapter 10, we indicated that modifying the moments of stuttering was an optional phase for that treatment level. Since most beginning stutterers develop spontaneous fluency, we think that only a few of these children need to learn how to modify any residual tense stutters. We do not believe this is true for many intermediate stutterers. Our experience suggests that many of these latter children have residual tense stutters and, therefore, can benefit from learning how to modify them.

Regardless of which fluency shaping program the intermediate stutterer completes, the DAF program or the fluency hierarchy, we use the procedures we described in Chapter 10 for modifying his moments of stuttering. We will only review these procedures here. The reader is referred to the earlier discussion for more detailed information.

As we indicated in our earlier discussion, we explain and model for the child that there are two ways to stutter on a word. There is the "hard" way and the "easy" way. The hard way resembles the child's typical remaining stutters. The easy way involves saying the word slowly by prolonging all the sounds in the word. It also involves using gentle onsets and soft articulatory contacts. We point out to the child that the easy way is similar to the way he talked when he was on the DAF machine or when he was talking slow in the early steps of the fluency hierarchy, whichever is appropriate.

Next, both we and the child put a number of these easy stutters voluntarily into our speech. We do these on nonstuttered words. We want the child to acquire the motor movements involved in using easy stutters. We also want the child to feel comfortable using them. By this time, some children may be turning their hard stutters into easy stutters. If they are not, we employ the following procedures.

We model for the child how this modification would look and sound. We begin by simulating the child's typical hard stutter, and then we come out of it with a slow, relaxed movement. We do this many times for the child. We then have the child join us as we simulate his hard stuttering, and in unison, we ease out of it, using a slow, relaxed movement. We want the child to feel what it is like to turn a hard stutter into an easy stutter. Finally, we signal the child when he is having a hard stutter, and he is to come out of it, using a slow, relaxed movement. With considerable support and practice along these lines, the typical intermediate stutterer can learn to modify his residual moments of stuttering.

By now, the child is speaking rather well in many situations, but some situations are probably still giving him some problems. We continue with the transfer procedures, but we now turn more of our attention toward reducing the child's negative feelings about his speech and toward eliminating any avoidance behaviors.

REDUCING NEGATIVE FEELINGS AND ATTITUDES AND ELIMINATING AVOIDANCES

Besides being an understanding and accepting listener for the child, we have four goals during this phase of treatment. First, we help the child cope with any teasing. In fact, if this has been a significant problem, we would have responded to it earlier. Second, we desensitize the child to any remaining fluency disrupters. Third, we help the child reduce his fear of stuttering by using a great deal of voluntary stuttering during therapy sessions. Fourth, we help the child eliminate his use of avoidance behaviors. This includes both word and situation avoidances. Let us deal with each of these goals in turn.

Coping with Teasing. We believe it is very important to eliminate any teasing the child may be receiving because of his stuttering, and we will be addressing this issue shortly when we discuss parent and classroom teacher counseling. However, regardless of how hard we try to eliminate this teasing, we know that it is impossible to eliminate all of it. Thus, we believe it is very important to give the child some defenses against the teasing he may receive.

We agree with Van Riper that the best defense against teasing is acceptance. For example, if the child can say, "I know I stutter, and I am going to speech class to get some help," or a similar statement, this will disarm most teasers. Nobody likes to tease someone from whom they can not get a rise. Fighting or running away, on the other hand, just reinforces the teasing behavior. Be that as it may, in our experience we find it difficult to get a child in this age range to calmly accept and admit his stuttering to his tormentors. When we have been successful, we have done the following things.

First, we explain to the child the importance of his calmly and openly admitting his stuttering to his teasers, rather than responding with embarrassment or anger. We explain how this type of response will usually discourage his teasers. We then explore with the child the sort of statement he could see himself making. The words he uses must be words with which he feels comfortable. Next, we do a great deal of role playing with the child. We play the role of the teaser, and his task is to calmly respond to our heckling with the type of statement he had chosen to use. We need to do this many times until the child feels comfortable with his response and until he can see himself actually doing this in a real-life situation. Finally, the day comes when he tries out his new behavior. We hope it works. If it does not, we are there to give him support and encouragement.

Desensitizing the Child to Fluency Disrupters. As we indicated earlier, the child is probably speaking rather well by now in many situations. Further, many of the child's fluency disrupters have already been eliminated or substantially reduced as part of our parent counseling. However, some fluency disrupters, because of their nature, can not be totally eliminated from the child's life. The child needs to learn to cope with these. For example, one young intermediate stutterer with whom one of the authors recently worked became very upset whenever he lost a competitive game. He got angry and cried. At these times, he also did not pay attention to his speech, and his stuttering increased. We felt it was important to desensitize this child to losing; after all, everybody loses sometime in his life. Other intermediate stutterers have other fluency disrupters, and we believe it is important to desensitize them to these, too.

We discussed our procedures for desensitizing the beginning stutterer to fluency disrupters in Chapter 10, and our procedures for the intermediate stutterer are identical. To refresh the reader's memory, however, we will briefly describe the procedures we used with the above young intermediate stutterer who hated to lose. This boy had completed the fluency hierarchy and was speaking very fluently in therapy. We told him we were going to play games, and we were going to play our hardest and try to beat him. We further told him he was to use his FEBS and be fluent, even if he were losing the game. We reinforced his fluency and reminded him to use his FEBS when he was not fluent. In the beginning, we lost more than we won, and his fluency was good. Gradually, we began to win more and more. At first, his fluency suffered, but we reminded him to use his FEBS. He did, and his fluency returned. Eventually, we were winning most of the time, but he was remaining fluent. He had learned to maintain his fluency, even though he was losing. He had also learned to become a better loser!

Using Voluntary Stuttering. At this point in treatment, the typical intermediate stutterer often has some residual moments of stuttering left in his speech during his daily activities. If we sense that he is embarrassed or fearful of these, we want to help him become more comfortable with these residual stutters.

We found that we could accomplish this if both we and the child put a number of relaxed, unhurried voluntary repetitions and prolongations into our speech. We do this while we are engaging in some enjoyable activity, such as playing the child's favorite game. We explain to the child why we are doing this. We explain that we can learn to remain calm and relaxed even though we are experiencing some stuttering. We then calmly model relaxed repetitions or prolongations and ask the child to imitate us. At first, this is on single words. Later, it will be during conversations. We go slowly. We do not push the child too rapidly to engage in this activity, especially if he is at all hesitant. We reinforce the child's attempts and praise him for his courage. We point out to the child how we are stuttering, but at the same time, we are remaining relaxed and comfortable. We engage in these activities only in the therapy room. We do not have the child use this voluntary stuttering outside of the therapy situation the way we do with the advanced stutterer. We find that, by experiencing these relaxed, voluntary stutters over and over again while engaging in a pleasant activity with an accepting clinician, the child loses much of the emotionality associated with his stuttering.

Eliminating Avoidances.   We believe it is important for the intermediate stutterer to eliminate or substantially reduce his use of avoidances. We begin by helping the child to understand that it is unwise for him to avoid certain words and situations because he is afraid of them. We point out that, the more he runs away from saying a specific word or talking in a given situation, the more afraid of that word or situation he becomes. We explain that it is better for him in the long run to say what he wants to say, even if he is afraid and even if he stutters. We go on to explain that, by confronting his fears, he overcomes them.

To help the child understand the above principles, we find it helpful to draw analogies between overcoming being afraid of saying certain words or talking in certain situations and overcoming some other fear in his life, preferably one he has previously conquered. For example, if the child recalls overcoming some other fear in his life, we have him tell us about how he did it. As he tells us about his victory, we point out to him how he confronted his fear and how he no longer is afraid. We also point out that he no longer avoids the old feared stimulus. We then draw an analogy to overcoming his fear and avoidance of certain words or certain speaking situations.

If the child does not recall overcoming some other fear in his life, we then make up a hypothetical situation. For example, we may talk about overcoming being afraid of jumping off the high diving board at the local swimming pool (Fig. 12.1). We suggest to the child that, if he wanted to overcome his fear of the high board, it would be best to start by just jumping off the side of the pool. When he became comfortable with this, he would then go off the low board. After becoming comfortable with the low board, he would then take on the medium high board. Eventually, he would reach the high diving board; and after jumping from it a number of times, he would find himself no longer afraid of it. There would also be no reason to avoid the high diving board any more either. We then explain to the child that we will use this same easy to hard strategy, or hierarchies, to help him overcome his speech fears and avoidances.

It is usually easier to help the child overcome his fear and avoidance of words than of situations. This is because we can provide the child with more support in confronting his word fears in the therapy situation than we can provide him in confronting his situation fears in his daily life. We can also use these feared words over and over again within the therapy situation. For example, we recall a young intermediate stutterer who quite consistently substituted "me" for "I." This was not a symptom of a language disorder. His parents reported that he had used "I" appropriately for a number of years before beginning to use this substitution. With this child, we began by saying "I" in unison with the child while we both used a slow, easy stutter on the word. We strongly reinforced his efforts. We then used "I" many, many times in carrier phrases while playing games. During these games, both the clinician and the child used easy stutters when saying the word. The child gradually regained his confidence in saying "I." Within a week or two,

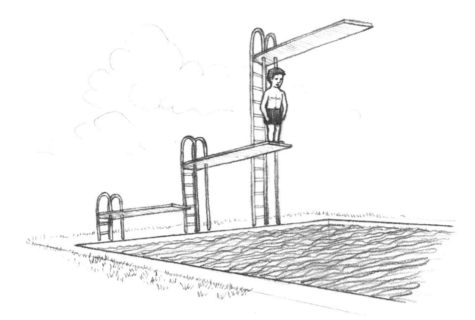

Figure 12.1. Using an easy to hard hierarchy to overcome fear and avoidance.

his avoidance of "I" was eliminated in the therapy situation, and his parents reported he was again using this pronoun appropriately at home.

Now, how do we help a child overcome his fear and avoidance of a speaking situation? To the degree that we are able in therapy, we sequence a series of speaking situations that leads up to and approximates the feared situation. For example, suppose a child was afraid to orally participate in his classroom. In this case and with the child's consent, we would bring one or two of the child's classmates into therapy. We would play the role of the classroom teacher and have this small group of two or three answer and ask questions. When the child felt comfortable doing this, we would then have three or four of his classmates come to therapy for a similar activity. Next, it may be helpful for the child and us to go to his classroom during a noon hour or a recess. After explaining our goal and therapy procedures to the classroom teacher, we would have the child sit at his desk and have his teacher ask him questions about his lessons. These activities are about as far as we can go in simulating the child's feared situation. Now, he needs to take the last step by himself. However, he has been successful in a number of situations that approximate his feared situation. He also has a classroom teacher who is sensitized to his problem and understands his therapy. The chances are that, after some initial ambivalence, he will be successful in overcoming his reluctance to talk in class.

MAINTAINING IMPROVEMENT

By this point in therapy, the child is usually speaking well in most situations. That is, he is having a great deal of spontaneous fluency in many situations and having either controlled fluency or acceptable stuttering in others. His speech fears and avoidances have been eliminated or significantly reduced. We do not dismiss the child from therapy at this point; rather, we gradually phase him out of intensive therapy. We see him for therapy on a weekly basis for a month or so, and then on a semimonthly basis for a month or so. Then, if things continue to go well, we see him for a series of reevaluations over the next 2 years. At first, these reevaluations are on a monthly basis, then a bimonthly basis, and finally, a per semester basis.

During these reevaluations, we obtain a sample of the child's speech and oral reading, and we interview him regarding how well he has been talking in everyday speaking situations. We also interview his parents and his classroom teacher regarding his talking at home and in school. If we find that the child's fluency has regressed or if he has begun to use avoidance behaviors again, we reenroll him in therapy. Our experience suggests that a number of these children may have one or two mild regressions before their fluency stabilizes. These regressions are often associated with the beginning of the school year or with transferring from one school to another.

When we bring the child back into therapy, it is usually for a month or two. During these "booster" sessions, the child may need to get his fluency enhancing or stuttering modification skills tuned up. He may need a brief refresher course on the importance of not avoiding, or he may just need an opportunity to talk to an understanding listener about his stuttering. In time, these regressions and our reevaluations become further apart. Finally, the day arrives to dismiss the child from treatment.

Clinical Procedures: Parent Counseling

Our counseling procedures for the parents of the intermediate stutterer are very similar to those we discussed in Chapter 8 for the parents of the beginning stutterer. The reader is referred to the earlier chapter for a review of that discussion. At this time, we will comment only upon the differences, many of which are self-explanatory, between the parent counseling procedures for the intermediate stutterer and the beginning stutterer.

As the reader will recall, we had four goals in mind when we counseled the parents of the beginning stutterer. We have the same goals, plus one additional one, when counseling the parents of the intermediate stutterer. The previous four goals are (a) explaining the treatment program and the parents' role in it, (b) explaining the possible causes of stuttering, (c) identifying and reducing fluency disrupters, and (d) identifying and increasing fluency enhancing situations. The additional goal is eliminating teasing. We will discuss each of the above goals in turn.

EXPLAINING THE TREATMENT PROGRAM AND THE PARENTS' ROLE IN IT

There are a few differences between counseling the parents of the intermediate and the beginning stutterer that we need to comment upon relative to this goal. First, when we explain the nature of the treatment program to the parents of the beginning stutterer, we explain the establishing and transferring fluency hierarchy to them. This may or may not be appropriate with the parents of an intermediate stutterer. As will be remembered, some intermediate stutterers go through this program, but others complete our DAF program instead. Thus, it is important to explain the appropriate program to the child's parents. Further, since we teach many intermediate stutterers to use easy stutters, we need to explain these to the child's parents.

Second, we tell the parents of the beginning stutterer that the therapy typically takes anywhere from 6 months to 2 years. Treatment for the intermediate stutterer usually takes longer. Our experience indicates that therapy typically takes from 1 to 3 years.

A third difference involves what the parents should tell their child about coming to speech therapy. We said that, many times, parents of beginning stutterers are told that they should not mention their child's stuttering to him. We stated that we believe this is an unwise approach. We believe this even more strongly with the intermediate stutterer. Since this child is very aware of his speech problem, his parents must have open, frank discussions with him about his stuttering and his therapy. We also suggested that the parents of the beginning stutterer tell their child that, with therapy, he will grow up talking like everybody else. This is usually true with the beginning stutterer, but it is not necessarily true with the intermediate stutterer. Thus, the parents of the intermediate stutterer should tell their child that, with therapy, he will learn to talk much better, but they should not promise him that he will talk normally.

Finally, we share information on spontaneous recovery with the parents of beginning stutterers. We indicated that between 50 and 80% of these children recover without any treatment and that, with treatment, these percentages go up. We do not believe that this is true with intermediate stutterers. Since we do not have data on spontaneous recovery with intermediate stutterers, we do not bring up this topic with their parents.

EXPLAINING THE POSSIBLE CAUSES OF STUTTERING

Everything we said in Chapter 8 relative to explaining stuttering to the parents of the beginning stutterer applies here as well. There is, however, one additional bit of information we need to add when we talk to the parents of an intermediate stutterer. We need to talk with them about their child's avoidance behaviors. We need to describe these behaviors to the parents. We need to explain how these word and situation avoidances are behaviors their child has learned to use to cope with the embarrassment and fear of talking. We also need to explain how, in therapy, we will be helping the child eliminate his use of these avoidance behaviors.

IDENTIFYING AND REDUCING FLUENCY DISRUPTERS

Since what we said in Chapter 8 about helping the parents of a beginning stutterer identify and reduce the fluency disrupters in their child's environment is also applicable to the parents of the intermediate stutterer, there is no need to repeat that information here. Based upon our experience, however, there is one qualifying statement we need to make. Since the stuttering of the intermediate stutterer is more firmly established than that of the beginning stutterer, decreasing the fluency disrupters in the intermediate stutterer's environment will have less positive impact upon his fluency than upon that of the beginning stutterer. This does not mean that the clinician does not attempt to do this; it only means that the clinician should expect more modest results.

IDENTIFYING AND INCREASING FLUENCY ENHANCING SITUATIONS

The information provided in Chapter 8 about helping the parents of the beginning stutterer identify and increase fluency enhancing situations is also applicable for the parents of the intermediate stutterer. There is no need to reproduce that material here. Again, however, we believe that these procedures are less effective with the intermediate stutterer.

ELIMINATING TEASING

If any of the intermediate stutterer's siblings are teasing him about his stuttering, his parents need to stop this. We have found the best way to do this is to have the parents have a serious talk with the sibling. The parents need to explain to the sibling that teasing makes the stuttering worse and must be discontinued. Usually, this is sufficient. If it is not, we have found it effective for us to talk to the sibling about the importance of not teasing a young stutterer. Having an adult, other than a parent, talk seriously about this matter often carries more weight with the child.

Clinical Procedures: Classroom Teacher Counseling

We believe it is very important to have the intermediate stutterer's classroom teacher involved in the child's treatment program (Fig. 12.2). After all, the teacher spends as much, if not more, waking time with the child than any other adult. We have four goals in mind when we are working with this classroom teacher. They are (*a*) explaining the treatment program and the teacher's role in it, (*b*) talking with the child about his stuttering, (*c*) coping with oral participation, and (*d*) eliminating teasing.

EXPLAINING THE TREATMENT PROGRAM AND THE TEACHER'S ROLE IN IT

We believe it is beneficial for the classroom teacher to have an overview of the child's treatment program. We explain to the teacher how we are helping the child increase his fluency and modify his stutters. We explain how we are attempting to help the child to be more comfortable with his stuttering and to eliminate his speech avoidance behaviors. We want the teacher to understand the rationale behind our procedures. We are careful to answer any questions the teacher may have. We believe that helping the teacher understand our goals will have at least two benefits. One, the teacher will have a better understanding of how to interact with the child and, two, will be better able to give us feedback regarding the child's fluency in the classroom.

We also explain the teacher's role in the child's therapy. That is, we explain why and how we would like the teacher to implement the last three of the above goals. In other words, we discuss why and how we would like the teacher to talk with the child about his stuttering, how to help him cope with oral participa-

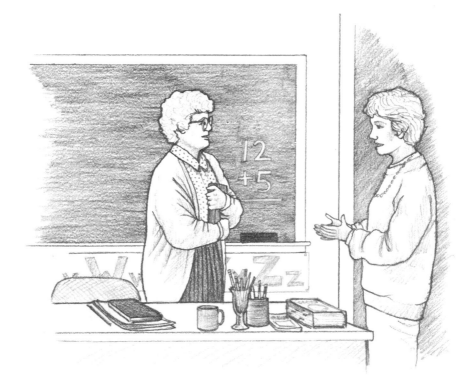

Figure 12.2.   It is important to have the classroom teacher involved in the child's treatment.

tion, and how to eliminate any teasing he may be receiving. We will discuss each of these below.

TALKING WITH THE CHILD ABOUT HIS STUTTERING

One of the authors recalls going all the way through school, from kindergarten through high school, without any teacher ever mentioning his stuttering. He stuttered severely year after year. Everyone knew he stuttered, but nobody ever acknowledged it. It was very uncomfortable.

We believe, along with Van Riper, that it is better for the classroom teacher to sit down with the intermediate stutterer and talk calmly with him about his stuttering. The teacher should let him know that she or he is aware of his stuttering and would like to help him in any way possible. The stutterer should be told that the teacher will not interrupt or hurry him when he is talking. Just this acknowledgment and acceptance of the child's stuttering by the teacher will make the child be more comfortable in the classroom.

COPING WITH ORAL PARTICIPATION

The teacher should also talk with the child about his oral participation in class. Again, like Van Riper, we believe it is important for the intermediate stutterer to orally participate in class, but it is also important for the child to feel comfortable in this participation. The teacher should ask for the child's input on this matter. Possibly some classroom procedure, such as calling on students in alphabetical order, is creating a great deal of apprehension for the stutterer and could be modified. Possibly he would prefer to be called on early so that his apprehension does not have the opportunity to build. With some understanding of the child's feelings and with some flexibility in procedures, most classroom teachers can help the intermediate stutterer become much more comfortable in his oral participation.

ELIMINATING TEASING

It is not unusual for stutterers in elementary or junior high school to be teased about their stuttering. If the classroom teacher becomes aware of this, she or he should attempt to stop it. As we previously indicated during our discussion of parent counseling, we believe the best way to do this is to have a serious talk with the young teaser. In other words, the teacher needs to explain to the child who is doing the teasing that his teasing is making the young stutterer's speech worse and that he needs to discontinue doing it immediately. The teacher should make it clear that this behavior will not be tolerated.

This concludes our integration of stuttering modification and fluency shaping therapies for the intermediate stutterer. Let us now review the clinical procedures of some other clinicians who also integrate procedures from these two approaches.

OTHER CLINICIANS

Hugo Gregory and June Campbell

Hugo Gregory and June Campbell (Gregory, 1984b, 1986a; Gregory & Campbell, 1988) refer to the intermediate stutterer as the "more confirmed school-aged stutterer." In terms of the speech behaviors targeted in therapy, they begin by using a less specific approach and then move to a more specific approach only if it is needed.

In their less specific approach, Gregory and Campbell do not attempt to modify the child's moments of stuttering. Rather, they model an "easy, relaxed approach with smooth movements" (ERA-SM) for the child. Gregory also uses ERA-SM with advanced stutterers. ERA-SM involves a slower rate of speech and smooth transitions from sound to sound and from word to word. These changes occur at the beginning of a word or phrase, not during the entire sentence. In other words, Gregory and Campbell are teaching the use of fluency enhancing skills at the beginning of an utterance. These clinicians also integrate work on ERA-SM with general body relaxation. They point out to the child that feelings of general body relaxation are being carried over into the movements involved in speech. In teaching ERA-SM, Gregory and Campbell take the child through a progression of tasks that begins with one-word responses and ends with longer, more complex ones. In going through this hierarchy, they use the following types of activities to elicit speech from the child: choral reading, reading alone, answering questions, describing pictures, and engaging in conversation.

If the child still has residual stutters associated with certain sounds or words, Gregory and Campbell employ their more specific approach. This involves teaching the child to modify individual moments of stuttering. To do this, they feign a stutter for the child and ask the child to imitate them. They then model a modification of this stutter and ask the child to imitate this modification. This may involve slowing down a repetition or easing the tension on a prolongation. Following this, Gregory and Campbell model the child's typical stutter and have the child imitate and experiment with ways to modify it. Eventually, this modification evolves into an easy, relaxed approach with smooth movements.

Gregory and Campbell also believe it is important to deal with the intermediate stutterer's feelings and attitudes about his speech. By being supportive and understanding listeners, they encourage the child to explore any area of concern he may have about his problem. Gregory and Campbell recommend that any discussions with the child be concrete and related to specific events. In addition, Gregory and Campbell may teach the child to use voluntary disfluency if he is overly sensitive about his speech. This involves putting normal disfluencies, such as revisions and insertions, into his speech. They want the child to realize that some disfluency is a normal part of talking.

In terms of transferring the new speech patterns into the child's environment, Gregory and Campbell teach the child's parents to model ERA-SM in their speech and to reinforce their child's use of it at home. They also work with the child's classroom teacher so that she or he understands the child's therapy and can be supportive of it. Finally, to help the child maintain his improvement, Gregory and Campbell recommend that the child have monthly rechecks for 12 to 18 months following intensive therapy.

MERYL WALL AND FLORENCE MYERS

We previously discussed Meryl Wall and Florence Myers' (1984) treatment procedures for the beginning stutterer in Chapter 10. As will be recalled, they believe that stuttering results from a lack of synergism between psycholinguistic, physiological, and psychosocial factors in children and that all three factors need to be taken into account in treatment. Because their clinical procedures for the intermediate stutterer include the procedures they use with the beginning stutterer, we will briefly describe these procedures at this time. For additional information, the reader may wish to review the discussion in Chapter 10. We will then describe the additional clinical procedures that we believe Wall and Myers would use in their treatment of the intermediate stutterer.

In their treatment of the beginning stutterer, Wall and Myers control the length and semantic-syntactic complexity of the child's utterances. They typically begin by eliciting one- or two-word utterances and then gradually build to conversation. The child needs to be fluent at one level of linguistic difficulty before he can move on to the next. During these activities, Wall and Myers provide the child with an "easy speech" model to facilitate fluency. This is characterized by a slow-normal rate, relaxed articulation, gentle voice onset, and slightly reduced volume. If the child still has stutters on some words, Wall and Myers will teach the child to modify these stutters. For example, they may teach the child to use a Van Riper pull-out. They will also share information about stuttering with the child's parents and help them reduce fluency disrupters in the home.

In addition to these treatment procedures for the beginning stutterer, Wall and Myers do several other things with the intermediate stutterer. They all deal with the psychosocial, or feelings and attitudes, aspects of the problem. First of all, they state that this child "knows" he stutters and that it is important to openly deal with this in therapy. They suggest that not acknowledging it would be insensitive. Wall and Myers believe the child will be relieved by this openness.

Second, Wall and Myers believe it is important to deal with the intermediate stutterer's word and situation fears and avoidances. They begin to work on these fears and avoidances after the child has developed some increased fluency and has gained some control over his blocks. In dealing with situation avoidances, Wall and Myers employ hierarchies. For example, if a child is afraid of reading aloud in front of his class, they role-play this situation with him in therapy. They have the child practice using pull-outs while standing up and reading to them in therapy. They then have some other children come to therapy with the child, and they have him practice using pull-outs while standing up and reading to these children. Finally, with the cooperation of the classroom teacher, Wall and Myers have the child use pull-outs while reading aloud to his entire class.

Third, Wall and Myers believe it is important to work on the intermediate stutterer's response to teasing. They deal with teasing through discussion and role-playing with the child. They take turns being the teaser and the teased. They help the child explore alternate ways to respond to being teased and help him gain insight into the motives of the teaser. Eventually, they want the child to be able to respond calmly with an appropriate statement that defuses the teaser.

SUMMARY OF INTEGRATION OF APPROACHES

At the beginning of this chapter, we stated that clinicians who integrate stuttering modification and fluency shaping therapies for the intermediate stutterer combine or modify their therapies for the advanced and/or beginning stutterer when working with the intermediate stutterer. In other words, they do not have a totally unique therapy for the intermediate stutterer. We also said that stuttering modification and fluency shaping therapies for the intermediate stutterer differ the most on two clinical issues: (a) the speech behaviors targeted in therapy and (b) the attention given to reducing negative feelings and attitudes. From the discussion of our treatment procedures and from the review of Gregory and Campbell's and Wall and Myers' clinical procedures, the reader should see that it is possible to combine or modify clinical procedures used with either advanced or beginning stutterers when working with the intermediate stutterer. The reader should also recognize that it is possible to do this with regard to the speech behaviors targeted in therapy and with regard to reducing negative feelings and attitudes. None of the above clinicians integrated their clinical procedures in exactly the same way, but they all did integrate procedures from both stuttering modification and fluency shaping therapies.

STUDY QUESTIONS

1/   List the 4 phases in Peters and Guitar's treatment for the intermediate stutterer. What is the goal for each of these phases?

2/   List and briefly describe the clinical procedures involved in Peters and Guitar's understanding stuttering phase.

3/   How do Peters and Guitar decide which fluency shaping procedure to use in the using fluency enhancing behaviors and modifying the moments of stuttering phase?

4/   What procedures do Peters and Guitar use to transfer the fluency out of the clinical setting in the using fluency enhancing behaviors and modifying the moments of stuttering phase?

5/   List and briefly describe the clinical procedures involved in Peters and Guitar's reducing negative feelings and attitudes and eliminating avoidances phase.

6/   Briefly describe the clinical procedures involved in Peters and Guitar's maintaining fluency phase.

7/   Describe Peters and Guitar's counseling with the parents of the intermediate stutterer.

8/   Describe Peters and Guitar's counseling with the classroom teacher.

Suggested Readings

Turnbaugh, K. R. & Guitar, B. E. (1981). Short-term intensive stuttering treatment in a public school setting. *Language, Speech, and Hearing Services in Schools, 12,* 107–114.
    This article describes an integrated treatment program for an intermediate stutterer in which the reducing negative feelings and attitudes and eliminating avoidances phase precedes the using fluency enhancing skills and modifying the moments of stuttering phase. This is the reverse of the sequence discussed in this chapter.

Wall, M. J. & Myers, F. L. (1984). Therapy for the child stutterer. In M. J. Wall & F. L. Myers, *Clinical management of childhood stuttering* (pp. 179–227). Baltimore: University Park Press.
    We already recommended this excellent chapter at the end of Chapter 10. We recommend it again as an example of how the clinician can integrate stuttering modification and fluency shaping procedures with the intermediate stutterer.

REFERENCES

Adams, M. (1977). A clinical strategy for differentiating the normally nonfluent child and the incipient stutterer. *Journal of Fluency Disorders, 2*, 141-148.

Adams, M. R. (1980). The young stutterer: Diagnosis, treatment and assessment of progress. *Seminars in Speech, Language and Hearing, 1*, 289-299.

Adams, M. R., & Hayden, P. (1976). The ability of stutterers and nonstutterers to initiate and terminate phonation during production of an isolated vowel. *Journal of Speech and Hearing Research, 19*, 290-296.

Adams, M. R., & Runyan, C. M. (1981). Stuttering and fluency: Exclusive events or points on a continuum? *Journal of Fluency Disorders, 6*, 197-218.

Alfonso, P.J., Story, R.S., & Watson, B.C. (1987). The organization of supralaryngeal articulation in stutterers' fluent speech production: A second report. *Annual Bulletin Research Institute of Logopedics and Phoniatrics, 21*, 117-129.

Allen, S. (1988). *Durations of segments in repetitive disfluencies in stuttering and nonstuttering children*. Unpublished manuscript, E.M. Luse Center, University of Vermont, Burlington, VT.

Andrews, G., Craig, A., Feyer, A.-M., Hoddinott, S., Howie, P., & Neilson, M. (1983). Stuttering: A review of research findings and theories circa 1982. *Journal of Speech and Hearing Disorders, 48*, 226-246.

Andrews, G. & Cutler, J. (1974). Stuttering therapy: The relation between changes in symptom level and attitudes. *Journal of Speech and Hearing Disorders, 39*, 312-319.

Andrews, G., & Harris, M. (1964). *The syndrome of stuttering*. Clinics in Developmental Medicine, no. 17. London: Spastics Society Medical Education and Information Unit in association with W. Heinemann Medical Books.

Andrews, G., Howie, P.M., Dozsa, M., & Guitar, B.E. (1982). Stuttering: Speech pattern characteristics under fluency-inducing conditions. *Journal of Speech and Hearing Research, 25*, 208-216.

Andrews, G. & Ingham, R. (1971). Stuttering: Considerations in the evaluation of treatment. *British Journal of Communication Disorders, 6*, 129-138.

Andrews, G., Morris-Yates, A., Howie, P., & Martin, N.G. (in press). The genetic nature of stuttering. *British Medical Journal*.

Bernstein, N.E. (1981). Are there constraints on childhood disfluency? *Journal of Fluency Disorders, 6*, 341-350.

Bernstein-Ratner, N., & Sih, C.C. (1987). Effects of gradual increases in sentence length and complexity on children's dysfluency. *Journal of Speech and Hearing Research, 52*, 278-287.

Bernthal, J. & Bankson, N. (1988). *Articulation and phonological disorders*. Englewood Cliffs: Prentice-Hall.

Berry, M.F. (1937). *The medical history of stuttering children*. Unpublished doctoral dissertation, University of Wisconsin, Madison.

Berry, M.F. (1938). Developmental history of stuttering children. *Journal of Pediatrics, 12*, 209-217.

Bloch, E.L. & Goodstein, L.D. (1971). Functional speech disorders and personality: A decade of research. *Journal of Speech and Hearing Disorders, 36,* 295-314.

Bloodstein, O. (1944). Studies in the psychology of stuttering: XIX. The relationship between oral reading rate and severity of stuttering. *Journal of Speech Disorders, 9,* 161-173.

Bloodstein, O. (1948). *Conditions under which stuttering is reduced or absent.* Unpublished doctoral dissertation, University of Iowa, Iowa City.

Bloodstein, O. (1950). Hypothetical conditions under which stuttering is reduced or absent. *Journal of Speech and Hearing Disorders, 15,* 142-153.

Bloodstein, O. (1958). Stuttering as an anticipatory struggle reaction. In J. Eisenson (Ed.), *Stuttering: A symposium.* New York: Harper & Row.

Bloodstein, O. (1975). Stuttering as tension and fragmentation. In J. Eisenson (Ed.), *Stuttering: A second symposium.* New York: Harper & Row.

Bloodstein, O. (1987). *A handbook on stuttering.* Chicago: National Easter Seal Society.

Boberg, E. (1984). Intensive adult/teen therapy program. In W. H. Perkins (Ed.), *Stuttering disorders.* New York: Thieme-Stratton.

Boone, D. (1983). *The voice and voice therapy.* Englewood Cliffs: Prentice-Hall.

Bouton, M.E., & Bolles, R.C. (1985). Contexts, event-memories, and extinction. In P.D. Balsam & A. Tomie (Eds.), *Context and learning.* Hillsdale, N.J.: Lawrence Erlbaum Associates.

Branigan, G. (1979). Some reasons why successive single word utterances are not. *Journal of Child Language, 6,* 411-421.

Brown, S.F. (1937). The influence of grammatical function on the incidence of stuttering. *Journal of Speech Disorders, 2,* 207-215.

Brown, S.F. (1938a). A further study of stuttering in relation to various speech sounds. *Quarterly Journal of Speech, 24,* 390-397.

Brown, S.F. (1938b). Stuttering with relation to word accent and word position. *Journal of Abnormal Social Psychology, 33,* 112-120.

Brown, S.F. (1938c). The theoretical importance of certain factors influencing the incidence of stuttering. *Journal of Speech Disorders, 3,* 223-230.

Brown, S.F. (1943). An analysis of certain data concerning loci of "stutterings" from the viewpoint of general semantics. *Papers from the Second American Congress of General Semantics, 2,* 194-199.

Brown, S.F. (1945). The loci of stutterings in the speech sequence. *Journal of Speech Disorders, 10,* 181-192.

Brown, S.F. & Moren, A. (1942). The frequency of stuttering in relation to word length during oral reading. *Journal of Speech Disorders, 7,* 153-159.

Brutten, G.J. (1970). Two-factor behavior theory and therapy. In *Conditioning in stuttering therapy: Applications and limitations.* Memphis: Speech Foundation of America.

Brutten, G.J. (1975). Stuttering: Topography, assessment and behavior change strategies. In J. Eisenson (Ed.), *Stuttering: A second symposium.* New York: Harper & Row.

Brutten, G.J. & Dunham, S. (1989). The Communication Attitude Test: A normative study of grade school children. *Journal of Fluency Disorders, 14,* 371-377.

Brutten, G.J. & Shoemaker, D. (1967). *The modification of stuttering.* Englewood Cliffs: Prentice-Hall.

Caruso, A.J. (1988). Childhood stuttering: A review of behavioral, acoustical, and physiological research. *Asha, 30,* 73. Abstract.

Clarke-Stewart, A. & Friedman, S. (1987). *Child development: Infancy through adolescence*. New York: John Wiley & Sons.

Colburn, N., & Mysak, E.D. (1982a). Developmental disfluency and emerging grammar. I. Disfluency characteristics in early syntactic utterances. *Journal of Speech and Hearing Research*, 25, 414-420.

Colburn, N., & Mysak, E.D. (1982b). Developmental disfluency and emerging grammar. II. Co-occurrence of disfluency with specified semantic-syntactic structures. *Journal of Speech and Hearing Research*, 25, 421-427.

Colcord, R.D., & Adams, M.R. (1979). Voicing duration and vocal SPL changes associated with stuttering reduction during singing. *Journal of Speech and Hearing Research*, 22, 468-479.

Conture, E. G. (1982). *Stuttering*. Englewood Cliffs: Prentice-Hall.

Conture, E.G. (1990). *Stuttering* (2nd ed.). Englewood Cliffs: Prentice-Hall.

Conture, E. & Fraser, J. (1989). *Stuttering and your child: Questions and answers*. Memphis: Speech Foundation of America.

Conture, E.G., McCall, G.N., & Brewer, D.W. (1977). Laryngeal behavior during stuttering. *Journal of Speech and Hearing Research*, 20, 661-668.

Conture, E., Rothenberg, R., & Molitor, R. (1986). Electroglottographic observations of young stutterers' fluency. *Journal of Speech and Hearing Research*, 29, 384-393.

Cooper, E. B. (1979). *Understanding stuttering: Information for parents*. Chicago: National Easter Seal Society.

Costello, J. M. (1980). Operant conditioning and the treatment of stuttering. *Seminars in Speech, Language and Hearing*, 1, 311-325.

Costello, J. M. (1983). Current behavioral treatments for children. In D. Prins & R. J. Ingham (Eds.), *Treatment of stuttering in early childhood: Methods and issues*. San Diego: College-Hill Press.

Cox, N.J., Seider, R.A., & Kidd, K.K. (1984). Some environmental factors and hypotheses for stuttering in families with several stutterers. *Journal of Speech and Hearing Research*, 27, 543-548.

Cross, D.E., & Luper, H.L. (1979). Voice reaction time of stuttering and nonstuttering children and adults. *Journal of Fluency Disorders*, 4, 59-77.

Crystal, D. (1987). Towards a "bucket" theory of language disability: Taking account of interaction between linguistic levels. *Clinical Linguistics and Phonetics*, 1, 7-22.

Cullinan, W.L., & Springer, M.T. (1980). Voice initiation times in stuttering and nonstuttering children. *Journal of Speech and Hearing Research*, 23, 344-360.

Curlee, R. (1980). A case selection strategy for young disfluent children. In W.H. Perkins (Ed.), *Strategies in stuttering therapy*. Seminars in Speech, Language, and Hearing. New York: Thieme-Stratton.

Curlee, R. F., & Perkins, W. H. (1969). Conversational rate control therapy for stuttering. *Journal of Speech and Hearing Disorders*, 34, 245-250.

Curlee, R. F., & Perkins, W. H. (1984). Preface. In R. F. Curlee & W. H. Perkins (Eds.), *Nature and treatment of stuttering: New directions*. San Diego: College-Hill Press.

Dalton, P., & Hardcastle, W.J. (1977). *Disorders of fluency*. New York: Elsevier.

Daly, D. (1986). The clutterer. In K. St. Louis (Ed.), *The atypical stutterer*. New York: Academic Press.

Darley, F.L. (1955). The relationship of parental attitudes and adjustments to the development of stuttering. In W. Johnson & R.R. Leutenegger (Eds.), *Stuttering in children and adults*. Minneapolis: University of Minnesota Press.

Darley, F. & Spriestersbach, D. (1978). *Diagnostic methods in speech pathology* (2nd ed.). New York: Harper & Row.

Davis, D.M. (1940). The relation of repetitions in the speech of young children to certain measures of language maturity and situational factors: Part II & III. *Journal of Speech Disorders, 5,* 235-246.

DeJoy, D.A., & Gregory, H.H. (1973). The relationship of children's disfluencies to the syntax, length, and vocabulary of their sentences. *Asha, 15,* 472. Abstract.

DeJoy, D.A., & Gregory, H.H. (1985). The relationship between age and frequency of disfluency in preschool children. *Journal of Fluency Disorders, 10,* 107-122.

Dell, C. (1979). *Treating the school age stutterer: A guide for clinicians.* Memphis: Speech Foundation of America.

DeNil, L. & Brutten, E. (in press). Speech-associated attitudes of stuttering and normally fluent children: A normative investigation. *Journal of Speech and Hearing Disorders.*

DiSimoni, F.G. (1974). Preliminary study of certain timing relationships in the speech of stutterers. *Journal of the Acoustical Society of America, 56,* 695-696.

Emerick, L. & Haynes, W. (1986). *Diagnosis and evaluation in speech pathology* (3rd ed.). Englewood Cliffs: Prentice-Hall.

Fibiger, S. (1971). Stuttering explained as a physiological tremor. *Quarterly Progress and Status Report, 2-3,* Speech Transmission Laboratory, Royal Institute of Technology, Stockholm, Sweden.

Flugel, F. (1979). Erhebungen von Personlichkeitsmerk-malen an Muttern stotternder Kinder und Jugendicher. *dsh Abstracts, 19,* 226.

Frankenburg, W.K., & Dodds, J.B. (1967). The Denver Developmental Screening Test. *Journal of Pediatrics, 71,* 181-191.

Fraser, J., & Perkins, W.H. (Eds.), (1987). *Do you stutter: A guide for teens.* Memphis: Speech Foundation of America.

Freeman, F.J. (1988). Gestural analysis of stuttering. *Asha, 30,* 121. Abstract.

Freeman, F.J., & Ushijima, T. (1975). Laryngeal activity accompanying the moment of stuttering: A preliminary report of EMG investigations. *Journal of Fluency Disorders, 1,* 36-45.

Freeman, F.J., & Ushijima, T. (1978). Laryngeal muscle activity during stuttering. *Journal of Speech and Hearing Research, 21,* 538-562.

Geschwind, N., & Galaburda, A.M. (1985). Cerebral lateralization: Biological mechanisms, associations, and pathology: I. A hypothesis and a program for research. *Archives of Neurology, 42,* 429-459.

Gibson, E. (1972). Reading for some purpose. In J.F. Kavanaugh & I. Mattingly (Eds.), *Language by ear and by eye.* Cambridge: MIT Press.

Glasner, P. & Rosenthal, D. (1957). Parental diagnosis of stuttering in young children. *Journal of Speech and Hearing Disorders, 22,* 288-295.

Goldman-Eisler, F. (1968). *Psycholinguistcs: Experiments in spontaneous speech.* New York: Academic Press.

Goodstein, L.D. (1956). MMPI profiles of stutterers' parents: A follow-up study. *Journal of Speech and Hearing Disorders, 21,* 430-435.

Goodstein, L.D., & Dahlstrom, W.G. (1956). MMPI differences between parents of stuttering and nonstuttering children. *Journal of Consulting Psychology, 20,* 365-370.

Gordon, P.A., Luper, H.L., & Peterson, H.A. (1986). The effects of syntactic complexity on the occurrence of disfluencies in 5 year old stutterers. *Journal of Fluency Disorders, 11,* 151-164.

Gottwald, S., & Starkweather, C.W. (1985. November). *The prognosis of stuttering*. Miniseminar presented at the meeting of the American Speech and Hearing Association, Washington.

Gottwald, S., & Starkweather, C.W. (1984. November). *Stuttering prevention: Rationale and method*. Short course presented at the meeting of the American Speech and Hearing Association, San Francisco.

Gray, J.A. (1987). *The psychology of fear and stress* (2nd ed.). Cambridge: Cambridge University Press.

Gregory, H. H. (1968). Application of learning theory concepts in the management of stuttering. In H. H. Gregory (Ed.), *Learning theory and stuttering therapy*. Evanston, IL: Northwestern University Press.

Gregory, H. H. (1979). Controversial issues: Statement and review of the literature. In H. H. Gregory (Ed.), *Controversies about stuttering therapy*. Baltimore: University Park Press.

Gregory, H. H. (1984a). Prevention of stuttering: Management of early stages. In R. F. Curlee & W. H. Perkins (Eds.), *Nature and treatment of stuttering: New directions*. San Diego: College-Hill Press.

Gregory, H. H. (1984b). Stuttering therapy for children. In W. H. Perkins (Ed.), *Stuttering disorders*. New York: Thieme-Stratton.

Gregory, H. H. (1986a). *Stuttering: Differential evaluation and therapy*. Austin, TX: Pro-Ed.

Gregory, H. H. (1986b). Environmental manipulation and family counseling. In G. H. Shames & H. Rubin (Eds.), *Stuttering: Then and now*. Columbus: Charles E. Merrill.

Gregory, H. H., & Campbell, J. H. (1988). Stuttering in the school-age child. In D. E. Yoder & R. D. Kent (Eds.), *Decision making in speech-language pathology*. Toronto: B.C. Decker.

Gregory, H. H., & Hill, D. (1980). Stuttering therapy for children. *Seminars in Speech, Language and Hearing, 1*, 351-363.

Guitar, B. (1976). Pretreatment factors associated with the outcome of stuttering therapy. *Journal of Speech and Hearing Research, 19*, 590-600.

Guitar, B. (1979). A response to Ingham's critique. *Journal of Speech and Hearing Disorders, 44*. 400-403.

Guitar, B. (1981). Stuttering. In J. Darby (Ed.), *Speech evaluation in medicine*. New York: Grune & Stratton.

Guitar, B. (1982). Fluency shaping with young stutterers. *Journal of Childhood Communication Disorders, 6*, 50-59.

Guitar, B., & Bass, C. (1978). Stuttering therapy: The relation between attitude change and long-term outcome. *Journal of Speech and Hearing Disorders, 43*, 392-400.

Guitar, B. & Conture, E. (undated). *If you think your child is stuttering . . .* Memphis: Speech Foundation of America.

Guitar, B. & Grims, S. (1977. November). *Developing a scale to assess communication attitudes in children who stutter*. Poster session presented at American Speech-Hearing-Language Association Convention, Atlanta, Georgia.

Guitar, B., Guitar, C., Neilson, P.D., O'Dwyer, N., & Andrews, G. (1988). Onset sequencing of selected lip muscles in stutterers and nonstutterers. *Journal of Speech and Hearing Research, 31*, 28-35.

Guitar, B., & Peters, T.J. (1980). *Stuttering: An integration of contemporary therapies*. Memphis: Speech Foundation of America. [publication no. 16]

Hall, J.W., & Jerger, J. (1978). Central auditory function in stutterers. *Journal of Speech and Hearing Research, 21*, 324-337.

Hammond, G.R. (1982). Hemispheric differences in temporal resolution. *Brain and Cognition, 1*, 95-118.

Haynes, W.O., & Hood, S.B. (1978). Disfluency changes in children as a function of the systematic modification of linguistic complexity. *Journal of Communication Disorders, 11*, 79-93.

Helm-Estabrooks, N. (1986). Diagnosis and management of neurogenic stuttering in adults. In K. St. Louis (Ed.), *The atypical stutterer*. New York: Academic Press.

Hill, H.E. (1954). An experimental study of disorganization of speech and manual responses in normal subjects. *Journal of Speech and Hearing Disorders, 19*, 295-305.

Hillman, R.E., & Gilbert, H.R. (1977). Voice onset time for voiceless stop consonants in the fluent reading of stutterers and nonstutterers. *Journal of the Acoustical Society of America, 61*, 610-611.

Hiscock, M., & Kinsbourne, M. (1977). Selective listening asymmetry in preschool children. *Developmental Psychology, 13*, 217-224.

Hiscock, M., & Kinsbourne, M. (1980). Asymmetry of verbal-manual time sharing in children: A follow-up study. *Neuropsychologia, 18*, 151-162.

Hoffman, P, Schuckers, G., & Daniloff, R. (1989). *Children's phonetic disorders: Theory and treatment*. Boston: College-Hill.

Howie, P.M. (1981). Concordance for stuttering in monozygotic and dizygotic twin pairs. *Journal of Speech and Hearing Research, 24*, 317-321.

Ingham, R.J. (1979). Comment on "Stuttering therapy: The relation between attitude change and long-term outcome." *Journal of Speech and Hearing Disorders, 44*, 397-400.

Jacobson, E. (1938). *Progressive relaxation*. Chicago: University of Chicago Press.

Jaffe, J., & Anderson, S.W. (1979). Prescript to Chapter 1: Communication rhythms and the evolution of language. In A.W. Siegman & S. Feldman (Eds.), *Of speech and time: Temporal speech patterns in interpersonal contexts*. Hillsdale, N.J.: Lawrence Erlbaum Associates.

Johnson, W. (1955). A study of the onset and development of stuttering. In W. Johnson & R.R. Leutenegger (Eds.), *Stuttering in children and adults*. Minneapolis: University of Minnesota Press.

Johnson, W. and associates (1959). *The onset of stuttering*. Minneapolis: University of Minnesota Press.

Johnson, W. *et al.* (1942). A study of the onset and development of stuttering. *Journal of Speech Disorders, 7*, 251-257.

Johnson, W., & Brown, S.F. (1935). Stuttering in relation to various speech sounds. *Quarterly Journal of Speech, 21*, 481-496.

Johnson, W., Darley, F., & Spriestersbach, D.C. (1952). *Diagnostic manual in speech correction*. New York: Harper & Row.

Johnson, W., & Inness, M. (1939). Studies in the psychology of stuttering: XIII. A statistical analysis of the adaptation and consistency effects in relation to stuttering. *Journal of Speech Disorders, 4*, 79-86.

Johnson, W., & Knott, J.R. (1937). Studies in the psychology of stuttering: I. The distribution of moments of stuttering in successive readings of the same materials. *Journal of Speech Disorders, 2*, 17-19.

Johnson, W. & Leutenegger, R.R. (Eds.). (1955). *Stuttering in children and adults*. Minneapolis: University of Minnesota Press.

Johnson, W., & Rosen, L. (1937). Studies in the psychology of stuttering: VII. Effects of certain changes in speech pattern upon frequency of stuttering. *Journal of Speech Disorders, 2,* 105-109.

Johnson, W., & Solomon, A. (1937). Studies in the psychology of stuttering: IV. A quantitative study of expectation of stuttering as a process involving a low degree of consciousness. *Journal of Speech Disorders, 2,* 95-97.

Kagan, J. (1981). *The second year: The emergence of self-awareness.* Cambridge, MA: Harvard University Press.

Kagan, J., Reznick, J.S. & Snidman, N. (1987). The physiology and psychology of behavioral inhibition in children. *Child Development, 58,* 1459-1473.

Kasprisin-Burrelli, A., Egolf, D.B., & Shames, G.H. (1972). A comparison of parental verbal behavior with stuttering and nonstuttering children. *Journal of Communication Disorders, 5,* 335-346.

Kent, L.R., & Williams, D.E. (1963). Alleged former stutterers in grade two. *Asha, 5,* 772. Abstract.

Kent, R.D. (1981). Sensorimotor aspects of speech development. In R.D. Alberts & M.R. Peterson (Eds.), *The development of perception: Psycho-biological perspectives.* New York: Academic Press.

Kent, R.D. (1983). Facts about stuttering: Neuropsychologic perspectives. *Journal of Speech and Hearing Disorders, 48,* 249-255.

Kent, R.D. (1984). Stuttering as a temporal programming disorder. In R.F. Curlee & W.H. Perkins (Eds.), *Nature and treatment of stuttering: New directions.* San Diego: College-Hill Press.

Kent, R.D. (1985). Developing and disordered speech: Strategies for organization. *ASHA Reports, 15,* 29-37.

Kent, R.D. & Perkins, W. (1984). Oral-verbal fluency: Aspects of verbal formulation, speech motor control and underlying neural systems. Unpublished manuscript.

Kenyon, E.L. (1942). The etiology of stammering: Fundamentally a wrong psycho-physiologic habit in control of the vocal cords for the production of an individual speech sound. *Journal of Speech Disorders, 7,* 97-104.

Kidd, K.K. (1977). A genetic perspective on stuttering. *Journal of Fluency Disorders, 2,* 259-269.

Kidd, K.K. (1984). Stuttering as a genetic disorder. In R.F. Curlee & W.H. Perkins (Eds.), *Nature and treatment of stuttering: New directions.* San Diego: College-Hill Press.

Kidd, K.K., Kidd, J.R., & Records, M.A. (1978). The possible causes of the sex ratio in stuttering and its implications. *Journal of Fluency Disorders, 3,* 13-23.

Kidd, K.K., Reich, T., and Kessler, S. (1973) *Genetics, 74,* (No.2, Part 2): s137.

Kinsbourne, M., & Hicks, R. (1978). Functional cerebral space: A model for overflow, transfer and interference effects in human performance: A tutorial review. In M. Kinsbourne (Ed.), *Asymmetrical function of the brain.* Cambridge: Cambridge University Press.

Kline, M.L., & Starkweather, C.W. (1979). Receptive and expressive language performance in young stutterers. *Asha, 21,* 797. Abstract.

Knott, J.R., Johnson, W., & Webster, M.J. (1937). Studies in the psychology of stuttering: II. A quantitative evaluation of expectation of stuttering in relation to the occurrence of stuttering. *Journal of Speech Disorders, 2,* 20-22.

Kramer, M.B., Green, D., & Guitar, B. (1987). A comparison of stutterers and nonstutterers on masking level differences and synthetic sentence identification tasks *Journal of Communication Disorders, 20,* 379-390.

Liberman, A.M., Cooper, F.S., Sharkweiler, D.S., & Studdert-Kennedy, M. (1967). Perception of the Speech Code. *Psychological Review, 74,* 431-461.

Lidz, T. (1968). *The person: His development throughout the life cycle.* New York: Basic Books.

Luchsinger, R. (1944). Biological studies on monozygotic and dizygotic twins relative to size and form of the larynx. *Archive Julius Klaus-Stiftung fur Verergungsforschung, 19,* 3-4.

Lund, N. & Duchan, J. (1988). *Assessing children's language in naturalistic contexts* (2nd ed.). Englewood Cliffs: Prentice-Hall.

Luper, H. L., & Mulder, R. L. (1964). *Stuttering: Therapy for children.* Englewood Cliffs: Prentice-Hall.

Mahr, G. & Leith, W. (1990). Psychogenic acquired stuttering. Manuscript submitted for publication.

Malecot, A., Johnston, R., & Kizziar, P.A. (1972). Syllabic rate and utterance length in French. *Phonetica, 26,* 235-251.

Martin, R., & Haroldson, S.K. (1979). Effects of five experimental treatments on stuttering. *Journal of Speech and Hearing Research, 22,* 132-146.

McClean, M., Goldsmith, H., & Cerf, A. (1984). Lower-lip EMG and displacement during bilabial dysfluencies in adult stutterers. *Journal of Speech and Hearing Research, 27,* 342-349.

McDearmon, J.R. (1968). Primary stuttering at the onset of stuttering: A reexamination of data. *Journal of Speech and Hearing Research, 11,* 631-637.

McFarland, D.H., & Moore, W.H. Jr. (1982. November). *Alpha hemispheric asymmetries during an electromyographic feedback procedure for stuttering.* Paper presented to the Annual Convention of the American Speech and Hearing Association.

McLoughlin, J. & Lewis, R. (1990). *Assessing special students* (3rd ed.). Columbus, OH: Merrill.

Merits-Patterson, R., & Reed, C.G. (1981). Disfluencies in the speech of language-delayed children. *Journal of Speech and Hearing Research, 24,* 55-58.

Meyers, S.C., & Freeman, F.J. (1985a). Interruptions as a variable in stuttering and disfluency. *Journal of Speech and Hearing Research, 28,* 428-435.

Meyers, S.C., & Freeman, F.J. (1985b). Mother and child speech rate as a variable in stuttering and disfluency. *Journal of Speech and Hearing Research, 28,* 436-444.

Milisen, R. (1938). Frequency of stuttering with anticipation of stuttering controlled. *Journal of Speech Disorders, 3,* 207-214.

Miller, J. (1981). *Assessing language production in children.* Baltimore: University Park Press.

Mineka, S. (1985). Animal models of anxiety-based disorders: Their usefulness and limitations. In A.H. Tuma & J. Mase (Eds.), *Anxiety and the anxiety disorders.* Hillsdale, N.J.: Lawrence Erlbaum Associates.

Moncur, J.P. (1952). Parental domination in stuttering. *Journal of Speech and Hearing Disorders, 17,* 155-165.

Moore, W.H., Jr. (1984). Central nervous system characteristics of stutterers. In R.F. Curlee & W.H. Perkins (Eds.), *Nature and treatment of stuttering: New directions.* San Diego: College-Hill Press.

Moore, W.H., Jr., & Haynes, W.O. (1980). Alpha hemispheric asymmetry and stuttering: Some support for a segmentation dysfunction hypothesis. *Journal of Speech and Hearing Research, 23,* 229-247.

Morgenstern, J.J. (1956). Socioeconomic factors in stuttering. *Journal of Speech and Hearing Disorders, 21,* 25-33.

Morrell, F. (1961). Electrophysiological contributions to the neural basis of learning. *Physiological Reviews, 41,* 443-494.

Murray, H.L., & Reed, C.G. (1977). Language abilities of preschool stuttering children. *Journal of Fluency Disorders, 2,* 171-176.

Neilson, M.D. (1980). *Stuttering and the control of speech: A systems analysis ap-*

proach. Unpublished doctoral dissertation. University of New South Wales, Kensington, Australia.

Neilson, M.D. & Neilson, P. (1987). Speech motor control and stuttering: A computational model of adaptive sensory-motor processing. *Speech Communication, 6,* 325-333.

Neilson, P.D., Neilson, M.D., & O'Dwyer, N.J. (1982). Acquistion of motor skills in tracking tasks: Learning internal models. In D.G. Russell & B. Abernethy (Eds.), *Motor memory and control: The Otago symposium, Dunedin, New Zealand, 1982*. Dunedin: Human Performance Associates.

Neilson, P.D., Quinn, P.T., & Neilson, M.D. (1976). Auditory tracking measures of hemispheric asymmetry in normals and stutterers. *Australian Journal of Human Communication, 4,* 121-126.

Netsell, R. (1981). The acquisition of speech motor control: A perspective with direction for research. In E. Stark (Ed.), *Language behavior in infancy and early childhood*. New York: Elsevier-North Holland.

Nittrouer, S., Studdert-Kennedy, M., & McGowan, R.S. (1989). The emergence of phonetic segments: Evidence from the spectral structure of fricative-vowel syllables spoken by children and adults. *Journal of Speech and Hearing Research, 32,* 120-132.

Nudelman, H.B., Herbrich, K.E., Hoyt, B.D., & Rosenfield, D.B. (1987). Dynamic characteristics of vocal frequency tracking in stutterers and nonstutterers. In: H.F.M. Peters & W. Hulstijn (Eds.), *Speech motor dynamics in stuttering*. New York: Springer-Verlag.

Pearl, S.Z., & Bernthal, J.E. (1980). The effect of grammatical complexity upon disfluency behavior of nonstuttering preschool children. *Journal of Fluency Disorders, 5,* 55-68.

Perkins, W. H. (1973a). Replacement of stuttering with normal speech: I. Rationale. *Journal of Speech and Hearing Disorders, 38,* 283-294.

Perkins, W. H. (1973b). Replacement of stuttering with normal speech: II Clinical procedures. *Journal of Speech and Hearing Disorders, 38,* 295-303.

Perkins, W. H. (1979). From psychoanalysis to discoordination. In H. H. Gregory (Ed.), *Controversies about stuttering therapy*. Baltimore: University Park Press.

Perkins, W. H. (1981). An alternative to automatic fluency. In *Stuttering therapy: Transfer and maintenance*. Memphis: Speech Foundation of America.

Perkins, W. H. (1984). Techniques for establishing fluency. In W. H. Perkins (Ed.), *Stuttering disorders*. New York: Thieme-Stratton.

Perkins, W. H. (1986). Postscript: Discoordination of phonation with articulation and respiration. In G. H. Shames & H. Rubin (Eds.), *Stuttering: Then and now*. Columbus: Charles E. Merrill.

Perkins, W., Rudas, J., Johnson, L., & Bell, J. (1976). Stuttering: Discoordination of phonation with articulation and respiration. *Journal of Speech and Hearing Research, 19,* 509-522.

Peters, H.F.M. & Hulstijn, W. (Eds.). (1987). *Speech motor dynamics in stuttering*. New York: Springer-Verlag.

Peters, T. J. (1987). *Handouts for the advanced stutterer*. Unpublished material, University of Wisconsin-Eau Claire, Center for Communication Disorders, Eau Claire, WI.

Peterson, H. & Marquardt, T. (1990). *Appraisal and diagnosis of speech and language disorders* (2nd ed.). Englewood Cliffs: Prentice Hall.

Pindzola, R., Jenkins, M., & Lokken, K. (1989). Speaking rates of young children. *Language, Speech, and Hearing Services in Schools, 20,* 133-138.

Platt, J. and Basili, A. (1973). Jaw tremor during stuttering block: An electromyographic study. *Journal of Communication Disorders, 6,* 102-109.

Premack, D. (1959). Toward empirical behavior laws: 1. Positive reinforcement. *Psychology Review, 66*, 219-233.

Prins, D. (1984). Treatment of adults: Managing stuttering. In R. F. Curlee & W. H. Perkins (Eds.), *Nature and treatment of stuttering: New directions.* San Diego: College-Hill Press.

Riley, G. (1972). A stuttering severity instrument for children and adults. *Journal of Speech and Hearing Disorders, 37,* 314-322.

Riley, G. & Riley, J. (1979). A component model for diagnosing and treating children who stutter. *Journal of Fluency Disorders, 4,* 279-293.

Riley, G. D. & Riley, J. (1983). Evaluation as a basis for intervention. In D. Prins & R. J. Ingham (Eds.), *Treatment of stuttering in early childhood: Methods and issues.* San Diego: College-Hill Press.

Riley, G. D. & Riley, J. (1984). A component model for treating stuttering in children. In M. Peins (Ed.), *Contemporary approaches in stuttering therapy.* Boston: Little, Brown & Company.

Roessler, R. & Bolton, B. (1978). *Psychosocial adjustment to disability.* Baltimore: University Park Press.

Roth, C., Aronson, A., & Davis, L. (1989). Clinical studies in psychogenic stuttering of adult onset. *Journal of Speech and Hearing Disorders, 54,* 634-646.

Rumelhart, D., McClelland, J., & the PDP Research Group. (1986). Parallel distributed processing: Explorations in the microstructure of cognition. Cambridge, MA: MIT Press.

Ryan, B. P. (1971). Operant procedures applied to stuttering therapy for children. *Journal of Speech and Hearing Disorders, 36,* 264-280.

Ryan, B. P. (1974). *Programmed therapy of stuttering in children and adults.* Springfield, IL: Charles C. Thomas.

Ryan, B. P. (1979). Stuttering therapy in a framework of operant conditioning and programmed learning. In H. H. Gregory (Ed.), *Controversies about stuttering therapy.* Baltimore: University Park Press.

Ryan, B. P. (1984). Treatment of stuttering in school children. In W. H. Perkins (Ed.), *Stuttering disorders.* New York: Thieme-Stratton.

Ryan, B. P. (1986). Postscript: Operant therapy for children. In G. H. Shames & H. Rubin (Eds.), *Stuttering: Then and now.* Columbus: Charles E. Merrill.

Sackeim, H.A. & Gur, R.C. (1978). Lateral asymmetry in intensity of emotional expression. *Neuropsychologia, 16,* 437-481.

St. Louis, K. (Ed.). (1986). *The atypical stutterer.* New York: Academic Press.

St. Onge, K. (1963). The stuttering syndrome. *Journal of Speech and Hearing Research, 6,* 195-197.

St. Onge, K., & Calvert, J.J. (1964). Stuttering research. *Quarterly Journal of Speech, 50,* 159-165.

Schindler, M.D. (1955). A study of the educational adjustments of stuttering and nonstuttering children. In W. Johnson & R.R. Leutenegger (Eds.), *Stuttering in children and adults.* Minneapolis: University of Minnesota Press.

Schwartz, M.F. (1974). The core of the stuttering block. *Journal of Speech and Hearing Disorders, 39,* 169-177.

Seeman, M. (1937). The significance of twin pathology for the investigation of speech disorders. *Archive gesamte Phonetik 1,* Part II, 88-92.

Shames, G. H., & Florance, C. L. (1980). *Stutter-free speech: A goal for therapy.* Columbus: Charles E. Merrill.

Shapiro, A.I. (1980). An electromyographic analysis of the fluent and dysfluent utterances of several types of stutterers. *Journal of Fluency Disorders, 5,* 203-231.

Shapiro, A.I., & DeCicco, B.A. (1982). The relationship between normal dysfluency and stuttering: An old question revisited. *Journal of Fluency Disorders, 7,* 109-121.

Sheehan, J.G. (1953). Theory and treatment of stuttering as an approach-avoidance conflict. *Journal of Psychology, 36,* 27-49.

Sheehan, J.G. (1970). *Stuttering: Research and therapy.* New York: Harper & Row.

Sheehan, J.G. (1974). Stuttering behavior: A phonetic analysis. *Journal of Communication Disorders, 7,* 193-212.

Sheehan, J.G. (1975). Conflict theory and avoidance-reduction therapy. In J. Eisenson (Ed.), *Stuttering: A second symposium.* New York: Harper & Row.

Sheehan, J. G., & Sheehan, V. M. (1984). Avoidance-reduction therapy: A response suppression hypothesis. In W. H. Perkins (Ed.), *Stuttering disorders.* New York: Thieme-Stratton.

Shields, D. (1989). *Dead languages.* New York: Knopf.

Shine, R. E. (1980). Direct management of the beginning stutterer. *Seminars in Speech, Language and Hearing. 1,* 339-350.

Silverman, E.-M. (1974). Word position and grammatical function in relation to preschoolers' speech disfluency. *Perceptual Motor Skills, 39,* 267-272.

Silverman, F.H. (1988). The "monster" study. *Journal of Fluency Disorders, 13,* 225-231.

Solomon, R.L., & Wynne, L.C. (1953). Traumatic avoidance learning: Acquisition in normal dogs. *Psychological Monographs, 67,* 1-19.

Stark, R., Tallal, C., & McCauley, R. (1988). *Language, speech and reading disorders in children.* Boston: Little, Brown.

Starkweather. C. W. (1980). A multiprocess behavioral approach to stuttering therapy. *Seminars in Speech, Language and Hearing, 1,* 327-337.

Starkweather, C.W. (1981). Speech fluency and its development in normal children. In N. Lass (Ed.), *Speech and language: Advances in basic research and practice.* (Vol. 4). New York: Academic Press.

Starkweather, C.W. (1982). Stuttering and laryngeal behavior: A review. *ASHA Monographs, 22.*

Starkweather, C.W. (1983). *Speech and language: Principles and processes of behavior change.* Englewood Cliffs: Prentice Hall.

Starkweather, C. W. (1985). The development of fluency in normal children. In *Stuttering therapy: Prevention and intervention with children.* Memphis: Speech Foundation of America.

Starkweather, C.W. (1986). Talking with the parents of young stutterers. In *Counseling stutterers.* Memphis: Speech Foundation of America.

Starkweather, C.W. (1987). *Fluency and stuttering.* Englewood Cliffs: Prentice Hall.

Starkweather, C.W., Hirschman, P., & Tannenbaum, R.S. (1976). Latency of vocalization onset: Stutterers versus nonstutterers. *Journal of Speech and Hearing Research, 19,* 481-492.

Starkweather, C.W. & Myers, M. (1979). Duration of subsegments within the intervocalic interval in stutterers and nonstutterers. *Journal of Fluency Disorders, 4,* 205-214.

Stemberger, J.P. (1982). The nature of segments in the lexicon: Evidence from speech errors. *Lingua, 56,* 235-259.

Stocker, B., & Usprich, C. (1976). Stuttering in young children and level of demand. *Journal of Childhood Communication Disorders, 1,* 116-131.

Studdert-Kennedy, M. (1987). The phoneme as a perceptuomotor structure. In A. Allport, D. McKay, W. Prinz, &

E. Scheerer (Eds.), *Language perception and production*. London: Academic Press.

Till, J.A., Reich, A., Dickey, S., & Sieber, J. (1983). Phonatory and manual reaction times of stuttering and nonstuttering children. *Journal of Speech and Hearing Research, 26*, 171-180.

Toscher, M.M., & Rupp, R.R. (1978). A study of the central auditory processes in stutterers using the Synthetic Sentence Identification (SSI) test battery. *Journal of Speech and Hearing Research, 21*, 779-792.

Tudor, M. (1939). *An experimental study of the effect of evaluative labeling on speech fluency*. Unpublished master's thesis, University of Iowa, Iowa City.

Turnbaugh, K. R. & Guitar, B. E. (1981). Short-term intensive stuttering treatment in a public school setting. *Language, Speech, and Hearing Services in Schools, 12*, 107-114.

Turnbaugh, K.R., Guitar, B.E., & Hoffman, P.R. (1979). Speech clinicians' attribution of personality traits as a function of stuttering severity. *Journal of Speech and Hearing Research, 22*, 37-45.

Umeda, N. (1975). Vowel duration in American English. *Journal of the Acoustical Society of America, 58*, 434-445.

Umeda, N. (1977). Consonant duration in American English. *Journal of the Acoustical Society of America, 61*, 846-858.

Van Riper, C. (1936). Study of the thoracic breathing of stutterers during expectancy and occurrence of stuttering spasm. *Journal of Speech Disorders, 1*, 61-72.

Van Riper, C. (1971). *The nature of stuttering*. Englewood Cliffs: Prentice Hall.

Van Riper, C. (1973). *The treatment of stuttering*. Englewood Cliffs: Prentice Hall.

Van Riper, C. (1974). Modification of behavior. In *Therapy for stutterers*. Memphis: Speech Foundation of America.

Van Riper, C. (1982). *The nature of stuttering* (2nd ed.). Englewood Cliffs: Prentice Hall.

Van Riper, C., & Hull, C.J. (1955). The quantitative measurement of the effect of certain situations on stuttering. In W. Johnson & R.R. Leutenegger (Eds.), *Stuttering in children and adults*. Minneapolis: University of Minnesota Press.

Wall, M.J. (1980). A comparison of syntax in young stutterers and nonstutterers. *Journal of Fluency Disorders, 5*, 345-352.

Wall, M. J., & Myers, F. L. (1984). *Clinical management of childhood stuttering*. Baltimore: University Park Press.

Webster, R. L. (1974). A behavioral analysis of stuttering: Treatment and theory. In K. S. Calhoun, H. E. Adams, & K. M. Mitchell (Eds.), *Innovative treatment methods in psychopathology*. New York: Wiley.

Webster, R. L. (1979). Empirical considerations regarding stuttering therapy. In H. H. Gregory (Ed.), *Controversies about stuttering therapy*. Baltimore: University Park Press.

Webster, R. L. (1980). Evolution of a target-based behavioral therapy for stuttering. *Journal of Fluency Disorders, 5*, 303-320.

Weiss, C., Gordon, M, & Lillywhite, H. (1987). *Clinical management of articulatory and phonologic disorders* (2nd ed.). Baltimore: Williams & Wilkins.

Weiss, D.A. (1964). *Cluttering*. Englewood Cliffs: Prentice Hall.

West, R. (1931). The phenomenology of stuttering. In R. West (Ed.), *A symposium on stuttering*. Madison, WI: College Typing Company.

Wexler, K.B. & Mysak, E.D. (1982). Disfluency characteristics of 2-, 4- and 6-year old males. *Journal of Fluency Disorders, 7*, 37-46.

Wiig, E. & Semel, E. (1984). *Language assessment and intervention* (2nd ed.). Columbus: Charles Merrill.

Williams, D.E. (1957). A point of view about stuttering. *Journal of Speech and Hearing Disorders, 22,* 390-397.

Williams, D.E. (1971). Stuttering therapy for children. In L.E. Travis (Ed.), *Handbook of speech pathology.* New York: Appleton-Century-Crofts.

Williams, D.E. (1979). A perspective on approaches to stuttering therapy. In H.H. Gregory (Ed.), *Controversies about stuttering therapy.* Baltimore: University Park Press.

Williams, D.E., Melrose, B.M., & Woods, C.L. (1969). The relationship between stuttering and academic achievement in children. *Journal of Communication Disorders, 2,* 87-98.

Wilson, D. (1979). *Voice problems in children.* Baltimore: Williams & Wilkins.

Wingate, M.E. (1964). Recovery from stuttering. *Journal of Speech and Hearing Disorders, 29,* 312-321.

Wingate, M.E. (1969). Sound and pattern in "artificial" fluency. *Journal of Speech and Hearing Research, 12,* 677-686.

Wingate, M.E. (1970). Effect on stuttering of changes in audition. *Journal of Speech and Hearing Research, 13,* 861-873.

Wingate, M.E. (1983). Speaking unassisted: Comments on a paper by Andrews *et al. Journal of Speech and Hearing Disorders, 48,* 255-263.

Wingate, M.E. (1988). *The structure of stuttering: A psycholinguistic approach.* New York: Springer-Verlag.

Winitz, H. (1961). Repetitions in the vocalizations and speech of children in the first two years of life. *Journal of Speech and Hearing Disorders, Monograph Supplement, 7,* 55-62.

Wood, F., Stump, D., McKeehan, A., Sheldon, S., & Proctor, J. (1980). Patterns of regional cerebral blood flow during attempted reading aloud by stutterers both on and off haloperidol medication: Evidence for inadequate left frontal activation during stuttering. *Brain and Language, 9,* 141-144.

Woods, C.L., & Williams, D.E. (1976). Traits attributed to stuttering and normally fluent males. *Journal of Speech and Hearing Research, 19,* 267-278.

Woolf, G. (1967). The assessment of stuttering as struggle, avoidance, and expectancy. *British Journal of Disorders of Communication, 2,* 158-171.

Yairi, E. (1981). Disfluencies of normally speaking two-year old children. *Journal of Speech and Hearing Research, 24,* 490-495.

Yairi, E. (1982). Longitudinal studies of disfluencies in two-year-old children. *Journal of Speech and Hearing Research, 25,* 155-160.

Yairi, E. (1983). The onset of stuttering in two- and three-year old children: A preliminary report. *Journal of Speech and Hearing Disorders, 48,* 171-178.

Yairi, E., & Lewis, B. (1984). Disfluencies at the onset of stuttering. *Journal of Speech and Hearing Research, 27,* 154-159.

Young, M.A. (1981). A reanalysis of "Stuttering therapy: The relation between attitude change and long-term outcome." *Journal of Speech and Hearing Disorders, 46,* 221-222.

Zenner, A.A., Ritterman, S.I., Bowen, S.K., & Gronhovd, K.D. (1978). Measurement and comparison of anxiety levels of parents of stuttering, articulatory defective, and normal-speaking children. *Journal of Fluency Disorders, 3,* 273-283.

Zimbardo, P.G. (1985). *Psychology and life* (11th ed.). Glenview, IL.: Scott, Foresman and Company.

Zimmerman, G.N. (1980). Articulatory dynamics of fluent utterances of stutterers and nonstutterers. *Journal of Speech and Hearing Research, 23,* 95-107.

NAMES INDEX

Subject Index

Page numbers in *italics* denote figures; those followed by "t" denote tables.